Laparoscopic Surgical Oncology

Theodore N. Pappas
Professor of Surgery, Duke University Medical Center, Durham, NC, USA

Emmanuel A. Leandros
Associate Professor of Surgery, Medical School, University of Athens, Greece

John P. Bramis
Associate Professor of Surgery, Medical School, University of Athens, Greece

PMP

PASCHALIDIS MEDICAL PUBLICATIONS

Notice

Medicine is an ever-changing science. As new research and clinical experiences broaden our knowledge, changes in treatment and drug therapy are required. The editor and the publisher of this work have checked with sources believed to be reliable in their efforts to provide information that is complete and generally in accord with the standards accepted at the time of publication. However, in view of the possibility of human error or changes in medical sciences, neither the editor nor the publisher nor any other party who has been involved in the preparation of publication of this work warrants that the information contained herein is in every respect accurate or complete, and they disclaim all responsibility for any errors or omissions or for the results obtained from use of the information contained in this work. Readers are encouraged to confirm the information contained herein with other sources. For example and in particular, readers are advised to check the product information sheet included in the package of each drug they plan to administer to be certain that the information contained in this work is accurate and that changes have not been made in the recommended dose or in the contraindications for administration. This recommendation is of particular importance in connection with new or infrequently used drugs.

PMP (Paschalidis Medical Publications, Ltd.).
14th, Tetrapoleos str., Athens, 115 27, Greece
Tel.: 003-210-7789125, 003-210-7793012, Fax: 003-210-7759421,
e-mail:
orders: Paschalidis@Medical-Books.gr
© information: GP@Medical-Books.gr, CP@Medical-Books.gr

LAPAROSCOPIC SURGICAL ONCOLOGY

Introduction

The focus of this book is the description of laparoscopic techniques as they are currently applied in surgical oncology.

The contemporary practice of medicine attempt to integrate the myriad scientific disciplines in the care of patients; the practice of surgery represents the quintessential example, in which knowledge of anatomy, physiology and pathology is applied to the treatment of disease processes. The laparoscopic surgeon dedicated to surgical oncology in particular must incorporate oncological and surgical principles to a greater extent than many other sub specialists.

For a textbook of this kind to be complete, it must include information on clinical diagnosis and preoperative patient care, in addition to a description of the technical maneuvers necessary to perform the particular operative procedure.

In this regard the authors have endeavored to include the information necessary to the formulation of clinical decisions. This is particularly important in this field, since a misjudged application of the laparoscopic techniques for a cancer patient could potentially compromise the oncological outcome. In addition, operative techniques are presented in detail, emphasizing the clinical setting and the scientific rationale for their undertaking, in hopes of instilling sound judgment in the novice and reinforcing it in the established practitioner.

Each chapter begins with a short discussion of clinical pathophysiology, covering treatment indications and options. The operative procedure follows and is discussed in enough detail to provide an understandable commentary for the accompanying illustrations. We wish to apologize for the steps or details that are omitted. With some procedures we do not use any drawings, whereas with others we give more pictures and details.

There is no doubt that a diversity of technical variations exists, in addition to those provided in this textbook. In fact, the authors have a different specialty or subspecialty training background allowing individual approaches to given clinical situations.

It is hoped that the procedures included herein will stimulate others to formulate newer operative innovations in this new surgical field, just as the authors have been stimulated to improved on the techniques originally learned from their mentors.

T. Pappas
E. Leandros
J. Bramis

PREFACE

Laparoscopy in minimally invasive surgery was a revolution in the history of Surgery of the last decade of the 20th century. This new approach has changed the boundaries of the traditional clinical practice and philosophy of Surgery.

Minimal invasive Surgery started with cholecystectomy, but soon was expanded to other areas of surgery as surgeons became familiar with the new technology. As a result of this, appendectomy, removal of stones from the common bile duct, herniorraphy became more popular for Laparoscopy.

Then they went on to apply to more advanced laparoscopic techniques such as splenectomy, antiflux procedures, colectomy, and morbid obesity and of course removal of other solid organs. Furthermore, Laparoscopy is now used widely in thoracic and heart surgery and in urology. We live in an era of rapid and major changes in medicine and especially in surgery. New types of equipment and devices have been discovered and used to facilitate surgeon's ability. One important thing nowadays is how to train residents to laparoscopic surgery.

General surgery training programme has a duty to do, to teach endoscopic skills. I appreciate that the teaching methods of laparoscopy is different from that of open surgery. We need more surgeons to do the advanced laparoscopic surgery safely, and I think it is an obligation of the leaders in this field to make training programs for those they are interested and deserve it. Certainly, a good book is a contribution to this direction.

I would like to congratulate the editors of this book, "Surgical Oncology" for the excellent job they have done to present a manual book of high level suitable for surgeons of various field. However, it will be helpful to any professional health-care. This book helps to distribute surgical knowledge about the use of laparoscopy in oncology. It is interesting to note the approach of laparoscopy to oncology has to pass from the "learing curve".

All writers are known for their special experience in laparoscopy, coming from different parts of the world which confirms Pasteur's View "Medicine without frontiers".

Surgical oncology is a fascinating field in laparoscopy and it can grow slowly and steadily step by step in order to obtain good results by carefully checking the "learning curve" in order to avoid complications.

This book will be of great help and guide for laparoscopic surgeons who practice oncology.

We must remember some procedures may not be amenable to laparoscopy or may need a certain number or size of ports, or may change to an open surgery for the safety of the patient. I always like to mention that surgeons should think also about the reduction of costs in Laparoscopy. We all know that is expensive.

The book is a contribution to the field of oncology, in an international level, easy to read and understand, with good pictures and drawings and I recommend it to all doctors interested in the subject. I feel proud to be able to make the introduction.

Basil Golematis
Emeritus Professor of Surgery
Hippokration Hospital

CONTENTS

EDITORS

Theodore N Pappas, *Professor of Surgery, Duke University Medical Center, Durham, NC, USA*

Emmanuel Leandros, *Associate Professor of Surgery, Medical School, University of Athens, Greece*

John P Bramis, *Associate Professor of Surgery, Medical School, University of Athens, Greece*

CONTRIBUTORS

J. Amaral, MD, *Department of Surgery, Brown University, Rhode Island, USA*

N. Alexakis MD, *Medical School, University of Athens, Greece*

M. Bau Mortensen MD, *Department of Surgical Gastroenterology, Odense University, Denmark*

SG de la Fuente MD, *Duke University Medical Center, Durham, NC, USA*

D. D'Ugo MD, *Department of Surgical Sciences, A. Gemelli Medical School, Catholic University of Rome, Italy*

J. Durup MD, *Department of Surgical Gastroenterology, Odense University, Denmark*

KH Fuchs MD, *Professor of Surgery, Department of Surgery, University of Wuerzburg, Germany*

M. Gagner, MD, *Professor of Surgery, Mount Sinai School of Medicine, New York, USA*

P. Gentileschi MD, *Mount Sinai School of Medicine, New York, USA*

I. Gomatos MD, *Department of Surgery, Hippokration Hospital, Athens Greece*

X. Jiao MD, *Division of Thoracic surgery, University of Maryland, Baltimore, USA*

N. Katkhouda MD, *Professor of Surgery, University of Southern California, Los Angeles, USA*

MM Konstadoulakis MD, *Assistant Professor of surgery, Medical School, University of Athens, Greece*

MJ Krasna MD, *Division of Thoracic surgery, University of Maryland, Baltimore, USA*

J. Marescaux MD, *Professor of surgery, University Louis Pasteur, Strasburg France*

H. Mohseri MD, *Division of Urology, University of Mississippi School of Medicine, Jackson, Mississippi, USA*

J. Mouiel MD, *Professor of Surgery, University of Nice, France*

IO Oikonomakis MD, *Department of surgery, 401 Military Hospital, Athens, Greece*

V. Pende MD, *Department of Surgical Sciences, A. Gemelli Medical School, Catholic University of Rome, Italy*

R. Persiani MD, *Department of Surgical Sciences, A. Gemelli Medical School, Catholic University of Rome, Italy*

A. Picciocchi MD, *Department of Surgical Sciences, A. Gemelli Medical School, Catholic University of Rome, Italy*

M. Sailer MD, *Department of Surgery, University of Wuerzburg, Germany*

WB Shingleton MD, *Division of Urology, University of Mississippi School of Medicine, Jackson, Mississippi, USA*

KM Smith MD, *Department of Surgery, University Louis Pasteur, Strasburg France*

LL Swanstrom MD, *Department of Surgery, Legacy Health System, Portland, Oregon, USA*

GN Tzimas MD, *Department of Surgery, Brown University, Rhode Island, USA*

DR Urbach MD, *Department of Surgery, Legacy Health System, Portland, Oregon, USA*

RM Walsh MD, *Department of Surgery, Cleveland Clinic Foundation, Cleveland, Ohio, USA*

SD. Wexner MD, *Professor of Surgery, Department of Colorectal surgery, Cleveland Clinic Florida, Weston, Florida, USA*

Aknowledgements
for coutribution - editorial assistance

Filippou Dimitrios, MD, PhD, *Department of General Surgery, Tzaneion Hospital, Athens, Greece*

Trigka Argiro, MD, *Anesthesiologist, Iaso General Hospital, Athens, Greece*

CHAPTER

Laparoscopic ultrasound in upper gastrointestinal cancer staging

1

Jesper Durup and Michael Bau Mortensen

Introduction

Besides having a correct diagnosis, accurate pretherapeutic staging and assessment of resectability in upper gastrointestinal malignancies (UGIM) are important in order to group the patients for different treatment strategies. One of the most important clinical tasks is to identify the patients that should not be operated. Unnecessary laparotomies in patients with non-resectable UGIM will increase mortality and morbidity as well as reduce the quality of life in their short remaining life time period.

In this chapter we will discuss the use of LaparoScopic UltraSound (LUS) regarding the pretherapeutic identification of non-resectable UGIM, and comment on the role of LUS and other imaging modalities in the staging and resectability assessment of UGIM.

History & Equipment

The main advantage of LUS is the possibility to place a high frequency ultrasound probe very close to the area of interest. This results in a highly detailed image that may provide important new information. This idea however, is not new. In 1964 Yamakawa[1] described the use of an A-mode, mechanical transducer, for laparoscopic ultrasound of the liver. But the equipment and image quality was not sufficient for clinical use. With the introduction of B-Mode, ultrasound prototypes for LUS were tested on the liver and the technical improvements resulted in equipment ready for clinical use.[2,3] The first probes used rotating mechanical transducers, and were rigid with a diameter of 10-12 mm. Electronic transducers attached to small diameter probes with flexible tips were then introduced in 1994.[4] Developments seen in the late nineties include probes with a tip which is flexible in all directions.[5] This feature should, at least theoretically, allow target visualization from different directions using the same trocar site. These electronic transducers are also e-

TABLE 1 Examples of dedicated LUS probes.

Company	Transducer	Characteristics	Frequency (MHz)
B-K Medical	8555	Curved array, semi-flexible, doppler	5.0 - 7.5
B-K Medical	8566	Curved array, multi-flexible, doppler, biopsy	5.0 - 7.5
Esaote	LP13A	Linear, semi-flexible, doppler	7.5 -10.0
ATL	Entos LAP L9-5	Linear, multi-flexible, doppler	5.0 - 9.0
Hitachi	EUP OL334	Curved array, multi-flexible, doppler	5.0 - 7.5
Sharplan	U Sight 92	Curved array, rigid	8.0
Aloka	UST 5536-7.5	Linear, semi-flexible	7.5

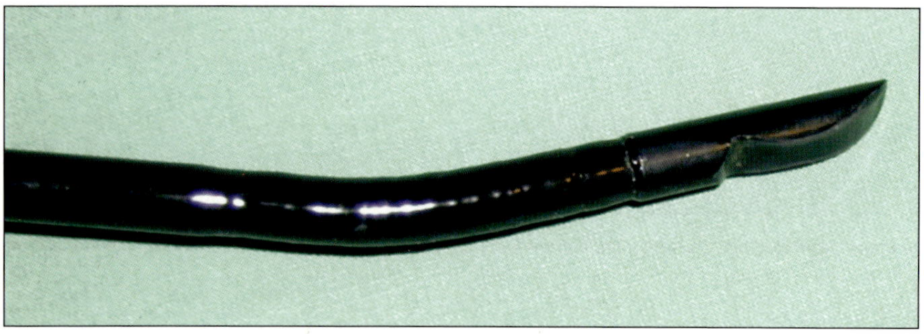

FIGURE 1. Tip of LUS probe. Curved array transducer (B-K Med 8555).

quipped with Doppler facilities as well as colour flow mapping (CFM), which can guide the differentiation between vascular and non-vascular structures. Finally, approaching the millennium, dedicated LUS probes with built-in biopsy guidance facilities have become available,[5] and the three-dimensional ultrasound technique has also been used and integrated in the LUS examinations.

Dedicated probes for LUS are equipped with ultrasound transducers with a frequency range from 5 to 7.5 MHz (Table 1). The transducer is designed with a curved or a linear array, and the transducer is placed at the tip of a long shaft (Figure 1). The diameter of the shaft is often between 9-11 mm and can be introduced through a standard laparoscopic port. The tip itself has to be flexible, and most commercial available probes now have flexible tips (Figure 2). The tip flexibility is important in order to get sufficient contact between the transducer and the target area/organ. Scanning of the dome of the liver illustrates why flexibility is important, especially as the insertion of additional abdominal trocars will give better access. As mentioned above the latest probes are four-way flexible like endoscopes. This should facilitate ultrasound examination of the target from different directions without moving the probe. However there are no studies that compare the two systems and the clinical value of using the four-way flexibility versus the two-way flexibility is uncertain.

Equipment for LUS guided biopsies is now available. The equipment consists of a needle stearing attachment device and a flexible steel needle, that can both be used with a standard LUS probe (Figure 3). Once the target is located, the biopsy system, is inserted and gently fixed to the tip of the probe. The target is located again, and the flexible biopsy needle is inserted under direct laparoscopic and ultrasonographic guidance. The needle can be traced ultrasonographically as it penetrates the target guided by a puncture line on the screen. The inner stylet is removed and the biopsy is taken. The handle on the biopsy needle can activate an automatic two-step procedure, where the first step is insertion of the inner needle and the second step is cutting a biopsy specimen over the insertion needle. After firing, the needle can be removed without withdrawing the probe from the target area. The automatic firing device is used for tru-cut biopsies using 19G or 20G needle sizes. A system for LUS guided fine-

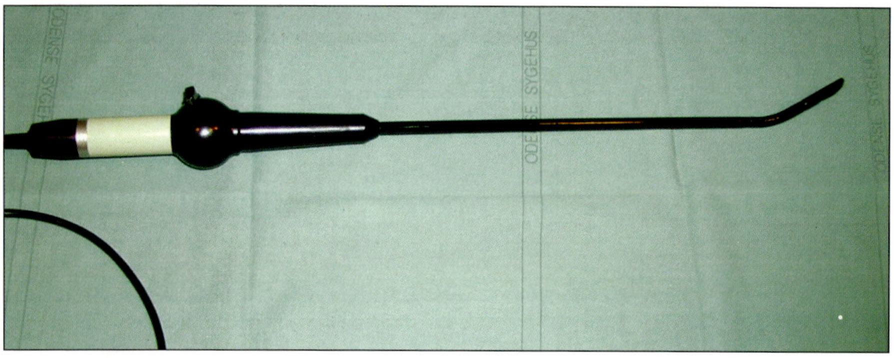

FIGURE 2. LUS Probe with two-way flexible tip. (B-K Med 8555).

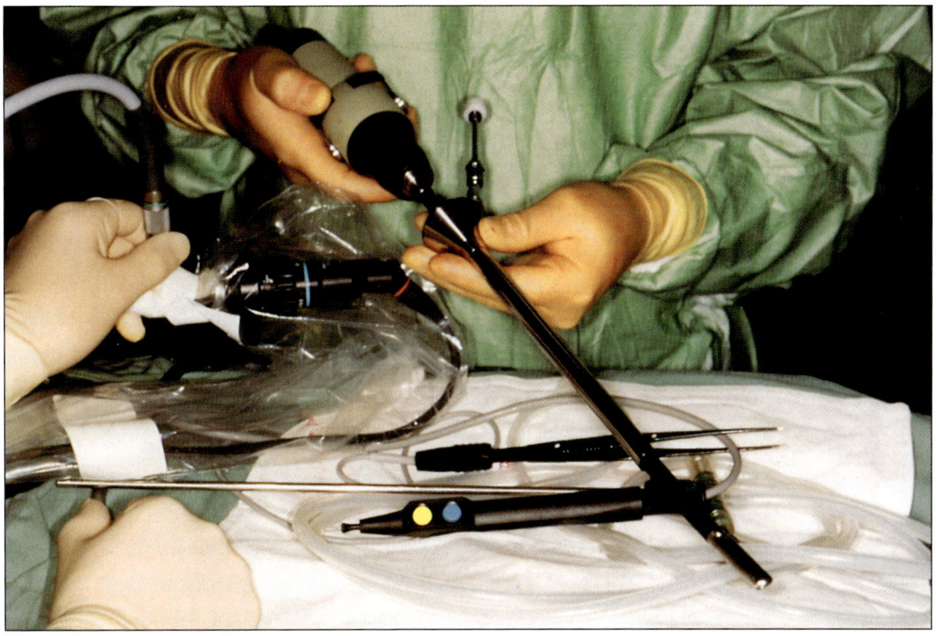

FIGURE 3. LUS four-way flexible probe with biopsy attachment. (B-K Med 8566).

needle aspiration biopsies has also been developed, - the only difference being the needle diameter (22G), and the lack of an automatic firing device. Although preliminary data suggest, that the LUS guided biopsy system is a quick and safe procedure with a high clinical impact the technique needs further evaluation in larger clinical trials.

The LUS probes can be connected to standard ultrasound (US) units. These units are often connected to a mixer unit that allows a picture feature on the laparoscopic monitor. A dedicated US unit for LUS is also available. This unit fits into the laparoscopic rag (Figure 4), and the mixer facility is build into the unit. A remote control can be placed at the operating table, allowing the surgeon to control the most important features at the US unit.

Most probes can only be disinfected with glutaraldehyde or similar products causing some problems in relation to environmental and hygiene regulations, but newer probes are also sterilizable in Sterris® or

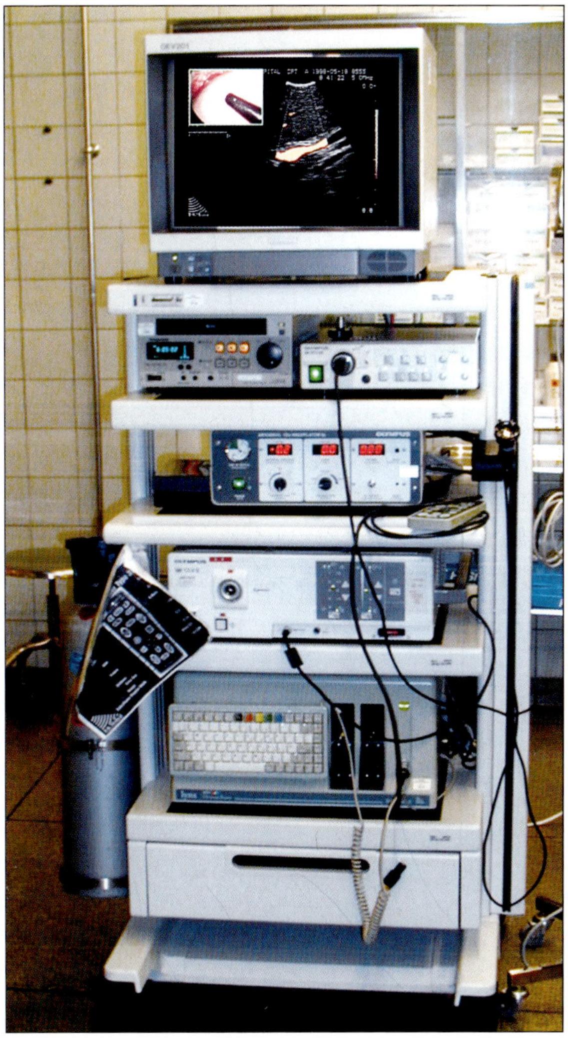

FIGURE 4. The laparoscopic rag with the US unit (B-K Med Lynx) at the lower shelter. Note the combined laparoscopic and ultrasound image on the monitor.

Sterrad® machines. Alternatively, the probe can be covered with sterile plastic or rubber condoms, but these tends to break during the procedure and can not be recommended due to risk of breaking sterility rules and due to poor image quality.

Future LUS probes will probably include such facilities as built-in systems for 3D-LUS and LUS guided treatment modalities (e.g. radioablation of hepatic tumors), and the transducer size will be reduced allowing even more minimal invasive LUS procedures.

Hepatic malignancies

LUS of the liver is easily performed. The probe is placed on the surface of the liver and the liver segments are systematically examined. Like intraoperative ultrasound LUS has a very high sensitivity in detecting hepatic tumors. Malignant tumors are often seen as dark (hypoechoic) round areas within the liver parenchyma, and their relation to the bile ducts and vessels are clearly visualized.

LUS can detect and outline additional liver tumors in patients who have primarily been assessed with CT-scan and external abdominal ultrasound. In an early study fifty patients with potential resectable liver tumors were examined. Laparoscopy demonstrated factors precluding curative resection in 23 patients (46%) but LUS identified liver tumors previously not visualized in 14 patients (33%).[6] Several studies have described the improved sensitivity for hepatic metastases with laparoscopy in comparison to CT scan and US,[7-9] but only few studies have systematically described the value of LUS. In a small study the sensitivity of CT scanning for hepatic metastases was reported as 0.55, and in the same group laparoscopy had a sensitivity of 0.67 and LUS a sensitivity of 0.82.[10] It has also been noted that the advantages of laparoscopy with LUS do not appear to decrease when advanced CT scanning methods such as triphasic spiral CT scanning have been used. Thus, in a study of 55 patients 221 lesions were seen on CT scan, but an additional 21 tumors (9.5%) in 11 patients (20%) were discovered by LUS. The size of these tumors ranged from 0.3 to 2.7 cm.[11]

For obvious reasons even trained surgeons are unable to palpate all intrahepatic tumors: In a blinded study 295 patients with colorectal tumors were examined by palpation, external and intraoperative ultrasound. The sensitivity and specificity for palpation was only 0.54 and 0.64, respectively, and external ultrasound, had figures of only 0.45 and 0.64. In comparison, and despite the fact that ultrasound specialists were not performing the intraoperative scannings, intraoperative ultrasound had a significantly higher sensitivity and specificity; - 0.62 and 0.64, respectively.[12]

Detection of all hepatic tumors is of high clinical importance in primary hepatic cancers and in colorectal cancer disease, because a precise mapping of the liver and of the location and number of metastases are essential regarding surgical treatment or alternative treatment modalities (e.g. radiofrequency ablation). However, as noted above, in UGIM patients the task of detecting and biopsing liver lesions is essential too, since these patients may not benefit from surgery if metastastic liver lesions are detected (see below).

Esophageal and Gastric Cancer

Endoscopic ultrasound (EUS) is the best modality for pretherapeutic loco-regional staging of esophageal cancer. EUS, however, is limited in its accuracy by stenotic or very large tumors, and superficial liver-metastases. Metastases in the right liver lobe and peritoneal carcinosis cannot be detected during EUS. Laparoscopy with LUS enables the visualisation and evaluation of abdominal lymph node stations as well as the liver in those patients where EUS is unable to pass the stenotic area. LUS cannot accurately TN-stage most esophageal cancers, simply because of the distance from the intraabdominal probe to the tumor. In a recent, prospective study the overall LUS accuracy regarding the T stage was 0.46, but when the tumor could be visualized by LUS the T staging accuracy rose to 0.93.[13] In a Dutch study CT, abdominal ultrasonography and EUS selected thirty-eight patients with esophageal cancer for curative resection. Laparoscopy changed the stage in 17% of the patients and LUS detected metastasis in 11%. But as there were problems concerning histological confirmation of LUS findings it was concluded that LUS was of limited value in staging of middle and lower esophageal cancer, but that it would have a potential use in patients with tumors that are located below the diaphragm.[14] This study appeared, however, prior to the development of dedicated systems for LUS guided biopsy.

If EUS, including the use of blind mini-probes, is unable to perform a complete loco-regional staging of tumors located in the thoracic esophagus, thoracoscopic ultrasonography (TUS) can be performed. TUS has only been described in the localization of lung nodules, but a mediastinal examination is certainly possible,[15] and TUS may tum out to be the thoracoscopic equivalent to LUS in patients with questionable resectability, both regarding primary tumors of the esophagus and malignant mediastinal tumors originating from the bronchus or lungs or mediastinal metastases.

Despite the fact that many stomach cancers are resected regardless of their stage, a complete pretherapeutic TNM staging and assessment of resectability should also be performed in these patients. Again, EUS is highly accurate for loco-regional staging, but it is also possible to achieve high accuracy concerning the T-staging of gastric cancer (especially T3 and T4 cancers) with LUS. A T stage accuracy as high as 0.81 has been reported, and this figure is similar to the EUS T staging accuracies EUS.[13] However, it is difficult to find and evaluate small cancers from the outer surface of the stomach, and the accuracy of LUS in T1 and T2 cancers still needs further evaluation, and so far they are probably better staged by EUS. Saline irrigation of the stomach through the nasogastric tube may facilitate the visualization of small gastric tumors.

The sensitivity for the detection of N1 and N2 lymph nodes with LUS is fair, and has been reported as high as 0.77.[13] The specificity, however, seems poor. LUS can easily visualize lymph nodes, but the main problem is to differentiate between benign and malignant nodes (Figure 5). The main purpose of LUS is to find suspicious lymph nodes that, if malignant, would change the therapeutic approach to the patient (Figure 6). Thus, these lymph nodes should be biopted and submitted for histopathological evaluation if these findings should have any kind of clinical impact.

The clinical impact of LUS has been evaluated in a study where 111 patients with gastric cancer were assessed by laparoscopy and LUS. The TNM stage was changed in 46% after the examination, with therapeutic consequences in 45 patients (41%). LUS was responsible for the change in 18% of the cases.[16]

It has been suggested that intensive staging in gastric cancer is not mandatory, but it is still a fact that many "resectable" tumors are found to be non-resectable during laparotomy. In a study more than one-third of the EUS staged T3 gastric cancers was either non-resectable or palliative treated,[17] and another study reported an only 21% curative resection rate out of 150 laparotomies for gastric cancer.[18]

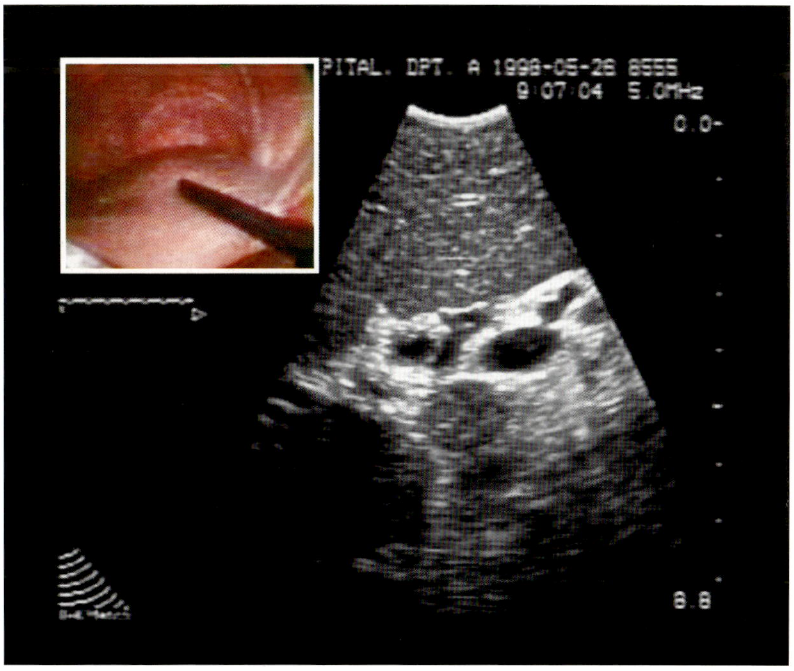

FIGURE 5. Enlarged lymph node in the hepato-duodenal ligament.

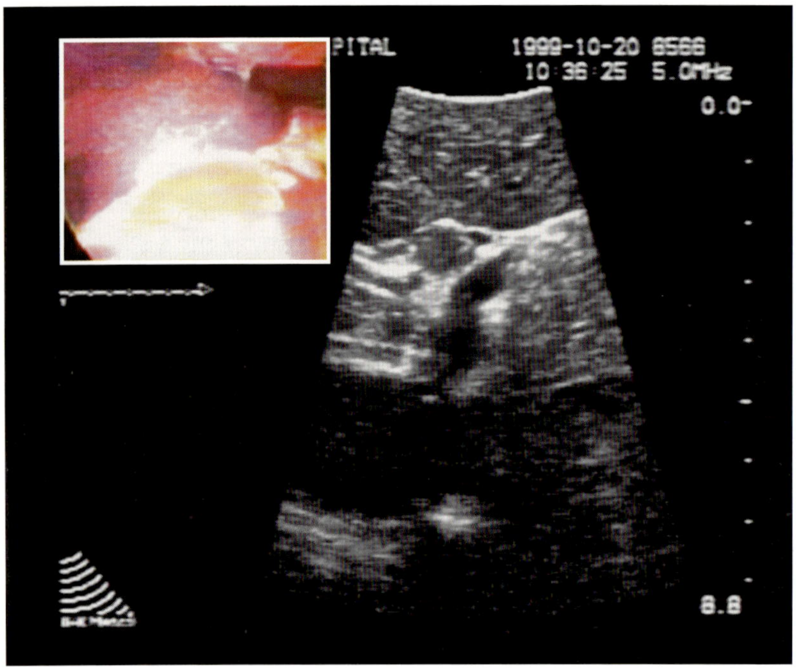

FIGURE 6. Lymph node (arrow) close to the coeliac trunc and left gastric artery.

Accurate assessment of resectability of gastric cancer can be performed with laparoscopy with LUS. Diagnostic laparoscopy visualizes even discrete peritoneal carcinosis and superficial hepatic metastases, and by adding information from LUS concerning the T and N stage nearly all non-resectable patients can be detected. Studies have found that laparoscopy and LUS can avoid futile laparotomy in 19-44% of patients who were found to be resectable by conventional imaging modalities.[16,19-22] Thus, it seems there is an indication for diagnostic laparoscopy with LUS before the final treatment decision in both gastric and esophageal cancer, especially in cases where EUS is inconclusive, or not available, or when other modalities have assessed the patient to be resectable. A strategy based on this combined approach also seem the most cost-effective.[23]

Pancreatic Cancer

Pancreatic tumors can be visualized and staged accurately with LUS. The tumor can be of mixed echogenecity but often presents as a hypoeccoic lesions with slightly irregular margins. In T staging the accuracy of LUS is approximately 0.85,[13,24] but the majority of tumors assessed with LUS are T2 and T3 and the accuracy in T1 pancreatic tumors has not been well evaluated for LUS. Vascular tumor invasion constitutes an important problem in pancreatic cancer. Vascular invasion (both arteries and veins) can be visualized by LUS, but it is of the utmost importance to have well established and specific criteria for the evaluation of vessel-tumor interfaces. The LUS criteria for tumor invasion into vessels are similar to those that are used during EUS. Direct signs of tumor invasion are loss of the normal hyperechoic vessel wall, tumor protruding into the lumen of the vessel or tumor circumferenting the entire vessel. If one or several of these findings can be demonstrated in two different (perpendicular) scanning angles, then the predictive value is close to 100%. Thus, if these criteria cannot be fulfilled, then the LUS procedure may suspect vessel invasion but final proof is lacking. Indirect signs of vessel invasion include change of flow (turbulence/direction of flow) within the vessel close to, or at, the suspected area, as well as the detection of collateral flow (e.g. small veins along the body of the pancreas in patients with tumorinvasion into the portal vein or the superior mesenteric vein). Whether the use of 3D-LUS and/or ultrasound contrast agents may increase the vessel invasion detection rate is still unclear.

Tumor infiltration of peripancreatic structures and organs can also be detected and evaluated during laparoscopy with LUS, however, there are areas in which interpretation may be difficult (e.g. tumor infiltration of the colon mesentery and the gastro-colic ligament).

Like other ultrasound modalities LUS cannot discriminate between pancreatitis and tumor, but multiple precise LUS guided tru-cut biopsies might diagnose these cases if an exact diagnose is warranted (se below).

The detection of malignant lymph nodes in pancreatic cancer is very important. Malignant lymph node infiltration reduces the survival considerably, and will often have an important influence on the therapeutic approach. The accuracy in N staging with LUS is reported to be app. 0.60-0.80, but the sensitivity for N1 nodes, are only between 0.33 and 0.71.[13,24-26] All studies so far have been evaluating lymph nodes based on ultrasonographically criteria of malignancy and not on LUS guided biopsies. Thus, it seems only fair to await studies including LUS guided biopsies before a final statement concerning LUS evaluation of the N stage can be given.

In most cases metastases can be discovered during laparoscopy alone. By adding LUS lymph nodes and hepatic metastases can be discovered without further laparoscopic dissection. The sensitivity and specificity of LUS regarding metastases in pancreatic cancer are very high[13,24-27] (Figure 7), and false positive diagnosis of metastases are rarely seen. As with the N stage histological confirmation is needed prior to abandoning an attempt for curative surgery.

In the assessment of local resectability the accuracy with laparoscopy and LUS are very high in all studies presented so far. Especially the combination of laparoscopy with LUS seem important: In a study the accuracy for laparoscopy alone was 0.34, but by adding LUS the accuracy rose to 0.89.[13] In another study where different imaging modalities was compared, the most accurate method for assessment of local resectability was EUS. But by adding laparoscopy and LUS an additional 26% with non-resectable cancers were discovered.[5]

The effectiveness of laparoscopic staging has been mentioned, but only a few studies have dealt with the economic aspect of different staging strategies. One study demonstrated that laparoscopy reduced hospitalization time and thus reduced the overall cost.[28] We have compared the different combinations of imaging modalities, including LAP, LUS and EUS, with regard to the diagnosis of non-resectable patients, and the actual costs for the detection of each non-resectable patient. The most cost effective single modality was EUS, and the most expensive strategy was the combination of CT+US+LAP. The EUS+LAP+LUS combination was the most cost-effective strategy in these 120 patients.[23]

LUS guided biopsies

Two methods for LUS biopsies are available: The LUS assisted biopsy procedure and the LUS guided biopsy procedure with dedicated equipment (Figure 3). The LUS assisted biopsy procedure is technically demanding as it includes free-hand biopsy with simultaneous ultrasound monitoring, but in a large study 186 patients were biopsied using this method. All patients had hepatocellular carcinomas and liver cirrhosis. The laparoscopy and biopsy procedure were performed under local anesthesia and slight sedation. LUS found additive liver tumors in 34% of all patients, and biopsy confirmed additional malignant tumors in 12% of all patients. Thus, LUS with biopsy changed the therapeutic approach in 18/23 (78%) of the patients with newly detected hepatic malignant tumors.[29]

The equipment for LUS guided biopsy has been

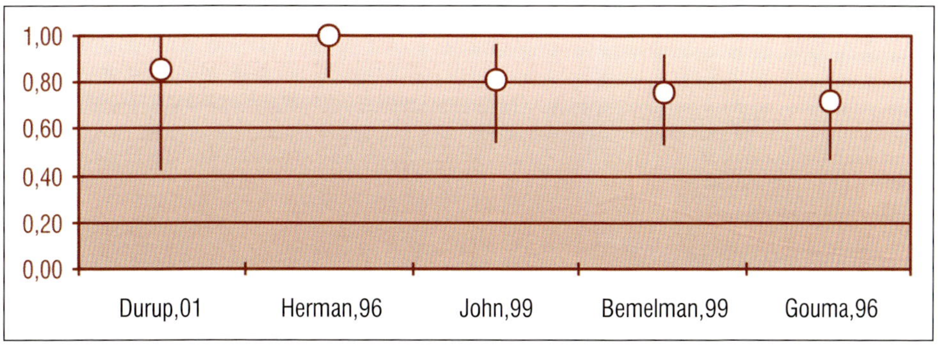

FIGURE 7. Sensitivity of M1 in PC with LAP+LUS

described,[5] but results concerning efficacy and safety, however, are still lacking. In a preliminary study we performed 44 biopsies in 20 patients using a new dedicated biopsy system for 19, 20 and 22G cytological or histological biopsies. The biopsy procedures lasted 16.3 minutes and no complications were seen. The obtained material was considered acceptable for analysis in 75%, but a specific diagnosis was only available in 65% of the patients. A large prospective and randomized study has now been initiated in order to obtain more experience with this new procedure.

The equipment for LUS guided biopsies also opens an interesting area for LUS guided treatment. In a study, LUS guided radiofrequency thermal ablation (RFA) was used to destroy hepatic tumors. Ten patients were treated, and total ablation was performed in 9. There were no complications.[30]

In a recent, but not randomized study, 84 patients with 231 hepatic lesions were treated with percutaneous, laparoscopic or operative RFA. The use of intraoperative ultrasound found additional hepatic tumors in 38% of the patients. After one-month follow-up with spiral CT scan, there was recurrence in 15 (18%) patients. There were 7 (8%) complications and one procedure related death. The majority of the complications were seen in the percutaneous RFA group.[31] Thus, LUS may aid in both selecting patients and guiding the treatment with RFA.

With equipment for interventional LUS available, we will probably see other treatment-related procedures in the future. LUS guided destruction of the celiac plexus in patients with non-resectable pancreatic cancer and intractable pain, or treatment of intra-abdominal abscesses or cysts, or the destruction of small pancreatic tumors such as insulinomas could become future indications for LUS guided therapy.

Complications

Although complications to diagnostic laparoscopy with LUS are reported low, a word of caution seems justified. In a review of the LUS literature, covering 5,285 patients with gastrointestinal malignancies that underwent staging laparoscopy, complications were reported in 159 cases (3%). There were 5 deaths (0.09%) associated with the procedure. Bleeding was the most common complication and was seen in 54 (1%) cases, while infection was seen in 31 (0.5%) cases. More serious complications were perforation of the intestine in 6 cases, and bile leakage after hepatic biopsies in 4 cases. In several studies, however, the rate of complication is not mentioned.. Diagnostic staging laparoscopy in local anesthesia has been reported to reduce the risk of complications: In a study where 136 patients underwent staging laparoscopy in local anesthesia the complication rate was 2%, and one patient having atrial fibrillation was the only cardiopulmonary complication.[32] In another study where 109 patients had staging laparoscopy under local anesthesia no complications were registered.[33]

Port site metastases (recurrence) have been described in several papers. In the above literature review 4 cases of port site metastases were identified. However, since 1978 more than 100 reports of metastases to laparoscopy wounds have been reported. This was also seen in cases where there was no mobilization performed, and in low stage cancer patients. But the majority of metastases reported have been in patients with advanced disease. The actual incidence of this problem is still unknown. Some authors have estimated the incidence in colorectal laparoscopic surgery at approximately 1 percent, but comparison between incidence in laparoscopic and conventional colectomy has not been performed.

In general, complications might be prevented if a blunt trocar and careful dissection are used, and minimal touch technique and careful exsufflation of carbondioxide or helium through the trocar and not through the wound may reduce the number of port site metastases. Use of small instruments in combination with the procedure performed in local anesthesia might reduce the cardiopulmonary complications, but the impact of specific precautions against different kinds of complications must await further trials.

Conclusion

Laparoscopic Ultrasound (LUS) in combination with

laparoscopy adds important clinical information in the staging of patients with upper gastrointestinal malignancies.

An accurate TNM staging and assessment of resectability of patients with gastric and pancreatic cancer can be accomplished with LUS, and distant metastases in lymph nodes and the liver can be imaged accurately for biopsy. The intraoperative ultrasound is superior to other modalities in diagnosing hepatic lesions.

Dedicated equipment for LUS and LUS guided biopsy is now available, and the frequency of reported complications following LUS and LUS guided biopsy seem to be low.

LUS should be a part of the staging algorithm of patients with upper gastrointestinal cancer, but more minimally invasive, accurate and safe methods such as endoscopic ultrasound, should always be performed prior to LUS.

Reference

1. Yamakawa,K. Yoshioka,S. Shirnizu,S. Laparoschography: an ultrasonic diagnosis under the laparoscopic observation. Japanese Medical Ultrasonic1964.2:26-28.
2. Aramaki, N., Yoshida, K., Yamashiro, Y., and Namihisa, T. Ultrasonic Laparoscopy. Scan J Gastroenterol 1982;17(suppl.78):185.
3. Fukuda, M., Mima, S., Tanabe, T., Haniu, T., Suzuki, Y., Hirata, K., and Terada, S. Endoscopic Sonography of the Liver--Diagnostic Application of the Echolaparoscope to Localize Intrahepatic Lesions. Scand J Gastroenterol Suppl. 1984;102:24-38.
4. Cavina, E., Goletti, O., and Buccianti, P. Echolaparoscopy: an Indispensable Procedure for Laparoscopic Surgery. Endosc.Surg.Allied.Technol. 1994;2:143-8.
5. Durup Scheel-Hincke, J., Mortensen, M. B., Pless, T., and Hovendal, C. P. Laparoscopic Four-Way Ultrasound Probe With Histologic Biopsy Facility Using a Flexible Tru-Cut Needle. Surg. Endosc. 2000;14(9):867-9.
6. John, T. G., Greig, J. D., Crosbie, J. L., Miles, W. F. A., and Garden, O. J. Superior Staging of Liver Tumors With Laparoscopy and Laparoscopic Ultrasound. Ann.Surg. 1994; 220(6):711-9.
7. Hunerbein, M., Rau, B., Hohenberger, P., and Schlag, P. M. The Role of Staging Laparoscopy for Multimodal Therapy of Gastrointestinal Cancer. Surg.Endosc. 1998; 12(7): 921-5.
8. O'Brien, M. G., Fitzgerald, E. F., Lee, G., Crowley, M., Shanahan, F., and O'Sullivan, G. C. A Prospective Comparison of Laparoscopy and Imaging in the Staging of Esophagogastric Cancer Before Surgery. Am.J.Gastroenterol. 1995;90(12): 2191-4.
9. Watt, I., Stewart, I., Anderson, D., Bell, G., and Anderson, J. R. Laparoscopy, Ultrasound and Computed Tomography in Cancer of the Oesophagus and Gastric Cardia: a Prospective Comparison for Detecting Intra-Abdominal Metastases. Br. J. Surg. 1989;76(10):1036-9.
10. Finch, M. D., John, T. G., Garden, O. J., Allan, P. L., and Paterson Brown, S. Laparoscopic Ultrasonography for Staging Gastroesophageal Cancer. Surgery 1997; 121(1):10-7.
11. Foroutani, A., Garland, A. M., Berber, E., String, A., Engle, K., Ryan, T. L., Pearl, J. M., and Siperstein, A. E. Laparoscopic Ultrasound Vs Triphasic Computed Tomography for Detecting Liver Tumors. Arch.Surg. 2000;135(8):933-8.
12. Rafaelsen, S. R., Kronborg, O., Larsen, C., and Fenger, C. Intraoperative Ultrasonography in Detection of Hepatic Metastases From Colorectal Cancer. Dis.Colon Rectum 1995; 38(4):355-60.
13. Durup, J. TNM staging and assessment of resectability of esophageal cancer, gastric cancer and pancreatic cancer using laparoscopic ultrasonography (LUS). Thesis. University of Southern Denmark; 2001.
14. Bemelman, W. A., Van Delden, O. M., van Lanschot, J. J., De Wit, L. T., Smits, N. J., Fockens, P., Gouma, D. J., and Obertop, H. Laparoscopy and Laparoscopic Ultrasonography in Staging of Carcinoma of the Esophagus and Gastric Cardia. J. Am. Coll. Surg. 1995;181(5):421-5.
15. Gossot, D., Colomer, S., Fourquier, P., Celerier, M., and Revillon, Y. Thoracoscopic Ultrasonic Localisation of Lung Nodules: Initial Results of an in-Vitro and in-Vivo Study. Endosc Surg 1994;2:153-5.
16. Feussner, H., Omote, K., Fink, U., Walker, S. J., and Siewert, J. R. Pretherapeutic Laparoscopic Staging in Advanced Gastric Carcinoma. Endoscopy 1999;31(5):342-7.
17. Bartlett, DL., Conlon, KCP., Gerdes, H., and Karpeh, MS. Laparoscopic Ultrasonography: The Best Pretreatment Staging Modality in Gastric Adenocarciniom? Case Report. Surgery 1995;118(3):562-6.
18. McCulloch, P. Should General Surgeons Treat Gastric Carcinoma? An Audit of Practice and Results, 1980-1985. Br. J. Surg. 1994;81(3):417-20.
19. Conlon, K. C. and Karpeh, M. S., Jr. Laparoscopy and Laparoscopic Ultrasound in the Staging of Gastric Cancer. Semin.Oncol. 1996;23(3):347-51.
20. Romijn, M. G., van Overhagen, H., Spillenaar Bilgen, E. J., Ijzermans, J. N., Tilanus, H. W., and Lameris, J. S. Laparoscopy and Laparoscopic Ultrasonography in Staging of Oesophageal and Cardial Carcinoma. Br.J.Surg. 1998;85(7): 1010-2.
21. Smith, A., John, T. G., Garden, O. J., and Brown, S. P. Role of Laparoscopic Ultrasonography in the Management of Patients With Oesophagogastric Cancer. Br.J.Surg 1999;86(8):1083-7.
22. Mortensen, MB., Durup Scheel-Hincke, J., Madsen, MR., Qvist, N., and Hovendal, C. Combined Endoscopic Ultrasonography and Laparoscopic Ultrasonography in the Pretherapeutic Assessment of Resectability in Patients With Upper Gastrointestinal Malignancies. Scand J Gastroent 1996;31(11):1115-9.

23. Mortensen,MB. Ainsworth,AP. Langkilde,LK. Durup Scheel-Hincke,J. Pless,T. Hovendal,CP.Cost-effectiveness of different diagnostic strategies in patients with non-resectable upper gastrointestinal tract malaignancies.Surg.Endosc. 2000.14: 278-281
24. John, T. G., Wright, A., Allan, P. L., Redhead, D. N., Paterson, Brown S., Carter, D. C., and Garden, O. J. Laparoscopy With Laparoscopic Ultrasonography in the TNM Staging of Pancreatic Carcinoma. World J.Surg 1999;23(9):870-81.
25. Bemelman, WA., Wit, LT., Delden, OM., Smits, NJ., Obertop, H., Rauws, EJA., and Gouma, DJ. Diagnostic Laparoscopy Combined With Laparoscopic Ultrasonography in Staging of Cancer of the Pancreatic Head Region. British Jounal of Surgery 1995;82:820-4.
26. Gouma, D. J., De Wit, L. T., Nieveen van Dijkum, E., Van Delden, O., Bemelman, W. A., Rauws, E. A. J., Van Lanschot, J. J. B., and Obertop, H. Laparoscopic Ultrasonography for Staging of Gastrointestinal Malignancy. Scand.J.Gastroenterol. 1996;31(suppl 218):43-9.
27. Herman, K. Intraoperative Ultrasound in Gastrointestinal Cancer. An Analysis of 272 Operated Patients. Hepatogastroenterology. 1996;43(9):565-70.
28. Westcott, C. J. and Pappas, T. N. Laparoscopy and Peripancreatic Neoplasia. World J.Surg. 1999;23(4):378-83.
29. Ido, K., Nakazawa, Y., Isoda, N., Kawamoto, C., Nagamine, N., Ono, K., Hozumi, M., Sato, Y., Kimura, K., and Sugano, K. The Role of Laparoscopic US and Laparoscopic US-Guided Aspiration Biopsy in the Diagnosis of Multicentric Hepatocellular Carcinoma. Gastrointest.Endosc 1999; 50 (4): 523-6.
30. Cuschieri, A., Bracken, J., and Boni, L. Initial Experience With Laparoscopic Ultrasound-Guided Radiofrequency Thermal Ablation of Hepatic Tumours. Endoscopy 1999;31(4):318-21.
31. Wood, T. F., Rose, D. M., Chung, M., Allegra, D. P., Foshag, L. J., and Bilchik, A. J. Radiofrequency Ablation of 231 Unresectable Hepatic Tumors: Indications, Limitations, and Complications. Ann.Surg.Oncol. 2000;7(8):593-600.
32. Sand, J., Mamela, K., Airo, I., and Nordback, I. Staging of Abdominal Cancer by Local Anesthesia Outpatient Laparoscopy. Hepatogastroenterology. 1996;43(12):1685-8.
33. Reddy, K. R., Levi, J., Livingstone, A., Jeffers, L., Molina, E., Kligerman, S., Bernstein, D., Kodali, V. P., and Schiff, E. R. Experience With Staging Laparoscopy in Pancreatic Malignancy. Gastrointest.Endosc 1999;49(4 Pt 1):498-503.

CHAPTER

2

Laparoscopic staging of gastric cancer

D. D' Ugo, V. Pende, R. Persiani, A. Picciocchi

1. Historical Overview

The concept of pneumoperitoneum was clinically introduced since the beginning of the 20th century. Jacobaeus, who first used the term "Laparoscopy" in 1911, pointed out the enormous clinical implications of this technique indicating that by using a laparoscope diagnoses of cirrhosis, tuberculous peritonitis and metastatic neoplasms could be confirmed.[1] With the further advances of video-endoscopy and the inclusion of television monitoring, current techniques of laparoscopy using improved imaging have led to the widest application in the diagnosis of abdominal malignancy.[2] During a "first historical phase" of such diagnostic experiences, a relevant number of authors was mainly concerned about the potential role of carbondioxide (CO_2) in the development of port-site metastases and peritoneal seeding after any kind of laparoscopic manipulation of a malignant disease.

Nduka and coworkers in 1994[3] focused their attention on three factors possibly involved in the pathogenesis of port-site metastases: at first, repeated passages of surgical instruments through the trocars could be responsible of the vehiculation of exfoliated viable tumor cells. Furthermore, continous manipulation of primary tumor caused by the lack of tactile sensibility during any laparoscopic operation could imply an increase of a possible tumor exfoliation process. At last a potential direct effect of pneumoperitoneum (tumor cell aerosolization) should be also considered. Isolated reports[4] indicated a possible role of smoke and debris produced by tissue electrocoagulation on the possible peritoneal diffusion of neoplastic cells. More recently, a number of papers have clarified the controversies in this field: animal studies clearly demonstrated that carbon-dioxide induced pneumoperitoneum does not represent a statistically significant risk factor in regards to port-site metastases[5], others stated that even if tumor cell aerosolization may eventually happen, it is only associated with high gas flow and a considerable concentration of viable neoplastic cells.[6,7] Recently, Pearlstone and coworkers anyhow reported that the incidence of port-site metastases does not show any statistically significant difference from the one described in cases of local tumor recurrence on surgical incisional wounds after open surgery for gastro-intestinal malignancies, suggesting that the biological behavior of cancer cells and not surgical manipulation nor pneumoperitoneum should be blamed as responsible for the pathogenesis of tumor implantation on any surgical scar.[8] Finally Reymond and coworkers have pointed out that the majority of port-site metastases are observed in patients who underwent laparoscopic procedures associated with poor protective measures (retrieval bag; gas flow relay control); it is the opinion of these authors that the variability in the incidence of port-site metastases, rainging from 0% to 21% as reported in different series, is dependant upon personal experience and technique of each individual surgical operator.[7] Therefore, at present, it may be concluded that port site metastases do not seem to represent any more a limiting factor towards a wider application of diagnostic laparoscopy for abdominal malignancies.

In regards to laparoscopic staging of gastric cancer, this technique has had quite different modalities of application throughout the world in recent years, mainly depending on diverse geographic sites with strikingly different social and economic enviroments. On one hand, Possik[9] in Brazil and Kriplani[10] in India have applied laparoscopic staging to the work-up of gastric cancer patients, especially with the aim of limiting an unacceptable high rate of exploratory laparotomies which in most series are associated with high post-operative morbidity and mortality and are certainly not beneficial to the general status of oncologic patients. On the other hand in the USA, Western Europe and Japan staging laparoscopy has been mainly adopted as a consequence of the increasing indications towards multimodal treatment plans. Main goal of laparoscopic exploration, under such circumstances, is the application of a more accurate staging modality compared with conventional imaging both for patients with technically unresectable gastric cancer and patients with locally advanced resectable disease, respectively to be treated by induction chemotherapy (with radiological or laparoscopic re-evaluation at the end of treatment) and by neo-adjuvant chemotherapy.[1]

One of the first important experiences concerning the use of laparoscopy for staging of gastric neoplasms was reported by Gross in 1984 on a series of 46 cases.[15] This report was followed by many others that will be discussed in the next paragraphs: at present a long list of published papers strongly suggests that laparoscopy is indeed capable to solve the majority of the problems related with gastric cancer staging, giving the unique opportunity of an accurate selection of patient subgroups on the base of their precise clinical stage and different prognosis, with the final goal of an individually "stage adapted" multimodal therapy.[9,10,16,17,18,19]

2. Techniques of Laparoscopy for Gastric Cancer Staging

Diagnostic Laparoscopy: Laparoscopic staging is generally performed under general anesthesia, although some authors reported experiences under local anesthesia.[20] Sometimes diagnostic laparoscopy is performed as a separate procedure, but in most cases this is performed immediately prior to a planned open operation.[21] The patient is placed supine on the operating table; in our hands access to the abdominal cavity is provided by means of an open cut-down technique, usually performed peri-umbilically, whilst the Verres needle technique is seldom used due to concerns related to vascular or visceral perforation. A 10-12 mm "Hasson"- type trocar is inserted below the umbilicus (Figure 1) into the peritoneal cavity and an angled 30° scope is placed to obtain a wider view of the entire supramesocolic area. Laparoscopic staging must be conducted following an "inverted TNM mode": this means evaluating the M factor first (Figure 2a-b), followed by the N and T factors (Figure 3). Prior to any maneouver of surgical staging (in absence of ascitic fluid that, if present, is invariably aspirated and examined for immediate cytology), 200 ml of normal saline are instilled into the peritoneal cavity: specimens for cytology are aspirated from the pelvis, subhepatic space and left upper quadrant.

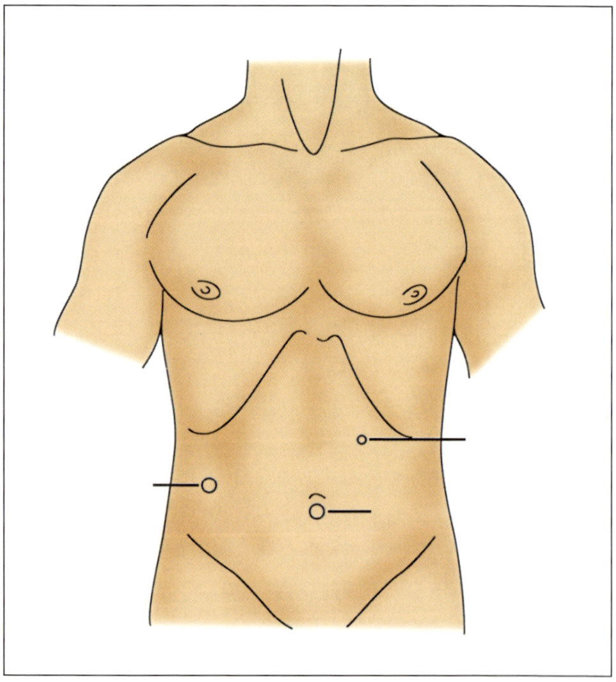

FIGURE 1. Trocar position during laparoscopy for gastric cancer.

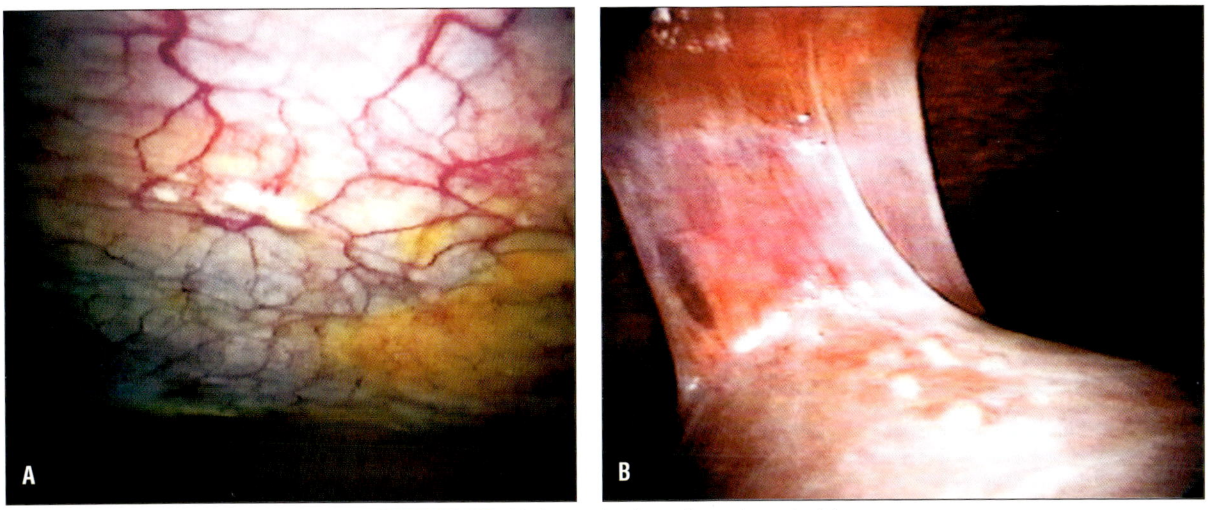

FIGURE 2A-2B. M factor (peritoneal carcinomatosis).

The parietal and visceral serosal surfaces of the peritoneum are inspected in a systematic fashion for malignant implants: discontinous tumor deposits can be identified and biopsied using endosurgical biopsy forceps. Placing the table in a Trendelemburg position facilitates the examination of the pelvis. In female patients the ovaries must be visualized in order to exclude Krukemberg metastases. The visible surfaces of omentum, diaphragm and liver are then inspected; a palpating probe is inserted through a second 5 mm port, usually placed at the left of the midline, in order to obtain a minimal manipulation of the left liver lobe and the small bowel.

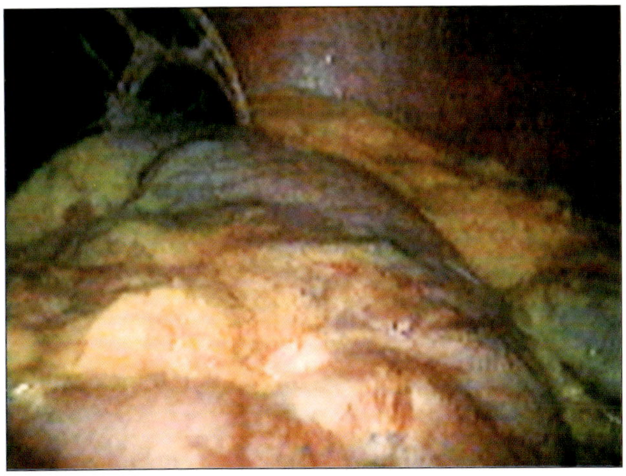

FIGURE 3. T factor (extra-serosal tumor infiltration).

Tilting the table facilitates the approach to the area of the stomach that is covered by the left liver lobe; before determining the extent of tumor infiltration on the gastric wall, the perigastric nodes are inspected along the greater and lesser curvature, on the gastro-hepatic ligament and at the hepatic hilum.

As far as staging of the N-factor is concerned, we differ from other authors in which we do not routinely perform lymphnode biopsy during preoperative laparoscopy; in fact, according to our protocol, the indication to a delayed surgical exeresis following a neoadjuvant chemotherapy is in most cases a consequence of T-staging, with the macroscopic evidence of an extra-serosal infiltration of the primary tumor. Some reports have shown the low accuracy of N-staging by a "plain" laparoscopic exploration, when it is not implemented by the use of laparoscopic ultrasonography (LUS).[21,22]

Furthermore, the most recent TNM classification of gastric carcinoma (fifth edition UICC, 1997) in regard lymphnode involvement (N1, N2 and N3) is based on the numeric count of metastatic nodes whereas the anatomic-topographic system - mutuated from the "Japanese" classification system- was previously adopted.[23] At present, this implies that only the removal and complete examination of at least 15 nodes is capable to establish if a node positive patient is indeed to be considered N1 or N2; nevertheless in rare circumstances a single-node biopsy may be important in the definition of the treatment strategy: this happens when preoperative imaging is strongly suggestive of a severe lymphnode involvement but laparoscopy does not demonstrate any extra-serosal primary tumor infiltration. In the light of a possible indication to an induction treatment under such circumstances (T1-2 tumors with a suspect of advanced N-staging at preoperative imaging with ultrasound or CT-scan) our attitude is to perform a single-node biopsy just to demonstrate the local advancement of the disease along with the certainty of nodal metastases.

Most of the tumors localized on the anterior wall of the stomach can be inspected without manipulation. The position for the placement of the third trocar is dictated as the anatomy becomes evident during the laparoscopic examination (this port is the one employed for LUS and/or a possible lesser sac endoscopy (Figure 1). When the tumor originates from the posterior wall or a posterior fixity is suspected, the posterior tumor mass may be lifted to test its mobility over the pancreatic body capsule in order to perform a **LESSER SAC ENDOSCOPY (LSE):** one of the probes may be thoroughly inserted behind the stomach through an avascular area of the gastro-colic ligament for a better staging accuracy (with a longer operative time). In most of the series, the mean operative time of this technique is 20 minutes.[21,22]

This technique was firstly experimented and "patented" in 1984 in the U.S.S.R:[24] according to the original description, the laparoscope is introduced into the lesser sac through a window created in the gastro-colic ligament attracted under laparoscopic control on the surface of the abdominal wall through a 1.5 to 2 cm mini-laparotomy incision (Figure 4). While the lesser sac is insufflated with the gas through the instrumental channel of the laparoscope or trocar sheath, all organs and ligaments forming the borders of the lesser sac are routinely inspected. Instrumental palpation, aspiration, puncture and forceps biopsy are performed through the instrumental channel of the laparoscope. The described method permitted a better inspection of the head, body and tail of the pancreas in respect to the classical approach.[24]

Extended Diagnostic Laparoscopy (EDL): This systematic technique was first applied in 1995 by some authors participating in the German Gastric Cancer Study Group. It includes a conventional laparoscopic staging with peritoneal and lesser sac exploration complemented by the use of LUS for a better appreciation of pancreas, liver and gastric wall thickness.

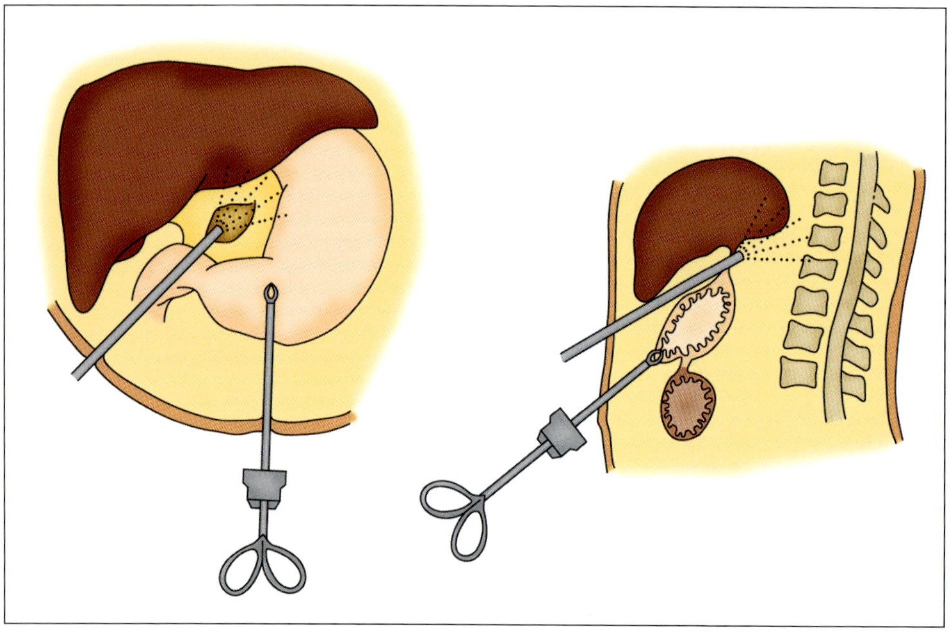

FIGURE 4. Lesser sac endoscopy technique.

Since standard laparoscopy is a two-dimensional modality, the lack of tactile sensation avoids the detection of small intraparenchymal liver lesions and palpatory assessment of the T-stage of the primary tumor. Intraoperative ultrasound has the potential to overcome this deficiency.[25] Initially developed for assessment of hepatic disease, LUS has recently been used in benign biliary tract disease and in staging of hepatic and pancreatic malignancy.[26,27,28]

Generally, a flexible-tip multifrequency (5-7.5 MHz/6-10 MHz) curved-array ultra-sound probe with color-flow Doppler capability, wich fits through a 12 mm port is used for LUS.[29,30] LUS is used to evaluate tumor size and extent, celiac and portal nodes, vascular invasion, involvement of contiguous structures and to perform a complete assessment of the liver. Biopsies of suspected metastatic lesions are taken under direct laparoscopic or ultrasonographic guidance using biopsy forceps or needle-aspiration.[31]

Feussner and co-workers[22] studied EDL in 111 gastric cancer patients: overall, detailed laparoscopy plus LUS altered the preoperative diagnosis in 46% of the patients (51/111) leading to changes in management in 45 (40.5%). LUS proved to be useful in confirming or excluding invasion and in revealing unsuspected liver metastases, and was responsible for a change in the diagnosis in 15.7% of the patients. The authors conclude that LUS should therefore always form an integral part of diagnostic laparoscopy.

3. Diagnostic Accuracy of Laparoscopy in Gastric Cancer: Clinical Experiences

The clinical role of US and CT for diagnosis of gastric cancer has been questioned because of their low accuracy in clinical staging: the high false-negative rate for CT has been confirmed by prospectives studies and it has be pointed out by some authors[9,10] that negative US or CT scans do not entirely exclude the possibility of liver or peritoneal malignancy.

Gross and colleagues[15] reported their experience with 46 gastric cancer patients: metastatic disease has been noted by laparoscopy in 27 of 46 cases (57%) that had been previously staged as M0 (Table 1).

Possik and associates[9] evaluated laparoscopic staging in 360 patients with gastric cancer. They demonstrated an accuracy of 89% for the detection of peritoneal dissemination and 96% for hepatic metastases.

More recently, Kriplani and Kaipur[10] performed preoperative staging laparoscopy as a separate procedure on a series of 40 patients who were considered resectable after ultrasonography (US) and computed tomography (CT) workup. Laparoscopy showed the presence of unsuspected metastatic disease in 13% and unresectable T4 cancer in 27.5% of the patients with an overall diagnostic accuracy of 92%.

Lowy[16] performed staging laparoscopy in 71 patients with potentially resectable gastric cancer

TABLE 1 Summary of laparoscopic studies and gastric cancer.

Author Year	# of pts	Preop. Imaging	M1 undetected disease (%)	Accuracy	Avoided exploratory laparotomies (%)
Gross 1984	46	NR*	57%	NR	NR
Possik 1986	360	US/Liver scint	34%	89% †96%	NR
Kriplani 1991	40	US/CT	13%	92%	NR
Lowy 1996	71	CT	23%	94% †33%	17%
Stell 1996	103	US/CT	NR	94% †99%	20%
Burke 1997	110	CT	37%	94%	22%
D'Ugo 1997	100	US/CT	21%	100%**	21%

* Not reported
† Top: peritoneal metastases; bottom: liver metastases
** Accuracy for M staging

as determined by current generation CT-scanning: in 16 (23%) of these patients, laparoscopy identified distant metastatic disease undetected by conventional staging; a surgical exploration was avoided in 12 of these patients.

Stell and co-workers[17] performed a prospective comparison of laparoscopy, ultrasonography and computed tomography in gastric cancer staging: with regards to detection of hepatic metastases they reported an accuracy of 99% for laparoscopy versus 76% and 79% respectively for US and CT; sensitivity by laparoscopy was 96% compared to 37% and 52% respectively by US and CT. In regards to peritoneal carcinomatosis the accuracy was 94% for laparoscopy, 84% for US and 81% for CT (sensitivity: 69% by laparoscopy vs 23% and 8% by US and CT).

In 1997 we prospectively compared[21,19] diagnostic accuracy of pre-operative laparoscopy with ultrasound and computed tomography respectively in a multicentric series of 70 cases and, more recently, in 100 gastric cancer patients: in the latter series laparoscopy detected 21 unsuspected metastatic cases out of 100 patients clinically considered as M0.

In regards to locally advanced tumors, laparoscopy showed a sensitivity of 69.7% for T3 and 89.6% for T4 tumors, significantly higher than US/CT staging (respectively 23.2% and 48.3%; $p<0.02$). Laparoscopy showed an accuracy of 100% for M staging with an overall TNM staging accuracy of 72% compared to 38% for US/CT.[6,20]

In their experience, Burke and colleagues[18] studied laparoscopy in a consecutive series of 110 gastric cancer patients: metastatic disease was demonstrated in 37% of patients who were considered to have localized gastric cancer by pre-operative CT or EUS. Laparoscopy accurately staged 94% of patients with respect to metastatic disease. A sensitivity of 84% and specificity of 100% has been noted in this study. Compared to patients that underwent an exploratory laparotomy only during the same time period, post-operative hospital stay was significantly reduced (1.4 days vs 6.5 days).

In summary it may be stated that laparoscopy is a relatively simple, well-tolerated and safe procedure; published reports and our data[19,21,34] support the belief that laparoscopy is a valuable technique in the staging of gastric cancer and confirm its important role in the detection of understaged metastatic disease compared to preoperative staging.

4. Clinical Implications of Staging Laparoscopy and Diagnostic - Therapeutic Protocols

Despite a decline in its incidence, gastric carcinoma remains one of the most common malignant tumor in the world.

In Europe and United States curative resection is performed in less than 60% of all gastric cancers since most patients have locally advanced or metastatic at presentation. Surgical therapy still represents the treatment of choice for gastric cancer, but -in regards to locally advanced tumors- surgery alone seems to have reached its limits concerning the rate of curative resections and long term survival.

Multimodal treatment options have preliminarily shown promising results, but a precise evaluation of these treatments is strictly dependant upon an accurate patient selection with a reliable staging of tumor extension, lymphnode involvement and site of distant metastases.[22]

In the recent past radiology played a prominent role in diagnosis and clinical staging of gastric malignancies; however computed tomography (CT), magnetic resonance (MR) and ultrasonography (US) lack sufficient accuracy in gastric cancer staging[32] and to date it is well known that locally advanced carcinoma of the stomach is often understaged by a conventional preoperative work-up based on US and CT which implies a high percentage of unhelpful exploratory laparotomies: perioperative complications invariably occur in 12 to 23% of such unresectable patients, with a reported mortality ranging up to 21%.[17,21,33]

To date, the introduction of video-laparoscopy and endoscopic ultrasonography (EUS) have radically modified conventional imaging methods for gastric cancer staging: video-laparoscopy has already shown significantly better results in regards to the detection of unstaged metastatic disease; preoperative laparoscopy in the prevention of unnecessary surgical exploration has been evaluated by previously discussed reports[9,10,17,30] and certainly represents a powerful diagnostic tool in the light of avoiding "open and close" operations,[34] since M+ disease should not be resected in the absence of obstruction or bleeding.[21] Moreover, there is some evidence that laparoscopy permits a more accurate staging of extraserosal tumors (T3-T4) and to date, an even more crucial task is given to preoperative laparoscopy: in fact, after 30 years of adjuvant treatment trials, it has been ascertained that patients who present with locally advanced but resectable disease (T3-4, any N, M0) have a low chance of cure after a complete surgical resection followed by an adjuvant chemotherapeutic regimen. Conversely, whereas a preoperative treatment protocol is applied, laparoscopy represents an useful tool for patient selection, ruling out any unhelpful delay of surgery in non advanced cases.[12,35] An increasing number of institutions throughout the world are consequently recommending neoadjuvant treatment protocols for locally advanced gastric cancer, provided that the disease is "properly staged".[36]

Some authors have pubblished their DECISION-MAKING flow-charts[18,16,19] in regards to patients selection for a possible enrollment in a preoperative chemotherapy trial: in all of them diagnostic laparoscopy plays a crucial role (Figure 5a-b-c).

It is our opinion that further trials on neo-adjuvant treatment both for resectable and unresectable gastric carcinoma are to be favoured. Nevertheless these experiences must be restricted to **Contnrolled studies,** that include a thorough enrollment of homogeneously selected cases thorough a constant application of laparoscopic staging modalities.

Recently some papers have focused on the impact of staging laparoscopy over the **Clinical Decision Making Process,** weighing the rate in which this procedure alters the clinical stage, thus determining a fall-back on the treatment strategy.[20,22]

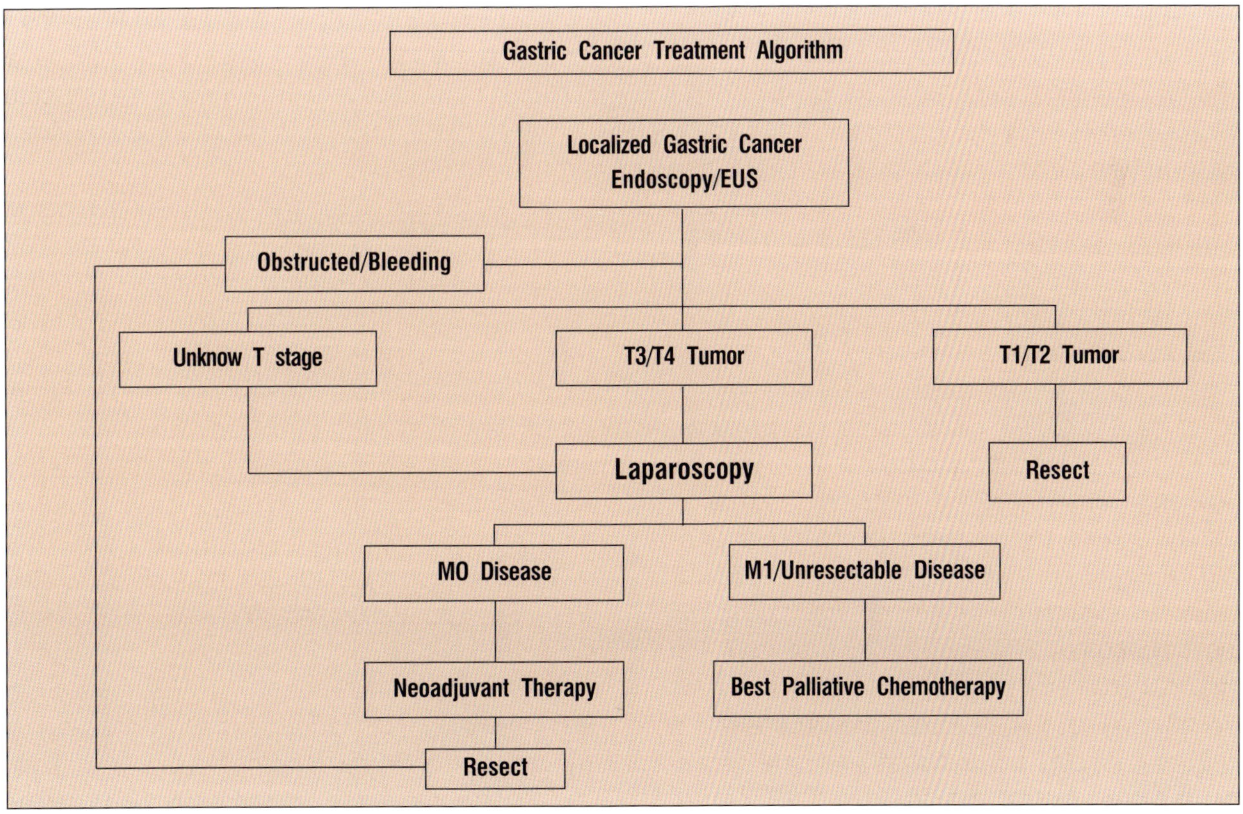

FIGURE 5A. Conlon K: Treatment algorithm for gastric cancer.

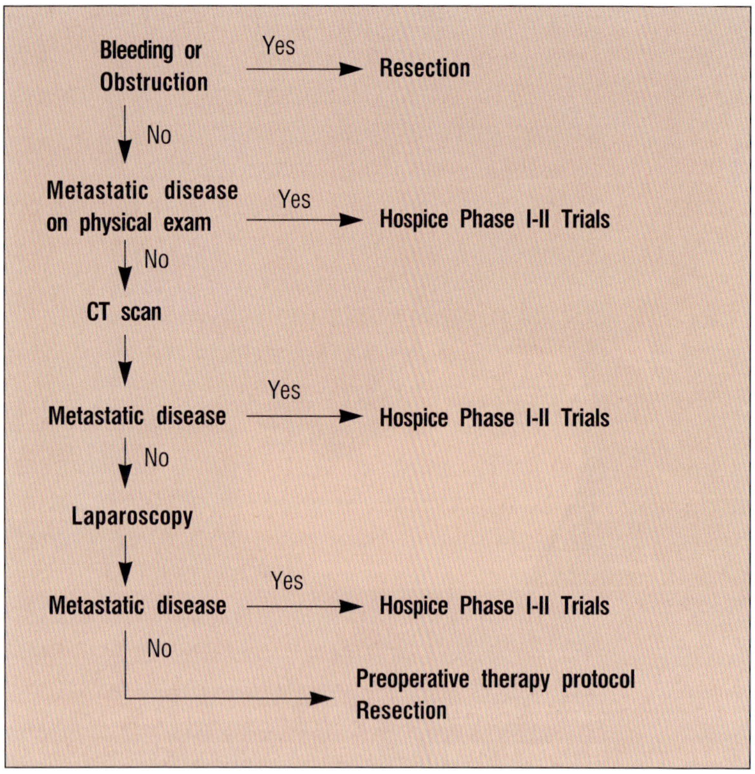

FIGURE 5B. Lowy A: Treatment algorithm for gastric cancer.

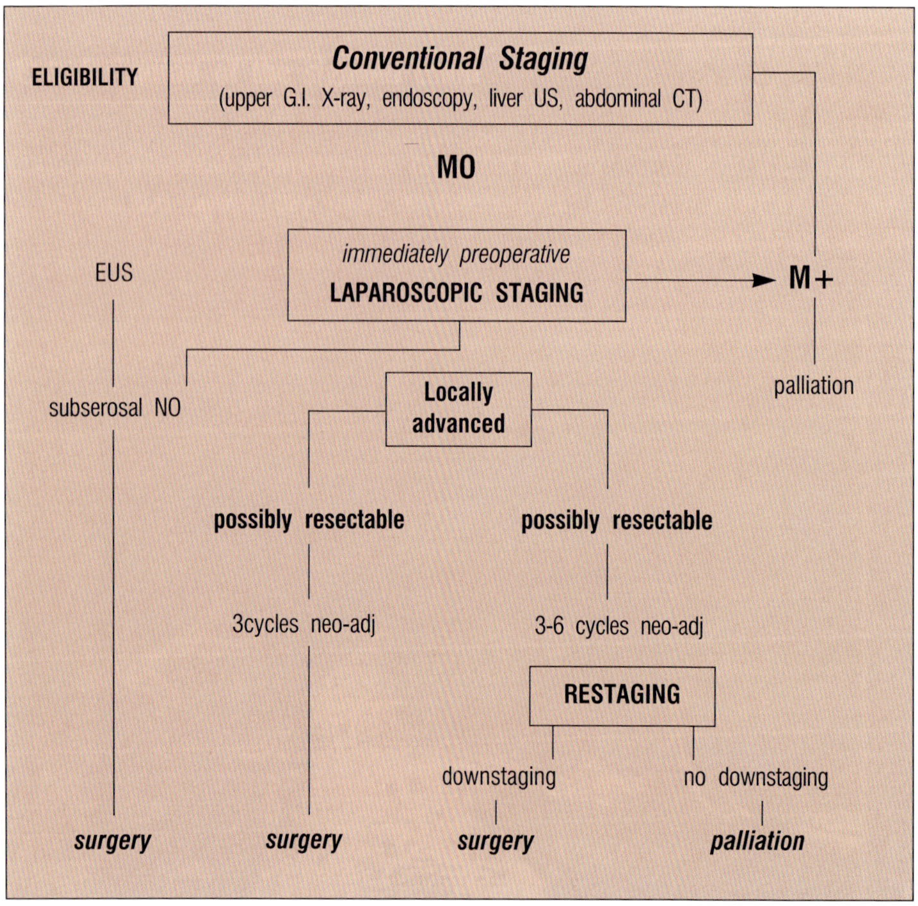

FIGURE 5C. D' Ugo D: Treatment algorithm for gastric cancer.

In our experience,[37] we have evaluated how frequently diagnostic laparoscopy modifies conventional clinical T and M staging and its consequent impact on treatment strategies for gastric cancer. In a subset of 91 gastric cancer patients, conventionally staged as M0 who underwent pretherapeutic laparoscopic staging, the results of laparoscopy modified the clinically established T and M values in 58.2% of cases: previously undetected metastases were evidenced in 13.1% of patients; T value was upgraded in 32% and downgraded in 13.1%.

Preoperative laparoscopy provided no additional findings compared with clinical stage in 54.9%, but it modified preoperative therapeutic strategy in 49/91 patients (53.8%) confirming a crucial role in staging gastric carcinoma.

5. Future Developments

Peritoneal Cytology: Burke and co-workers had examinaned the therapeutic impact of peritoneal lavage cytology obtained at the time of laparoscopic staging.[18] Laparoscopic washings were obtained from 127 consecutive patients with gastric cancer. A correlation between the extent of disease and prevalence of positive cytology was noted. No patient with early disease (T1-2,M0) was noted to have positive cytology. In contrast, 10% of patients with T3-4,M0 and 59% of patients with M1 disease were noted to have positive cytology.

Significantly, even in the absence of macroscopic metastatic disease, patients with positive cytology had a prognosis identical to those with macroscopically obvious metastatic disease, indicating that positive lavage cytology indicates microscopic peritoneal metastatic disease. It is the opinion of the authors of this report that, as these patients behave in a manner identical to patients with macroscopic peritoneal or hepatic metastases, they should therefore be staged as M1.

Ribeiro and colleagues recently reported similar results in a study of 49 consecutive patients with gastric cancer who underwent laparoscopic staging.[38] Lavage cytology was performed when ascites was absent. In the absence of macroscopic peritoneal carcinomatosis, positive cytology was noted in 29%. Positive cytology was correlated with the depth of invasion, histological subtype, advanced Borrmann class and stage IV tumors. They suggested that cytology added sensitivity to the laparoscopic examination and that it may therefore significantly alter the therapeutic approach.

Second Look Laparoscopy: As far as the efficacy of any kind of pre-surgical induction therapy is concerned, a crucial point is establishing precise criteria for an accurate evaluation of the tumor response after preoperative treatment.

In our series of neo-adjuvant chemotherapy for locally advanced RESECTABLE gastric carcinoma,[39] evaluation of the response is preliminarily performed by morphometric comparison of pretreatment imaging (endoscopy + CT scan + laparoscopic staging) with immediately preoperative imaging and intraoperative tumor restaging; all patients belonging to this cathegory do infact undergo surgery. Under such circumstances (resectable advanced disease) primary objectives of the multimodal treatment are the increase of R0-resection rate and possibly an amelioration of long-term survival; second look laparoscopy is therefore not applied in this patient group.

On the other hand, whereas preoperative chemotherapy is applied to similarly locally advanced but TECHNICALLY UNRESECTABLE cancers, second look laparoscopy may represent a powerful tool in ruling out from an unhelpful delayed exploration those patients who did not respond to medical treatment and do not deserve palliation for stenosis or bleeding.

Laparoscopic Palliation of Unresectable Gastric Cancer

Patients with incurable malignant disease presenting with distal gastric obstruction have a very poor prognosis. A few decades ago, the only therapeutic possibility for palliation and relief from symptoms (gastric outlet obstruction and or jaundice) was gastroentero-anastomosis and/or bilio-enteric anastomosis via laparotomy.[40] This operation, though providing satisfying functional results, remains quite invasive. It is related to a considerable period of hospitalization and to pain, discomfort and possible complications: open gastroenterostomy for palliation of malignancies has been associated with delayed gastric emptying in up to 16% with a morbidity and mortality rate respectively of 25% and 8-17%.[41] The effort to reduce operative trauma in unresectable cancer patients resulted in development of minor access or laparoscopic palliative operations. While laparoscopic surgery for malignant disease with curative intention has already been reported through many controversies,[42] palliative laparoscopic procedures are certainly of special benefit for patients who generally have a very short life expectancy. Some of the advantages offered by laparoscopic palliative surgery are: a reduced pain, a short recovery and a short hospital stay, allowing the surgical procedure to interfere as little as possible with quality of life. Therefore, several authors have started to perform gastroenterostomy routinely via laparoscopic access.[43,44]

Brune and co-workers,[45] performed laparoscopic gastrojejunostomy (lap-GEA) in 16 patients with gastro-intestinal malignancies. Laparoscopic gastrojejunostomy was performed as an antecolic isoperistaltic side-to-side anastomosis with a 30 mm Endo-GIA stapler with an enterostomy 25 cm below the gastrojejunostomy to assure sufficient biliary drainage from the afferent loop and avoid exposure of the gastric anastomosis to bile acids.

6. Conclusions

Immediately preoperative staging laparoscopy is a safe, simple, and relatively cheap procedure at most medical institutions. In regards to locally advanced gastric cancer, our data support the belief that to date laparoscopy plays two fundamental roles: on one hand, it undoubtedly represents the most specific method for detecting previously unsuspected M+ disease, thus sparing unresectable cases from unnecessary surgical exploration. On the other hand, following the increasing application of neoadjuvant treatment protocols for stage IIIa-IIIb tumors, we have seen that laparoscopy permits the most reliable and accurate selection of T3 and T4 cases, avoiding an unhelpful delay of surgery in non advanced cases. Accurate staging by preoperative video-laparoscopy allows for a more homogeneous evaluation of the treatment results in the context of research studies; finally, the application of "second-look" laparoscopy in se-lected cases may offer a chance to verify a possible tumor downstaging and to detect the sites of residual disease after neoadjuvant treatment.

References

1. Jacobaeus HC. Kurze Ubersicht uber meine Erfahrungen mit der Laparoskopie. Munch Med Wochenschr 58:2017-2019, 1911.
2. Greene FL. Laparoscopy in malignant disease. Surg Clin North Am 72 (5):1125-1136, 1992.
3. Nduka CC, Monson JRT, Menzies-Gow N et al. Abdominal wall metastases following laparoscopy. Br J Surg 81: 648-652, 1994.
4. Taffinder NJ, Champault G. Port site metastases sfter laparoscopic colorectal surgery for cure of malignancy. Br J Surg 83:133 (Letter), 1996 .
5. Ishida H, Murata N, Yamada H et al. Influence of trocar placement and CO2 pneumoperitoneum on port site metastases. Surg Endosc 14(2): 193-197, 2000.
6. Wittich P, Marquet RL, Kazemier G et al. Port site metastases after CO laparoscopy. Is the aerosolization of tumor cells a pilotal factor? Surg Endosc 14(2): 189-192, 2000.
7. Reymond MA, Schneider C, Kastl S et al. The pathogenesis of port site recurrences. J Gastrointest Surg 2(5): 406-414, 1998.
8. Pearlstone DB, Feig BW, Mansfield PF. Port site recurrences after laparoscopy for malignant disease. Semin Surg Oncol 16(4): 307-312, 1999.
9. Possik RA, Franco EL, Pires DR, et al.: Sensitivity, specificity and predictive value of laparoscopy for the staging of gastric cancer and for the detection of liver metastases. Cancer 58:1-6, 1986.
10. Kriplani AK, Kapur BML: Laparoscopy for pre-operative staging and assessment of operability in gastric carcinoma. Gastrointest Endosc 37(4):441-443, 1991.
11. Rougier P, Lasser P, Ducreux M et al. Preoperative chemotherapy in gastric cancer. Ann Oncol 5 (suppl 3): 59, 1994.
12. Fink U, Stein HJ, Schuhmacher C et al. Neoadjuvant chemotherapy for gastric cancer: un update. World J Surg 19: 509-516, 1995.
13. Wilke H, Preusser P, Fink U et al. Preoperative chemotherapy in locally advanced and unresectable gastric cancer: a phase II study with etoposide, doxorubicin and cisplatin. J Clin Oncol 7: 1318-1326, 1989.

14. Plukker JT, Mudler NH, Sleijfer DTH et al. Chemotherapy and surgery for locally advanced cancer of the cardia and fundus. Phase II study with methotrexate and fluoruracil. Br J Surg 78: 955, 1991.
15. Gross E, Bancewicz J, Ingram G. Assessment of gastric cancer by laparoscopy. Br Med J (Clin Res Ed) 288: 1577, 1984.
16. Lowy AM, Mansfield PF, Steven D et al. Laparoscopic staging for gastric cancer. Surgery 119 (6): 611-614, 1996.
17. Stell DA, Carter CR, Stewart I, et al.: Prospective comparison of laparoscopy, ultrasonography and computed tomography in the staging of gastric cancer. Br J Surg 86:1260-1262, 1996.
18. Burke EC, Karpeh MS, Conlon KC, et al.:Laparoscopy in the Management of gastric adenocarcinoma. Ann Surg 225(3): 262-267, 1997.
19. D'ugo DM, Persiani R, Caracciolo F, et al. Selection of locally advanced gastric carcinoma by preoperative staging laparoscopy. Surg Endosc 11:1159-1162, 1997.
20. Yano M, Tsujinaka T, Shiozaki H et al. Appraisal of treatment strategy by staging laparoscopy for locally advanced gastric cancer. World J Surg 24:1130-1136, 2000.
21. D'ugo DM, Coppola R, Persiani R, et al. Immediately preoperative laparoscopic staging for gastric cancer. Surg Endosc 10:996-999, 1996.
22. Feussner H, Omote K, Fink U, et al. Pretherapeutic laparoscopic staging in advanced gastric carcinoma. Endoscopy 31(5):342-347, 1999.
23. Sobin LH, Fleming ID. TNM classification of malignant tumors, fifth edition (1997). Union Internationale Contre le Cancer and the American Joint Commettee on Cancer. Cancer 80 (9): 1803-1804, 1997.
24. Charukhchyan SA., Lucas GW. Laparoscopy and lesser sac endoscopy in gastric carcinoma operability assessment. Am Surg 64:160-164, 1998.
25. Ascher SM, Evans SRT, Zeman RK. Laparoscopic cholecystectomy: intraoperative ultra-sound of the extra-hepatic biliary tree and the natural history of postoperative transabdominal ultrasounds fndings. Semin Ultrasound 14: 331-337, 1993.
26. Marugiah M, Paterson-Brown S, Winsdor JA et al. Early experience of laparoscopic ultrasonography in the management of pancreatic carcinoma. Surg Endosc 7: 119-124, 1993.
27. Cuesta MA, Mejer S, Borgstein PJ et al. Laparoscopic ultrasonography for hepato-biliary and pancreatic malignancy. Br J Surg 80: 1571-1574, 1993.
28. John TG, Greig JD, Carter DC et al. Carcinoma of the pancreatic head and periampullary region: tumor staging with laparoscopy and laparoscopic ultrasonography. Ann Surg 221: 156-164, 1995.
29. Velasco JM, Rossi H, Hieken TJ, et al. Laparoscopic ultrasound enhances diagnostic laparoscopy in the staging of intra-abdominal neoplasms. Presented at 42th Annual Meeting - Midwest Surgical Association, Galena, Illinois - August 15-18, 1999.
30. Conlon KC, Karpeh MS. Laparoscopy and laparoscopic ultrasound in the staging of gastric cancer. Seminars in Oncology 23(3):347-351, 1996.
31. Van Dijkum JN, De Wit LTH, Van Delden OM, et al. Staging laparoscopy and laparoscopic ultrasonography in more than 400 patients with upper gastrointestinal carcinoma. J Am Coll Surg 189(5):459-465, 1999.
32. Halpert RD, Feczko PF. Role of radiology in the diagnosis and staging of gastric malignancies. Endoscopy 25: 36-45, 1993.
33. Wanebo HJ, Kennedy BJ, Chmiel J et al. Cancer of the stomach. A patient care study by the American College of Surgeon. Ann Surg 218(5): 583-592, 1993.
34. Picciocchi A, D'ugo D, Ronconi P, et al.: The impact of staging laparoscopy on the treatment of locally advanced gastric cancer. J Exp Clin Cancer Res 16(2):84-86, 1997.
35. Sendler A, Dittler HJ, Feussner H. Preoperative staging of gastric cancer as a precondition for multimodal treatment. World J Surg 19(4): 501-508, 1995.
36. Siewert JR, Maruyama K. What's new in gastric cancer? (Editorial). World J Surg 19: 483, 1995.
37. Persiani R, Pende V, Picciocchi A et al. Laparoscopic staging of gastric carcinoma; diagnostic and therapeutic implications. Proceedings of 8th International Congress of E.A.E.S.- Nice, June 28-July 1, 2000.
38. Ribeiro U, Gama-Rodrigues JJ, Bitelman B et al. Value of peritoneal lavage cytology during laparoscopy staging of patients with gastric carcinoma. Surg Laparosc Endosc 8: 132-135, 1998.
39. D'Ugo D, Persiani R, Pende V et al. Neoadjuvant chemotherapy for locally advanced gastric cancer: results on an ongoing phase II study. Proceedings of 4th International Gastric Cancer Congress - New York, April 29-May 2, 2001.
40. Watanapa P, Williamson RCN. Surgical palliation for pancreatic cancer: developments during the pat two decades. Br J Surg 79: 1348, 1992.
41. De Roij PD, Rogatko A, Brennan M. Evaluation of palliative surgical procedures in unresectable pancreatic cancer. Br J Surg 78: 1053-1058, 1991.
42. Goh PMY, Kum CK. Laparoscopic BII gastrectomy: a review. Surg Oncol 2 suppl 1: 13-18, 1993.
43. Nathanson LK. Laparoscopic colecosto-jejunostomy and gastroenterostomy for malignant disease. Surg Oncol 2 suppl 1: 19-24, 1993.
44. Sosa JL, Zalewski M, Puente I. Laparoscopic gastro-jejunostomy technique: case report. Laparoendosc Surg 4: 215-220, 1994.
45. Brune IB, Feussner H, Neuhaus H et al. Laparoscopic gastrojejunostomy and endoscopic biliary stent placement for palliation of incurable gastric outlet obstruction with cholestasis. Surg Endosc 11: 834-837, 1997.

CHAPTER

Laparoscopic surgery for gastric cancer 3

M.M. Konstadoulakis, I.P. Gomatos

Introduction

Minimally invasive surgery combines modern technology with surgical innovation. It was first introduced in 1988, and progressively gained increasing momentum and acceptance by both the public and medical communities. Advanced technology has allowed surgeons to apply minimal access techniques to a wide variety of surgical procedures. These innovative procedures accomplish the traditional goals of surgery (diagnosis, staging, removal and repair of disease states) with small incisions and decreased psychological trauma. Moreover, today's advanced digital technology allows magnification of the laparoscopic surgery site up to 20 times actual size, permitting surgeons to see anatomical structures in exquisite detail. As a result, the list of minimally invasive surgical procedures is increasing on a daily basis. Currently, the application of laparoscopic techniques to general surgical procedures has revolutionized the field of general surgery. Furthermore, the application of laparoscopic techniques has been expanded to the era of surgical oncology to include staging and diagnostic procedures as well as curative and palliative resections.

The official history of laparoscopic gastric surgery begins in 1992, when Goh et al. performed the first entirely laparoscopic distal gastrectomy with a Billroth II reconstruction on a patient with chronic gastric ulcer[1,2,3,4,5]. Despite being controversial, laparoscopic curative resection for advanced gastric cancer has been performed at multiple institutions with encouraging early results. Up to day more than 1000 gastrectomies have been laparoscopically performed mainly for benign gastric tumors and low-grade malignant neoplasms[6,7,8]. Furthermore, there are several studies that advocate the use of laparoscopic palliative gastrectomies or gastric bypass for patients with advanced or metastatic disease. Among the many reasons for the slow acceptance of the above procedures are the technical skills required to perform laparoscopic gastrectomies, and the fear that laparoscopic surgery cannot accommodate basic oncological principles of open surgery. Moreover, certain aspects of curative gastrectomy (like a more extended lymph node dissection) cannot be easily performed by the classical laparoscopic surgical means. In order to apply the advantages of minimally invasive surgery in gastric surgery, we need to resolve the problems of GI tract reconstruction, radical cancer surgery and removal of larger specimens. The development of new technologies such as the hand-assist device, allow surgeons a better access of internal structures, making laparoscopy a safe option for a growing list of more complex surgical procedures.

One significant profit of minimally invasive surgery is that patients prefer it over an extended open procedure. This preference is followed by some major benefits. Surgical incision represents the primary source of pain, infection and psychologic stress, which often discourage patients, leading them to delay the performance of a needed operation. Such a delay in treatment may allow the disease to advance to a point where it is either incurable or the operation is made more difficult, resulting in an increased risk of complications or death. This risk is significantly increased in candidates for tumor resection. The ability to perform conventional operations through small incisions is sufficiently enticing to many patients so that they are agreeable to undergo surgery earlier in the course of their disease when an operation will be potentially easier and more effective.

Some of the benefits laparoscopic gastric surgery may offer to the patients are the following:

1. Three or four small scars instead of one large abdominal scar.
2. Shorter hospital stay.
3. Reduced postoperative pain.
4. Shorter recovery time and a more rapid return to daily activities, including work.
5. Better Survival? It seems from the results from retrospective or prospective but not randomized trials that laparoscopic gastrectomies for gastric cancer offer at least the same benefits with open gastric surgery.

Today, the use of laparoscopic surgery is gaining increasing acceptance in staging and treatment of gastric cancer. Unfortunately, despite the event that laparoscopic gastrectomy has been shown to be safe and effective in many retrospective series, there are no prospective randomized control trials comparing it to conventional open resection. There are several applications for laparoscopic gastric surgery today. Theses are staging, curative resections and palliative procedures.

Indications for Laparoscopic Gastrectomy

Laparoscopic gastrectomy is currently being applied for a growing list of benign and malignant diseases even though the precise indications have not been clarified yet. Several techniques for laparoscopic gastric resection have evolved during the past years. The most widely perfomed procedures may be classified as follows:

1. Laparoscopic partial or total gastrectomy with intracorporeal reconstruction of the GI tract.
2. Laparoscopic-assisted partial or total gastrectomy with extracorporeal reconstruction of the GI tract.
3. Laparoscopic-assisted partial or total gastrectomy with reconstruction of the GI tract by the Hand Assisted Laparoscopic System (H.A.L.S.).

The indications for laparoscopic gastrectomy regarding gastric cancer are still evolving. Early gastric cancer, is considered to be suitable for laparoscopic resection. Early gastric tumors involving the submucosa require gastrectomy with removal of the greater omentum and level-1 lymph nodes. Gastric tumors involving the muscularis propria, (T2 and T3) require a more extensive regional dissection. Although this procedure can be performed laparoscopically, there is concern on the adequacy of the omentectomy and nodal clearance by the laparoscopic approach and thus minimally invasive techniques cannot be regarded as standard practice. Despite concerns, an increasing number of surgeons advocate curative laparoscopic gastrectomy to treat this subset of tumors, with comparable results to traditional open procedures. Fixation of the tumor to the pancreas and celiac axis suggests inoperability indicative of a palliative bypass procedure. A laparoscopically performed palliative procedure can be performed for locally advanced disease with severe symptoms. These procedures will be discussed in a following paragraph. Although hepatic metastases and/or the presence of peritoneal deposits confirm incurability, they do not preclude palliative resection unless there is extensive involvement.

Laparoscopic Staging and Decision-Making for Gastric Cancer

Cancer staging is of paramount importance in planning the treatment approaches for patients with localized and advanced disease. Precise staging assessment identifies patients with potentially resectable localized tumors from patients with advanced disease or distant metastases. In view of the increasing alternatives for neoadjuvant therapy and nonoperative palliative procedures, physicians are obligated to ensure that each patient receives the most appropriate treatment with minimal morbidity and in a cost effective manner. In the past, it was not unusual for patients with gastric malignancies to come to laparotomy after conventional preoperative staging only to have metastases discovered during abdominal exploration. Preoperative imaging methods like CT, MRI or PET are associated with suboptimal diagnostic accuracy regarding metastatic disease. Surgeons introduced laparoscopic staging for gastric cancer in an attempt to decrease the incidence of this problem. The technical refinement of the laparoscope over the past decade and the enhancement of technique made laparoscopy the ideal tool for the definitive diagnosis and staging of malignancy especially for detecting metastases that are not found by standard preoperative staging.

Staging of gastric cancer can be accomplished by the evaluation of some inherent characteristics, such as gastric serosal infltration, lymph node involvement, adherens to adjacent structures, peritoneal carcinomatosis, ascites and the presence of liver metastases. The identification of advanced nodal, peritoneal, or hepatic disease is important prior to undertaking celiotomy. The major purpose of laparoscopy is to assess perigastric lymph nodes and to look for superficial peritoneal and hepatic masses that have not been identified by conventional imaging studies. Using a combination of laparoscopy and CT or MRI, at least 90% of unresectable tumors can be identified, without the need for exploratory celiotomy.

Liver represents the most common site of extragastric metastases. Metastatic disease of the liver is the most common indication for laparoscopic assessment, since many of the hepatic metastases are usually situated on its surface. Furthermore, the recent application of laparoscopic ultrasound has aided in the identification of tumors deep to Glisson's capsule. Examination of the abdomen by laparoscopic ultrasound was introduced as an adjunct to laparoscopy because it can detect intraparenchymal lesions such as intrahepatic metastases, as well as enlarged lymph nodes, and vascular invasion by tumor[9]. In contrast with traditional imaging studies, which often underestimate the involvement of the liver, laparoscopic approach has a higher sensitivity and specifity, which becomes critically important in tumor staging and surgical decision-making.

Preoperative laparoscopic evaluation in patients with gastric cancer may also aid in identifying those in whom the disease is disseminated throughout the abdomen, thus precluding a potential curative resection. It permits us to observe directly sites, such as the subphrenic space and the Douglas pouch, where peritoneal metastases are frequently present but are usually missed during conventional laparotomy. Because of the natural progression of the disease, the risk of finding peritoneal implants at the time of laparotomy after an otherwise, unremarkable CT scan, ranges between 25 and 37%. Since, few patients with M1 disease actually develop surgical bleeding or significant gastric outlet obstruction prior to death, a strong argument can be made for laparoscoping all patients with advanced gastric cancer. Staging laparoscopy should be performed for all patients at high risk for peritoneal metastasis, such as patients with large undifferentiated or multifocal tumors. Some authors suggest that a cytologic investigation of peritoneal washings should be performed as well, if other examinations are negative. Carcinoma cells may be obtained from the free peritoneal cavity even when the peritoneum itself is grossly free of metastatic implants. The positive cytology of free cancer cells in the abdominal lavage fluid is an independent prognostic factor for T2 and T3/4 patients with no apparent peritoneal seeding during surgery.

How We Do It

Regarding the technique for staging laparoscopy, the CO_2 pneumoperitoneum is established through a Veress needle in the umbilicus and kept constant at 12 mm Hg. Two to three trocars are then introduced, according to the scheme illustrated in (Figure 1). Regardless of the intervention performed, the first step in any laparoscopic procedure for biopsy-proven gastric malignancy consists of a complete and extensive exploration of the peritoneal cavity. At this time, we search for undetected implants and visceral metastases, which could require us to modify the operative strategy. The exploration, which is carried out with the aid of an ultrasound probe, requires access to the lesser sac

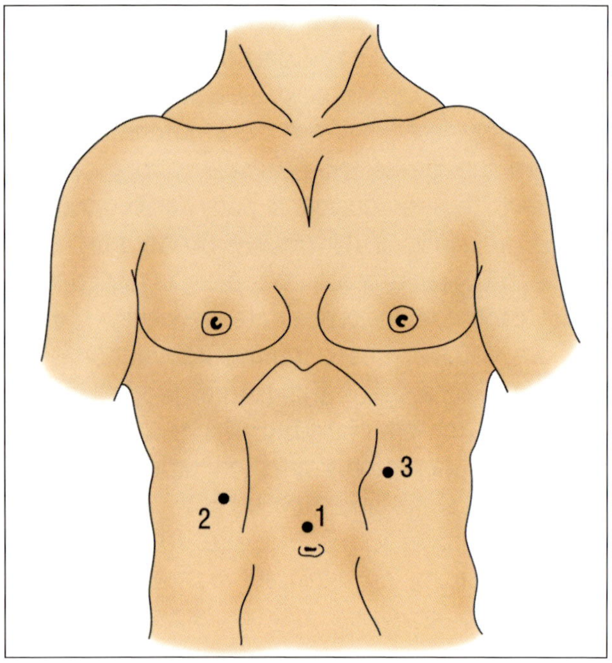

FIGURE 1. Trocar placement for staging laparoscopy.

cavity. It is followed by a standardized lymph node sampling at the level of the left gastric artery, including the greater gastric curvature, the supra and infrapyloric nodes, the splenic artery, and the splenic hylum. All retrieved material is sent for immediate analysis.

After the completion of the abdominal explration the surgeon decides on the appropriate curative or palliative procedure. In the presence of positive N1 nodes (according to the UICC classification system) or T3 lesions, it is more advisable to use a laparoscopy-assisted approach instead of a totally laparoscopic approach. In the presence of previously undetected or laparoscopy-confirmed M1 lesions we do not consider the patient eligible for curative surgery. In these cases we prefer to perform a palliative gastrectomy, which can be accomplished either by the conventional open approach or by a combined laparoscopic procedure. In both cases the decision is made on the basis of the surgeon's personal experience and the patient's clinical status. The existing trends in laparoscopic surgery suggest that all measures are taken to minimize tumor manipulation or gastric rupture. Macroscopically advanced gastric tumors presenting posterior gastric fixity, pancreatic penetration or colonic invasion are usually referred for palliative management.

Still there are several important technical aspects regarding diagnostic laparoscopy that have to be defined. The first controversial issue is the timing of the procedure. It can be either a separate procedure, or performed immediately before the planned curative surgery. Another unresolved debate is the extent of the procedure. It ranges from inspection only, with biopsy of suspicious lesions, to extensive dissection, use of LUS, and peritoneal cytology sampling[10]. Furthermore, irresponsible usage of surgical laparoscopy is not beneficial for the doctor or for the patient. In fact, in addition to the morbidity and mortality related to surgical procedures, dissemination of tumor cells as a consequence of biopsies or other tumor manipulations could occur. Port-site metastases following diagnostic laparoscopy have been well described in the literature[11]. Beyond any doubt surgical laparoscopy constitutes a step forward in surgical methodologies and contributes to improved preoperative staging, especially for peritoneal carcinomatosis with a sensitivity ranging between 87% and 92%[12,13]. Although, the available evidence regarding laparoscopic staging is all retrospective, it is of sufficient consistency to indicate that this diagnostic procedure adds to the primary staging altering the clinical stage of the disease and hence the management of the individual patient. Furthermore, we can perform needle aspiration or biopsy of perigastric masses if a tissue diagnosis has not previously been obtained. Thus, it should be used if therapeutic benefits can be gained, as is true for neoadjuvant chemotherapy. Otherwise, benefits and risks must be evaluated carefully.

Laparoscopic Gastrectomy

In laparoscopic gastrectomy two options for patient positioning are available: (1) The patient lying in the supine position with head-up tilt, with the surgeon operating from the right side of the surgical table, and (2) The patient lying in the supine position with head-up tilt and abduction of the lower limbs, with the surgeon operating between the abducted lower limbs of the patient. The second option is easier and more comfortable for the surgeon and is the position that gives the best ergonomic layout for hand-assisted laparoscopic gastric surgery.

The sites of the access ports for laparoscopic gastrectomy vary depending on the surgical approach used. The optical port is placed at the umbiliqus and the other operating ports are shown in (Figure 2). A 30° forward-oblique telescope is favored by a number of surgeons while other surgeons prefer a forward-viewing variety.

Laparoscopic partial gastrectomy includes the following steps.

1. Mobilization of the greater curvature.
2. Sling elevation of the stomach.
3. Ligation of the right gastric artery.
4. Ligation of the left gastric vessels in continuity.
5. Gastric resection.
6. Reconstruction of the GI tract.

For a Billroth I procedure we maintain duodenal continuity until the stomach is ready for resection.

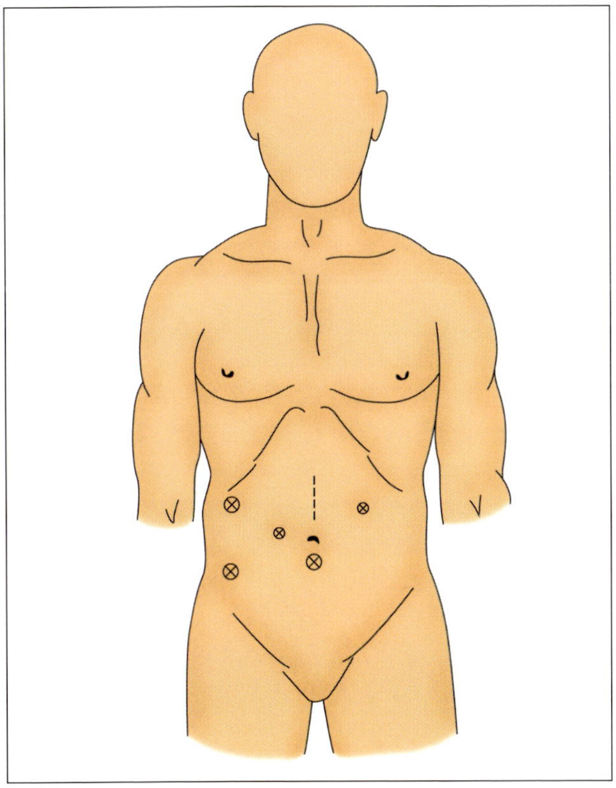

FIGURE 2. Port locations for laparoscopic or laparoscopically assisted gastrectomy. The dashed line indicates the site of mini-laparotomy.

At this point we make the first application of the endoscopic stapler vertically from the lesser curvature. The second and third applications are at an angle to the first application so that the transection line reaches the lesser curvature more proximally.

In order to perform a Billroth II laparoscopic gastrectomy, the duodenum is divided with an endoscopic linear stapler well beyond the pylorus. The staple line is carefully inspected and reinforced with interrupted sutures when necessary. The proximal transection site of the stomach is selected before performing the gastrectomy and the appropriate sites on the greater and lesser curvatures are cleared of fat and blood vessels. The stomach is transected vertically from the greater to the lesser curvature, using the endoscopic linear stapler. Usually, three applications of the 3.0-cm endoscopic linear stapler (blue cartridge) are necessary. In both cases, the specimen is removed through a small midline laparotomy.

Laparoscopic total gastrectomy is usually performed for early gastric tumors situated at the middle and upper third of the stomach as well as for gastric lymphomas. The technique is similar to that for laparoscopic distal gastrectomy with these important differences:

1. The mobilization of the greater curvature involves detachment of the entire greater omentum from the transverse colon.
2. Division of the lesser omentum.
3. Sling elevation of the stomach.
4. Hiatal dissection with mobilization of the abdominal esophagus and bilateral truncal vagotomy.
5. Dissection of the celiac axis with division of the left gastric artery at its origin and division of the left gastric (coronary) vein.
6. Ligature of the right gastric artery.
7. Duodenal mobilization and transection.
8. Proximal transection, removal of specimen and reconstruction through upper midline minilaparotomy or through the hand-assisted wound.

The reconstruction of the continuity of the GI tract after laparoscopic gastrectomy can be performed intracorporeally (by staplers, suturing, or both), or extracorporealy through an upper midline minilaparotomy. In the latter instance, the protected minilaparotomy serves as the route for extraction of the resected specimen as well.

Intracorporeal Reconstruction of the GI Tract: Intracorporeal GI tract reconstruction is usually performed in palliative distal gastrectomy for incurable cancer. In these cases after the closure of the duodenal stump, we perform an intracorporeal antecolic stapled gastro-jejunostomy.

Extracorporeal GI Tract Reconstruction: Reconstruction after distal Billroth II gastrectomy for cancer, is best performed with an open Roux-en-Y anastomosis through the minilaparotomy, while reconstruction after distal Billroth I gastrectomy for benign disease is performed with a sutured gastroduodenostomy through a minilaparotomy.

After total gastrectomy, the reconstruction of the GI tract is performed by placing a purse-string suture (2-0 prolene) at the cut end of the esophagus. We then introduce the anvil of the circular stapler into the lumen of the esophagus and tie the purse string over the stem. A classical Hunt-Lawrence Roux-en-Y is created from the upper jejunum using the established open surgical techniques. The pouch is then stapled to the esophagus in standard fashion.

Hand-Assisted Laparoscopic Gastrectomy

Hand-assisted laparoscopic surgery (HALS) is a recent development of minimally invasive technique that allows insertion of the surgeon's non-dominant hand into the abdomen while pneumoperitoneum is maintained[14]. This development has greatly expedited complex laparoscopic surgery, and gastric operations are not an exception. Established advantages of HALS include the ability to reproduce an operative setting which is similar to that of open surgery retaining at the same time most benefits of the laparoscopic approach[15,16,17]. In open surgery, the nondominant hand of the surgeon is mainly used to retract, palpate, and expose tissue. It allows for excellent exploration, proper exposure, finger dissection, quality suturing needed for the completion of a GI tract anastomosis and meticulous hemostasis. The presence of the surgeon's hand inside the abdomen is useful when tactile feedback is a crucial component of the procedure, to enhance its safety or to make it quicker[18]. Procedures like gastrectomies for gastric tumors that would not be technically feasible by pure laparoscopy or that would involve substantial risk for the patient can now be considered by Hand assisted laparoscopic surgery with a lower degree of complexity and increased safety margin[19,20,21,22,23,24,25,26]. Furthermore the retrieval of the specimen from the abdomen is easier. In our Department we have employed this technique in a group of patients with early gastric cancer. Briefly, the technique we use is the following.

Patient Set-Up (Laparoscopic Hand Assisted Gastric Surgery)

Irrespective of the hand-assisted device used, the optimal position of the surgeon when using one of these systems is between the patient's lower limbs held abducted on stirrups (i.e., French position). The patient is positioned in the supine position with head-up tilt and abduction of the lower limbs, while the surgeon is operating between his legs. The main monitor is positioned at the head of the table. This arrangement is easier and more comfortable for the surgeon but may increase calf vein compression and subsequently the risk of deep venous thrombosis (DVT), especially if leg stirrups are used. DVT prophylaxis with subcutaneous heparin and graduated compression stockings is recommended as well as antibiotic prophylaxis.

Hand-Assist Device Placement

Choosing a site for the placement of hand-assist devices such as the HandPort should wait until the abdomen has been insufflated. The distortion of the abdominal wall under pneumoperitoneum would change the ultimate position and length of any incision attempted prior to insufflating. A site is then chosen in the high left upper quadrant just lateral to rectus abdominus. We believe that the optimal position of the hand is one that allows for triangulation with the other laparoscopic instruments and therefore substitutes for a typical port site in standard laparoscopy. The length of incision correlates mainly with the breadth of the surgeon's palm. This length also approximates the size of the surgeon's glove (7-8 cm for most surgeons). The incision is then carried full thickness. Loss of pneumoperitoneum will occur at this stage.

The ultimate hand-assist device placement can be modified according to the surgeon's dominant hand. In our description, we have chosen to introduce our right hand for hand-assistance and use our left hand to handle laparoscopic instruments. Conceptually, a right- handed surgeon may prefer to introduce his/her non-dominant hand through a mirror image set up while operating from the patient's left side. Either should allow good exposure and functional assistance. From the ergonomic perspective, the hand assist devices work best if the surgeon uses his non-dominant hand inside the abdomen whilst his dominant hand manipulates the endoscopic instrument introduced through a standard laparoscopic port. Thus the relative location between the hand-access device and the operating (dominant hand) port and the telescopic port is crucial. For right handed surgeons, the optimal placement of the hand access device for laparoscopic gastrectomy is through a transverse incision (5 7cm, depending on the surgeon's hand size) placed just to the right of the midline just above the umbilicus. The operating port is placed 5.0cm to the left and at the level of the umbilicus. The optical cannula is situated in the left upper quadrant at the same level as the hand assist device. This results in off-axis viewing, it provides acceptable imaging of the operative field especially if an oblique 30 telescope is used so that the optical axis-target angle is about 90° [21]. Additional ports for assisting instruments are placed on either side high up in the left and right upper quadrants. The hand assist device is also used for extraction of the specimen, and when appropriate for the reconstruction of the continuity of the GI tract.

Laparoscopic Palliative Surgery for Gastric Cancer

Palliative surgical procedures for gastric cancer have been designed to alleviate symptoms such as intestinal obstruction, bleeding, or the inability to take in nutrition in settings where the cancer may not be able to be removed due to advanced disease. These procedures dramatically improve the quality of life and allow other treatments, such as chemotherapy, immunotherapy or radiotherapy to be administered. Recently, laparoscopic surgery has been successfully introduced as an alternative approach in order to alleviate symptoms of gastric cancer patients presenting with inoperable tumors. Patients with unresectable gastric tumors and no evidence of metastatic disease can be expected to survive 5-6 months without any treatment. A minimally invasive approach allows for a quicker recovery and quicker start of non-surgical therapy than the open, traditional method. Laparoscopically performed gastrostomy, jejunostomy and gastric bypass are the most commonly performed laparoscopic palliative procedures today.

Percutaneous endoscopic gastrostomy and jejunostomy tube placement have long been considered the standard way for supplying enteral nutrition when oral intake is not possible. Both procedures are associated with high incidence of aspiration. A distally placed tube in the jejunum decreases the chance of this morbid complication. Nevertheless, when percutaneous endoscopic gastrostomy is indicated but cannot be done for technical reasons, laparoscopic enteral access is desirable. This technique is very demanding from the average surgeon to duplicate, involving nonstandard anchoring techniques of the bowel to the abdominal wall. Nevertheless it has already been used as a routine alternative procedure for open surgery in specialized centers with satisfying results, since it allows early mobilization of an already severely ill patient with minimal trauma. Using a mini-laparoscope less than a quarter inch in diameter, this operation is done to create a small hole in the small intestine for the insertion of a feeding tube. It is a safe and cost-effective operation to gain access to the small intestine.

Another palliative procedure for locally advanced gastric cancer involves bypassing the diseased part of the GI tract with gastrojejunostomy. Management of malignant duodenal obstruction has traditionally been by operative gastrojejunostomy. Nevertheless, this procedure is associated with significant morbidity and mortality. Since, laparoscopy provides a new option for early discharge, an increasing number of surgeons perform a laparoscopic-assisted gastrojejunostomy with encouraging early results. The above technique has already been used successfully to surgically treat morbid obesity and its numerous comorbidities. Previous reports suggests that laparoscopic gastric bypass is associated with less I.C.U. care, shorter hospital stays, fewer wound infections and fewer incisional hernias. Still, the procedure requires longer operative time and has a higher rate of anastomotic strictures. Gastric cancer patients with advanced disease are therefore perfect candidates for a laparoscopic palliative procedure.

Complications

Every kind of surgical intervention is associated with possible complications. Although laparoscopic surgery carries a far lower complication rate compared to conventional open procedures, it has been reported that about 2 to 4% of patients who undergo laparoscopic surgery will experience a complication. Severe bleeding, the risk of infection, postoperative pneumonia or blood clots forming in the deep veins in the legs are some of the most common complications associated with laparoscopic surgery. These risks are reduced by the use of antibiotics, pneumatic stockings, and laparoscopic techniques, which allow the patient to be active more quickly after surgery. Other complications such as wound infection and incisional hernia can easily be avoided by the experienced surgeon. There are also complications specific to the type of minimal invasive surgery. Damage to organs such as the bowel, spleen or liver may occur during laparoscopic gastrectomy. If these damages are not identified by the surgical team during surgery, they may result in serious infections.

Furhtermore, laparoscopic partial and total gastrectomy bear some rare, even unique complications, which are not so often encountered by surgeons performing conventional open gastric procedures. We present some of the most significant postoperative complications encountered in patients who have been laparoscopically treated for gastric malignancies worldwide.

i) ***Pneumothorax.*** Pneumothorax can occur, if the pleura is damaged during the mobilization of the mediastinal esophagus. Carbon dioxide then insufflates into the pleural space, which results into tension pneumothorax. Placement of a chest tube corrects the cardiopulmonary compromise but may cause desufflation of the pneumoperitoneum through the chest drain. If this happens, intermittent occlusion of the chest drain allows completion of the operation.

ii) Bleeding from the suture line is another significant postoperative complication. In our experience postoperative oozing is not uncommon after intracorporeally stapled gastrojejunal anastomosis (18%), while it is less frequent (5%) after hand-sutured anastomosis. Blood transfusion is usually required, and the haemorrhage generally stops without any further complications.

iii) Trocar site metastasis represents a significant issue concerning laparoscopic surgical treatment for malignancies. Many clinicians have reported the development of trocar site metastasis after the performance of laparoscopic colorectal or gallbladder surgery[27,28]. In these reports, most of the initial malignancies seemed to be in an advanced stage in which the cancer extended beyond the serosa or a rupture of the affected organ took place during surgery. Although some report that pneumoperitoneum with carbon dioxide may increase the risk of tumor implantation, its mechanism and possibility in clinical practise is still controversial[28,29]. In most gastric cancer cases, laparoscopic surgical treatment is indicated for early gastric cancer, which is still limited within the gastric wall. Furthermore, in order to avoid the risk of implanting cancer tissue, the resected specimen is cautiously isolated in a special specimen bag immediately after resection. For 8 years Balli et al. followed their colectomies for cancer and did not report a single port site recurrence in 320 cases. Their principles for avoiding this complication included: a) Fixation of trocars to the abdominal wall, b) "No touch technique" c) High vascular ligation, d) Intraoperative colonoscopy and intraluminal irrigation with 5% iodine povidone, e) Specimen isolation before extraction from the abdominal cavity, f) Intraperitoneal and trocar-site irrigation with a tumoricidal solution. The application of the above principles in laparoscopic gastrectomy may prove valuable in reducing the incidence of this complication.

iv) Twenty-five percent of the patients who are submitted to intracorporeal reconstruction of the GI tract deal with the poor functional results of the anastomosis. Vomiting and bile reflux are the most common manifestation of this problem. A re-operation is usually suggested to improve the patients' symptoms.

All the above problems can be dealt with either intraoperatively, or on a second look laparoscopy. Whenever there is difficulty with visualization, or the surgeon comes across other complications which cannot be laparoscopically amended it is indicated to convert to a conventional open technique. Although laparoscopic gastrectomies are more complicated procedures, than laparoscopic cholecystectomies, their conversion rate does not differ from the classical 1-10%, constituting them the treatment of choice for a setting of carefully selected patients. Of course a greater number of routinely performed laparoscopic gastrectomies is needed in order to draw valid conclusions regarding the morbidity and mortality of this procedure.

Summary

A controversial issue regarding curative laparoscopic resections for gastric cancer is whether they offer the ability to achieve equal tumor reduction with classical open procedures. A careful selection of the candidates to be submitted in this type of surgery determined by careful preoperative staging, appears to be essential, since the indications are still evolving, due to the rapid development of modern surgical techniques and equipment. Several studies report comparable oncologic outcomes in open and laparoscopic operations for colorectal malignancies. It is believed that if performed by experts, laparoscopic gastrectomy is as safe as conventional "open" surgery in carefully selected cases. Furthermore, with the advent of new laparoscopic instruments, laparoscopic gastric resections appear to be technically feasible providing early postoperative recovery together with adequate lymph node dissection for patients with preoperative diagnosis of intramuscular gastric cancer.

D_1 gastrectomy is eminently feasible through the laparoscopic or the laparoscopically assisted approach. The hand-assisted technique greatly expedites the execution of this surgery. Hand-access devices enable the introduction of the surgeon's assisting hand, which is used for effective atraumatic display and controlled traction of tissues during dissection. Our operative times for purely laparoscopic total gastrectomy averaged 6.5 hours, and 4 hours for subtotal gastrectomy. We are fairly confident that hand-assistance will allow us to reduce our operative times substantially (perhaps by as much as 50% or greater). The hand assist method should also allow for greater control that should result in fewer conversions. The other potential benefits of the hand-assisted approach remain to be determined.

Regarding laparoscopic D_1 gastrectomy, Reyes et al.[30] in a retrospective case-matched study, conducted on 36 gastric cancer patients, reported that totally laparoscopic partial gastrectomy is an excellent alternative to the traditional open approach which is associated with a more rapid return of intestinal function and a shorter hospital stay.

D_2 gastrectomy has also been performed laparoscopically. Azagra et al[1] reported nine D_1 and three D_2 total gastrectomies. In this study one major intraoperative complication (i.e., damage to the common hepatic artery) and one postoperative death (8%) were reported. Eleven people were alive at a mean follow-up of 27.5 months, but two developed hepatic metastases.[31,32,33]. Another study conducted by Goh et al[34] included 4 patients with advanced gastric cancer and revealed that laparoscopic radical gastrectomy for moderately advanced cancers can produce good results in terms of safety and oncologic adequacy. Since the benefits from this procedure are unclear, the existing concerns regarding the extent of lymphadenectomy and the possibility of tumor dissemination are justifiable.

Whatever the merits of the laparoscopic approach, established oncologic principles governing resections for neoplastic disease must not be overlooked in the adoption of the laparoscopic approach for the surgical management of these patients. The caution against laparoscopic D_2 gastrectomy is justified, and this procedure cannot be regarded as routine unless performed in centers with significant experience in this approach. Laparoscopically-assisted D_1 gastrectomy for stage I and II tumors is more acceptable and may be beneficial in elderly patients. For advanced gastric tumors with liver and/or lung metastases, palliative laparoscopic gastrectomies or bypss procedures definitely have advantage over the open techniques.

In a recent study, Adaschi et al.[35] analyzed and compared the hospital charges between laparoscopic-assisted gastrectomy and conventional open gastrectomy. Laparoscopy-assisted Billroth I gastrectomy appeared to be less expensive than conventional open Billroth I gastrectomy because the postoperative recovery period and the hospital stay were shorter. In patients who undergo gastrectomy, the additional costs of the disposable instruments can be fully offset by the lower charges for ward and meal and nursing care associated with laparoscopic gastrectomy. It appears that laparoscopic gastric surgery can decrease the cost of a Billroth I gastrectomy by avoiding the costs of a prolonged period of postoperative hospitalization.

Laparoscopic gastric resections are in the evaluation stage in terms of indications and techniques used, and the reported data are largely made up of case reports and small series. Thus, definitive conclusions on benefits, risks, morbidity and long-term outcome are not feasible. In order to obtain real answer to the superiority of the laparoscopic approach to the open surgery, a prospective randomized study concerning long-term survival is awaited. Nevertheless, taking into consideration the increasing frequency of minimally invasive procedures for gastric malignancies, it appears that in the near future more results regarding laparoscopic gastrectomies will be available.

References

1. Azagra JC, Goergen M, De Simone P, et al. Minimally invasive surgery for gastric cancer Surg Endosc 1999;13:351-357
2. Goh PMY, Tekant Y, Kum CK et al. Totally intra-abdominal laparoscopic Billroth II gastrectomy. Surg Endosc 1992;6:160
3. Goh PMY, Tekant Y, Isaac J, et al. The technique of laparoscopic Billroth II gastrectomy. Surg Endosc Laparosc 1992;2:258-260
4. Goh PMY Cum CK. Laparoscopic Billroth II gastrectomy: a review. Surg Oncol 1992;2(Suppl I): 13-18
5. Goh PMY. Laparoscopic Billroth II gastrectomy. Semin Laparosc Surg 1994;1:171-181
6. Kitano S, Simoda K, Miyahara M, et al. Laparoscopic approaches in the management of patients with early gastric carcinomas. Surg Endosc Laparosc 1995;5:359-362
7. Ohashi S. Laparoscopic intraluminal (intragastric) surgery for early gastric cancer: a new conceptin laparoscopic surgery. Surg Endosc 1995;9:169-171
8. Takechi K. Amodified technique for endoscopic mucosal resection of small early gastric carcinomas. Endoscopy 1992;24:804
9. Smith A, Finch MD, John TG, et al. Role of laparoscopic ultrasonography in the management of patients with oesophagogastric cancer. Br J Surg 1999;86:1083-7
10. Rosin D, Brasesco O, Rosenthal RJ. Laparoscopy for gastric tumors. Surg Oncol Clin N Am. 2001;10:511-529
11. J.R. Siewert, Invited Commentary. World J. Surg. 2000;24: 1135
12. Kriplani AK, Kapur BM. Laparoscopy for preoperative staging and assessment of operability in gastric carcinoma. Gastrointest Endosc 1991;37:441-443
13. Possic RA, Franco EL, Pires DR, et al. Sensitivity, specifity and predictive value of laparoscopy for the staging of gastric cancer and for the detection of liver metastases. Cancer 1986; 58:1-6
14. Meijer DW, Bannenberg JJ, Jakimowicz JJ. Hand-assisted laparoscopic surgery: an overview. Surg Endosc 2000;14:891-895
15. HALS Study Group. Hand-assisted laparoscopic surgery vs standard laparoscopic surgery for colorectla disease: a prospective randomized trial. Surg Endosc 2000;14:896-901
16. Memon MA, Fitzgibbons Jr RJ. Hand-assisted laparoscopic surgery (HALS): a useful technique for complex laparoscopic abdominal procedures. J Laparoendosc Adv Surg Tech 1998;8:180-184
17. Southern Surgeons' Club Study Group. Handoscopic surgery: a prospective multicenter trial of a minimally invasive technique for complex abdominal surgery. Arch Surg 1999; 134: 477-485
18. Naitoh T, Gagner M, Garcia-Ruiz A, et al. Hand-assisted laparoscopic digestive surgery provides safety and tactile sensation for malignancy or obesity. Surg Endosc 1999;13:157-160
19. Bleier JI, Krupnick AS, Kreisel D, et al. Hand-assisted laparoscopic vertical banded gastroplasty: early results. Surg Endosc 2000;14:902-907
20. Cuschieri A. Laparoscopic hand-assisted surgery for hepatic and pancreatic disease. Surg Endosc 2000;14:991-996

21. Darzi A. Hand-assisted laparoscopic colorectal surgery. Surg Endosc 2000;14:999-1004
22. Kolvenbach R. Hand-assisted laparoscopic aortoiliac surgery. Arch Surg 2000;135:854-859
23. Patterson EJ, Gagner M, Salky B, et al. Laparoscopic pancreatic resection: single-institution experience of 19 patients. J Am Coll Surg 2001;193:281-287
24. Tanaka M, Tokuda N, Koga H, et al. Hand assisted laparoscopic radical nephrectomy for renal carcinoma using a new abdominal wall sealing device. J Urol 2000;164:314-318
25. Targarona EM, Balague C, Trias M. Hand-assisted laparoscopic splenectomy. Semin Laparosc Surg 2001;8:126-134
26. Wolf JSJ, Tchetgen MB, Merion RM. Hand-assisted laparoscopic live donor nephrectomy. Urology 1988;52:885-887
27. Alexander RJT, Jaques BC, Mitchell KG. Laparoscopically assisted colectomy and wound recurrence. Lancet 1993;341:249-250
28. Cirocco WC, Schwartzman A, Golub RW. Abdominal wall recurrence after laparoscopic colectomy for colon cancer. Surgery. 1994;116:842-846
29. Whelan RL, Sellers GJ, Allendorf JD, et al. Trocar site recurrence is unlikely to result from aerosolization of tumor cells. Dis Colon Rectum 1996;39(10S): S7-13
30. Reyes CD, Weber KJ, Gagner M, et al. Laparoscopic vs open gastrectomy. Surg Endosc 2001;15:928-931
31. Hayashi K., Munakata Y. Laparoscopy assisted antral gastrectomy with regional lymph node dissection. Surg Endosc 1997;11:502-505
32. Watson DI, Devitt PG, Game PA. Laparoscopic Billroth II gastrectomy for early gastric cancer. BR J Surg 1995;82:661-662
33. Goh PMY, Alponat A, Kum CK et al. Early international results of laparoscopic gastrectomies. Surg Endosc 1997;11:650-652
34. Goh PM, Khan AZ, So JB, et al. Early experience with laparoscopic radical gastrectomy for advanced gastric cancer. Surg Laparosc Endosc Percutan Tech 2001;11:83-87
35. Adachi Y, Shiraishi N, Ikebe K, Aramaki M, Bandoh T, Kitano S. Evaluation of the cost for laparoscopic-assisted Billroth I gastrectomy. Surg Endosc 2001 ;15:932-936

Addendum

A decade after the introduction of therapeutic laparoscopy for gastric malignancies, laparoscopic surgery has been gaining steadily increasing acceptance, offering patients postoperative pain reduction, earlier hospital discharge, and earlier return to work. However, until recently, many doubts had been expressed regarding the ability of a minimally invasive laparoscopic procedure to satisfy all the oncologic criteria met during conventional open gastrectomy for the treatment of gastric cancer patients. In a prospective study conducted by Dulucq et al.[1], minimally invasive laparoscopic gastrectomy proved to accommodate well established oncologic principles, allowing tumor-free margins and sufficient extensive lymph node dissection, just as the conventional open procedure.

Further substantial evidence regarding the role of laparoscopic assisted gastrectomy for distal gastric cancer with respect to resectability and long-term outcome, has been also presented in a study conducted by Huscher et al.[2]. The study is the first prospective randomized trial addressing 5-year outcome in patients undergoing laparoscopic or the conventional open subtotal gastrectomy for distal gastric cancer. The treatment policy applied by the authors, included open or laparoscopic subtotal gastrectomy with D2 lymphadenectomy, with the exception of high-risk patients, where a D1 lymphatic dissection was performed in order to reduce postoperative complications. In this latter group, a Billroth II retrocolic gastrojejunostomy was also chosen instead of a Roux-en-Y reconstruction, with the intention to shorten the operative time. The laparoscopic approach did not preclude an oncologically correct resection of the gastric tumor, allowing for extended lymphadenectomy, whenever needed. Moreover, neither 5-year overall survival, nor 5-year disease-free survival rates were influenced by the surgical approach applied, confirming the radicality of the laparoscopic resection. As in other laparoscopic procedures, important operative and postoperative advantages were observed including lower intraoperative blood loss, earlier resumption of oral intake, and earlier discharge from the hospital. In a similar prospective study, Mockiki et al.[3]

demonstrated that laparoscopic assisted gastric resection can be an equally effective curative measure for patients suffering from early gastric cancer. It appears that in experienced hands, laparoscopic-assisted subtotal gastrectomy for distal gastric cancer is a feasible and safe alternative to open, standard gastric resection, with similar short- and long-term results that testify to the oncologic radicality of the procedure. However, laparoscopic gastric surgery is demanding from a technical point of view, especially when a D2 lymphadenectomy is performed. The caution however, against laparoscopic D2 gastrectomy is justified, since this procedure cannot be regarded as routine unless performed in centers with significant experience in this approach.

1. Dulucq JL, Wintringer P, Perissat J, Mahajna A. Completely laparoscopic total and partial gastrectomy for benign and malignant diseases: a single institute's prospective analysis. J Am Coll Surg 2005;200:191-197
2. Huscher CG, Mingoli A, Sgarzini G, Sansonetti A, Di Paola M, Recher A, Ponzano C. Laparoscopic versus open subtotal gastrectomy for distal gastric cancer: five-year results of a randomized prospective trial. Ann Surg 2005;241:232-237.
3. Mochiki E, Kamiyama Y, Aihara R, Nakabayashi T, Asao T, Kuwano H. Laparoscopic assisted distal gastrectomy for early gastric cancer: Five years' experience. Surgery 2005;137:317-322

CHAPTER

Basic principles of laparoscopic colonic surgery 4

S.D. Wexner, I.N. Oikonomakis

Introduction

Laparoscopic surgery, first employed by gynecological surgeons more than 15 years ago,[1] has recently gained worldwide acceptance by the surgical community for the treatment of a wide spectrum of surgical ailments.[2] Much of the enthusiasm has resulted from the reported decreased postoperative pain and the shorter hospitalization of patients undergoing laparoscopic procedures enabling a rapid return to work and a reduction in overall cost.[3-8] In addition, improved cosmesis compared to that attained after laparotomy, challenged surgeons to apply this new technique first to cholecystectomies,[9] then to more complicated procedures such as colectomies.

Indications and Contraindications

Potential indications for laparoscopic intestinal procedures are the same as for laparotomy including both benign and malignant diseases.[10-23] Accumulated experience and technological advancements have continuously expanded the frontiers of laparoscopic colonic surgery to include more difficult and demanding procedures. Table 1 lists the most common surgical conditions amenable to laparoscopic management. It should be emphatically noted that regardless of the type of procedure or the diagnosis, basic surgical principles must be followed for a successful outcome to be achieved. One should not compromise long established surgical principles in order to facilitate the technique nor should the surgeon change traditional judgment to facilitate laparoscopy. Colorectal laparoscopic surgery includes a variety of special features and challenges the surgeon with unique technical difficulties and risks which differentiate the entire endeavor from other abdominal procedures.

Laparoscopic colorectal surgery requires frequent repositioning of the surgeon, instruments, and television monitors. Thus, additional time may be needed as compared to single quadrant laparoscopic procedures. During laparoscopic colectomy many large, often calcified vessels encased in mesenteric fat require ligation. This step is time consuming and potentially hazardous. This is an inverse relationship between time and experience as rapid mechanical devices such as the endoscopic linear cutting stapler are more expensive than are other suturing methods. After having removed the specimen through an incision, a circumferentially intact, well vascularized, tension free anastomosis must be fashioned.

The potential benefits of laparoscopic surgery - reduced pain, length of hospitalization, earlier return to normal activity, and a better cosmetic result- are less significant than is the cure of the disease.

In the light of these views adequate exposure, proper visualization and meticulous hemostasis are mandatory. Mobilization is achieved as in conventional surgery by careful traction and countertrac-

TABLE 1 Indications for laparoscopic intestinal surgery.

Condition	Proposed procedure (Laparoscopic = L; Assisted = A)
Colonic neoplasia (adenoma or carcinoma)	Segmental resection with intracorporeal (L) or extracorporeal (A) anastomosis
Rectal carcinoma	Abdommoperineal excision with colostomy (L)
Familial Adenomatous Polyposis	Subtotal colectomy (L or A) with ileorectal anastomosis or restorative proctocolectomy with (A) ileoanal reservoir
Hartmann's procedure with either Brooke ileostomy or end colostomy	Closure of ileostomy or colostomy by ileoproctostomy or colostomy (L)
Inflammatory bowel disease (Crohn's disease or mucosal ulcerative colitis)	Segmental or subtotal colectomy with or without a stoma (L or A) or total proctocolectomy (A)
Diverticulitis	Segmental resection with anastomosis with or without proximal stomas (L or A) or Hartmann's procedure (L)
Ischaemic colitis	Segmental or subtotal colectomy (L or A)
Colonic haemorrhage	Segmental or subtotal colectomy (L or A)
Trauma	Segmental resection or primary repair or diversion (L or A)
Colonic inertia	Subtotal colectomy with ileorectal anastomosis (L or A)
Rectal prolapse	Laparoscopic rectopexy, sigmoid colectomy with rectopexy (L or A)
Volvulus	Laparoscopic fixation of the sigmoid, sigmoid colectomy (L or A)
Various	Stoma (L)

tion to facilitate division of retroperitoneal attachments. This component is significantly facilitated by the ultrasonic scalpel.

Diffuse fecal peritonitis should be viewed as a relative contraindication to laparoscopic bowel resection. A number of other conditions remain relative contraindications such as large inflammatory phlegmons, advanced locally invasive carcinomas, morbid obesity, and extensive abdominal adhesions. Although all of these challenges can be technically overcome, such efforts prolong operative time and may increase risk.[24]

There are two reasons for conversion-pre-emptive and reactive. The former type of conversion is undertaken when the surgeon does not have optimal visualization due to either adhesions or excessive bleeding due to tissue friability. In this case, the abdomen is opened to permit better visualization and clarification of the anatomy. The latter type of conversion is effected when an injury has resulted presumably from inadequate visualization due to either adhesions or excessive bleeding. Patients who undergo a preemptive conversion tend to fare well whereas patients who have undergone a reactive conversion tend to have significant postoperative complications and a prolonged hospital stay. It is certainly in the best interest of the patient to make the decision to convert early in the procedure and to do so in a pre-emptive rather than a reactive manner. Accordingly, all patients are both counseled and consented for the eventuality of a laparotomy.[25,26]

Preoperative preparation and initiation of procedure

Preoperative preparation is the same whether laparoscopy or laparotomy is planned.[27,28] The standard mechanical bowel preparation is undertaken with 2, 45cc doses of sodium phosphate. Oral and parenteral broad-spectrum antibiotics are administered. As previously mentioned, patients are informed about and consented for the possibility of a laparotomy. In addition, they are also informed about and consented for the possible need of intraoperative colonoscopy to localize lesions.[29,30,31]

Contingent upon the type of pathology, the patient may also be counseled and preoperative marked by an enterostomal therapist for either an ileostomy and/or colostomy. The surgeon should take caution and counsel and mark patients for stomas in a liberal fashion in case of this eventuality. Potential indications include, but are not limited to, Crohn's disease, diverticulitis, and rectal carcinoma.

After induction of adequate general and endotracheal anesthesia, a nasogastric tube and an indwelling bladder catheter are inserted to hopefully minimize, respectively, the risks of injury to the stomach and bladder during trocar insertion and to enhance visualization during the procedure. The patient is placed in a supine modified lithotomy position in Alien stirrups (Alien Medical Inc., Bedford Heights, OH). The flexion of both knees should be limited to no more than 15 degrees. Sequential compression stockings are activated prior to commencement of the procedure. In cases where significant retroperitoneal and/or pelvic inflammation and/or sizable and/or fixed masses are suspected, intraoperative ureteric catheter placement is planned. Once again, patients are informed of this decision and after the various risks, benefits, alternatives, and possible complications are explained to them prior to surgery, they sign consent forms for this procedure. In these instances, the urologist would perform cystoscopy with insertion of bowel or ureteric catheters after the induction of general or endotracheal anesthesia, patient positioning, and nasogastric tube placement, but prior to placement of any trocars. In our experience, this procedure adds approximately 15 minutes and has not, in the last 13 years during laparotomy or laparoscopy, been associated with any significant complications[32]. Conversely, it has significantly facilitated localization of the ureters on numerous occasions including cases of terminal ileal Crohn's disease, diverticulitis, enterovesical, colovesical, or colovaginal fistula, and abscess.

The skin is prepared and the abdomen and pelvis draped in case of conversion to a laparotomy is required. The first cannula is generally introduced through a 1 cm vertical incision, either immediately cephalad or caudad to the umbilicus. The vertical incision facilitates subsequent elongation in case of conversion to laparotomy or for specimen extirpation in case of a successful laparoscopic procedure. A Veress needle is preferred but if the patient has had a prior midline incision, then the Hasson technique[33] is utilized. After the audible and palpable click, the saline "drop" test, and the slow gradual raise in intraperitoneal pneumoperitoneum are noted, the Veress needle is removed and replaced by a 10 mm port. If a Hasson technique is utilized, then a 10 mm port would be utilized from the onset of the procedure. All ports are 10mm in diameter so that the camera can be inserted through any port, when necessary.[34] For left sided procedures, two or three additional right-sided ports are placed and for right-sided procedures, the converse is true. Generally, in patients who have not had prior surgery and who are relatively thin, an iliac fossa and a paraumbilical port on the contralateral side of the pathology are sufficient. However, in patients who are obese or who have had prior adhesions, a third upper quadrant contralateral port may be useful. In cases of significant adhesions, it may be necessary to alter port placement merely to achieve adhesiolysis. However, it is generally helpful for the surgeon to have the specific pattern of port placement with which the entire team is familiar to facilitate and help ensure the safety of these laparoscopic procedures.

Instruments

10 mm diameters ports and 10mm diameter instruments are used (Figures 1). In general, most colectomies can be performed with two "atraumatic" grasping clamps, a 10 mm diameter ultrasonic dissector (harmonic scalpel; Ethicon Endosurgery Inc., Cincinnati, OH), and a 30 mm vascular endoscopic linear stapler (Ethicon Endosurgery, Inc., Cincinnati, OH) (Figure 2). Optional additional equipment may include 10 mm diameter electrocautery scissors, a 10 mm diameter clip applier, and a 10 mm diameter anvil grasping (modified Allis) clamp (Ethicon Endosurgery, Inc., Cincinnati, OH) (Figure 3).

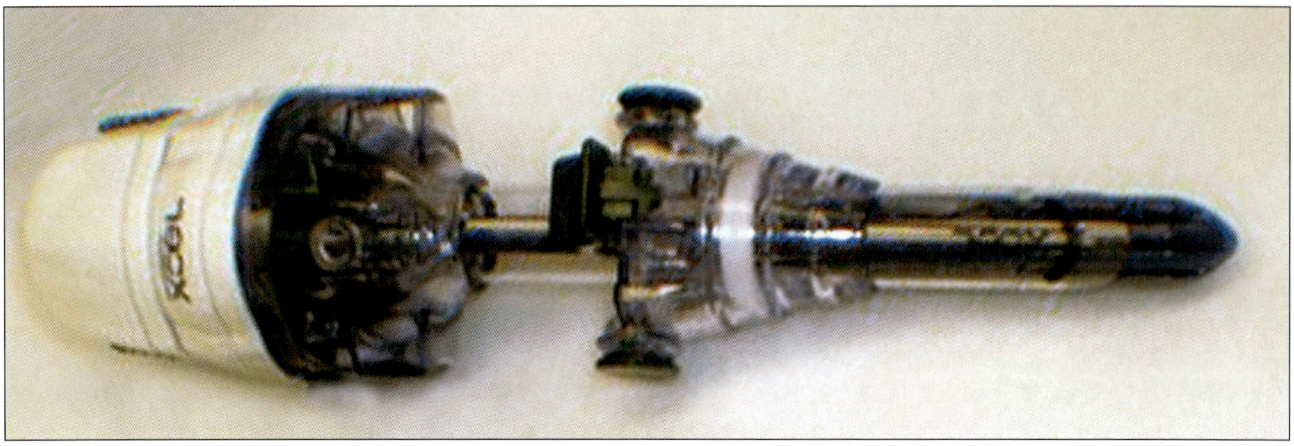

FIGURE 1. 10 mm diameter port.

Technical Tips

1. The surgeon and assistant(s) should strive to work on a straight line rather than backwards or an inverted fashion (Figure 4). A 30-degree telescope may be useful in this regard.
2. Despite the fact that many instruments are labeled as "atraumatic", they may cause significant injury to the bowel. Such injuries can be particularly salient in case of suboptimal bowel preparation or malignancy. In the former instance, intraperitoneal contamination can result in disastrous postoperative sequelae whereas in the latter situation, tumor cell seeding could well be hypothesized as being encouraged. Accordingly, the instruments must be used in a delicate manner. While some surgeons advocate grasping the mesentery rather than the bowel, we are reluctant to recommend this maneuver because of the potential for mesenteric hemorrhage in our large population of inflammatory bowel disease patients. Thus, we do prefer grasping the bowel in a gentler manner. The entire working length of the instrument and the grasped bowel must be clearly visualized on the monitors at all times during the procedure. Since most of the operations are performed with only three ports, it is relatively easy for the surgeon to manipulate the ultrasonic scissors with one hand and the instrument for traction with the other, while the assistant holds the camera. In obese patients or in patients with a redundant colon, additional traction or countertraction may be supplied by the assistant to the fourth port.

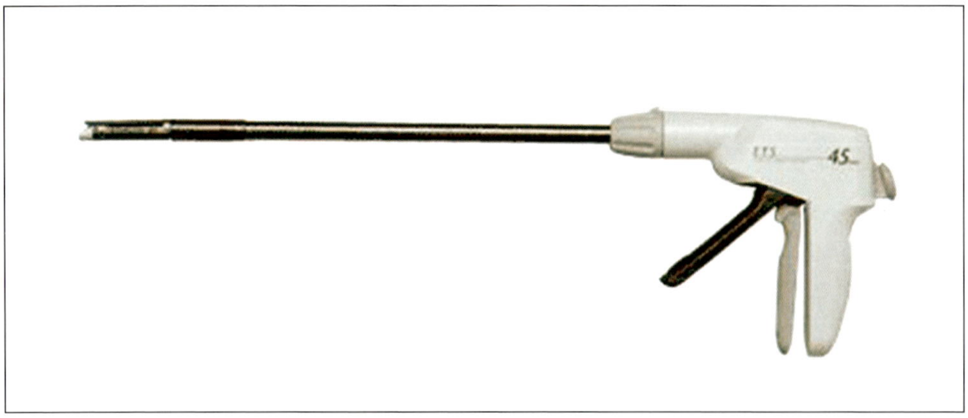

FIGURE 2. Linear stapler.

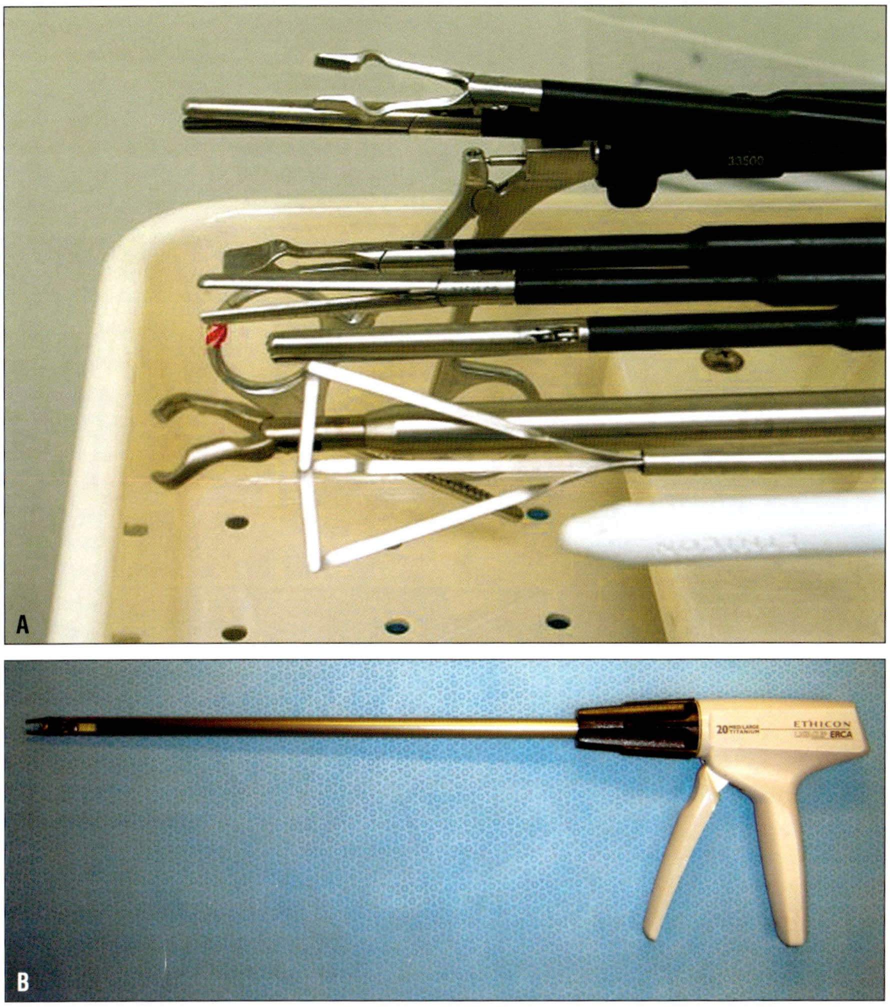

FIGURE 3. **A** Various types of laparoscopic clamps. **B** Clip applier.

3. All ports should be carefully placed with consideration for the epigastric vessels and for any subsequent stoma or drain placement. These port sites can frequently be "recycled" as either port or drain sites, if indicated.

After significant experience has been gained, the vast majority of laparoscopic colorectal procedures can be performed for virtually all diagnoses in a safe and efficient manner with relatively few instruments and ports.

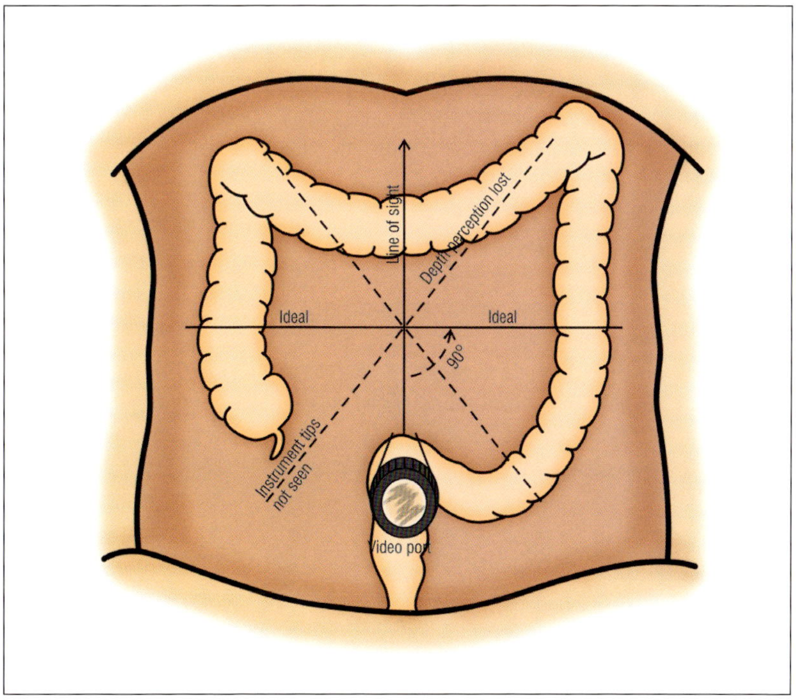

FIGURE 4. Optimal angles for instrument operation.

References

1. Vecchio R, Macfayden BV, Palazzo F. History of laparoscopic surgery. Panminerva Med 2000;42(1):87-90.
2. Cuschieri A. The spectrum of laparoscopic surgery. World J Surg 1992;16:1089-1098.
3. Wexner SD, Moscovitz ID. Laparoscopic colectomy in diverticular and Crohn's disease. Surg Clin North Am 2000; 80(4): 1299-319.
4. Fazio VW, Lopez-Kostner F. Role of laparoscopic surgery for treatment of early colorectal carcinoma. World J Surg 2000;24(9):1056-1060.
5. Talac R, Nelson H. Laparoscopic colon and rectal surgery. Surg Oncol Clin N Am 2000;9(l):l-12.
6. Senagore AJ, Luchtefeld MA, Mackeigan JM, Mazier WP. Open colectomy versus laparoscopic colectomy: are there differences? Am Surg 1993;59:549.
7. Scoggin SD, Frazee RC, Snyder SK, et al. Laparoscopic assisted bowel surgery Dis Colon Rectum 1993; 36: 747.
8. Tate JJT, Kwok S, Dawson JW, et al. Prospective comparison of laparoscopic and conventional anterior resection.Br J Surg 1993;80:1396.
9. Dubois F. Laparoscopic cholocystectomy. historical perspective and personal experience. Surg Laparosc Endosc 1991;1 (1):52-57.
10. Corman ML (Ed). Colon & Rectal Surgery 4th ed. Philadelphia: Lippincott-Raven, 1998.
11. Saclarides TJ, Ko ST, Airan M, Dillon C, Franklin J. Laparoscopic removal of large colonic lipoma: report of a case. Dis Colon Rectum 1991;34:1027-1029.
12. Berman IR. Sutureless laparoscopic rectopexy for procidentia: technique and implication. Dis Colon Rectum 1992;35:689-693.
13. Miller R, Roe AM, Eltnnghan & Espiner HJ. Laparoscopic fixation of sigmoid volvulus Br J Surg 1992;79:435.
14. Almqvist PM, Bohe M, Montgomery A. Laparoscopic creation of loop ileostomy and sigmoid colostomy. Eur J Surg 1995;161:907-909.
15. Regatas F, Siebra J, Rodrigues L, et al. Laparoscopically assisted colorectal anastomoses post Hartmann's procedure. Surg Laparosc Endosc 1996;6:l-4.
16. Wexner SD (Ed). Laparoscopic Colorectal Surgery. New York: Wiley-Liss, Inc, 1999.
17. Kockerling F, Scheidbach H, Schneider C, Barlehner E, Kohler L, Bruch HP, Konradt J, Wittekind C, Hohenberger W. Laparoscopic abdominoperineal resection, early postoperative results of a prospective study involving 116 patients. The Laparoscopic Colorectal Surgery Study Group. Dis Colon Rectum 2000;43(11):1503-1511.
18. Nelson H, Sargent JD, Wieand HS, et al. A Comparison of Laparoscopically Assisted and Open Colectomy for Colon Cancer. N Engl J Med 2004; 350: 2050-9.
19. Veldkamp R, Gholghesaei M, Bonjer HJ, et al. Laparoscopic resection of colon cancer. Surg Endosc 2004; 18: 1163-1185.
20. Leung KL, Kwok PYS, Lam CWS, et al. Laparoscopic resection of rectosigmoid carcinoma: prospective randomized trial. Lancet 2004; 363: 1187-92.
21. Lacy MA, Garcia-Valdecasas CJ, Delgado S, et al. Laparoscopy - assisted colectomy versus open colectomy for treatment of non-metastatic colon cancer: a randomized trial. Lancet 2002; 359: 2224-29.
22. Cera SM, Wexner SD. Minimally invasive treatment of colon cancer. Cancer J 2005 Jan-Feb; 11(1): 26-35.
23. Da Silva GM, Borjesson L, Wexner SD. Laparoscopy for colorectal cancer. Semin Laparosc Surg 2004 Mar; 11(1): 3-12.
24. Keighley MRB, Williams NS (Eds). Surgery of Anus, Rectum and Colon. London: W.B. Saunders, 1997.
25. Schwandner O, Schiedeck TH, Bruch H. The role of conversion in laparoscopic colorectal surgery. Do predictive factors exist? Surg Endosc 1999;13(2):151-156.
26. Krook MM, Targarona EM, Garriga J, Cerdan G, Trias M. Applicability of laparoscopic surgery for colorectal disease. J Laparoendosc Adv Surg Tech A 2000;10(5):263-268.
27. Wexner SD, Beck DE. Sepsis prevention in colorectal surgery. In Fielding LP, Goldberg SM (eds) Operative Surgery: Colon, Rectum and Anus (5th edn) Oxford: Butterworth Heinemann, 1993.
28. Butts JD, Woford ET. Timing of perioperative antibiotic administration AORN J 1997;65(1):109-15.
29. Larach SW, Vayer AG, Williamson PR, Goldstein E. Laparoscopic assisted colectomy: experience during the learning curve. Coloproctology 1993;15:38-41.
30. Reissman P, Teoh T-A, Piccirillo M, Nogueras JJ, Wexner SD. Colonoscopic assisted laparoscopic colectomy. Surg Endosc 1994;8.1352-1353.
31. McDermott J, Devereaux D, Caushaj P. Pitfall of laparoscopic colectomy: an unrecognized synchronous carcinoma. Dis Colon Rectum 1994;37:602-603.
32. Cohen SM, Wexner SD. Laparoscopic colorectal resection for cancer: the Cleveland Clinic Florida experience. Surg Oncol 1993;2:35-42.
33. Hasson HM. A modified instrument and method for laparoscopy. Am J Obstet Gynecol 1971;110:886-887.
34. Beck DE, Wexner SD (Eds). Fundamentals of Anorectal Surgery 2nd ed. London, WB Saunders, 1998.

CHAPTER

5

Laparoscopic right hemicolectomy

S.D. Wexner, I.N. Oikonomakis

Introduction

All patients scheduled for laparoscopic right hemicolectomy undergo preoperative evaluation and counseling and intraoperative positioning and port placement as described previously in this textbook.

Technique

After the first port has been placed in either the supra or infraumbilical location (Figure 1), the additional 2 to 3 ports are placed on the left side, one in the left iliac fossa, one in the left paraumbilical region, and the third (optional) port in the left upper quadrant. The third (optional) port is used in patients who are obese or who have extensive antecedent adhesions. The surgeon stands on the patient's left side and the assistant between the legs or next to the surgeon so that all work can be accomplished in parallel.

The patient is generally positioned in a steep Trendelenburg and left side down position so that gravity can facilitate the dissection.[1] Prior to commencing the dissection, the entire small bowel should be inspected from the ileocecal valve to the duodenojejunal flexure. In particular, since many modified right hemicolectomies (ileocolic resections) are undertaken for patients with Crohn's disease,[2] it is important to assess and measure the length of the small bowel. Small bowel assessment should be carefully undertaken by gently passing the bowel in a "hand over hand" technique wherein the surgeon controls both of the "atraumatic" clamps and the assistant focuses the camera. As the evaluation of the bowel proceeds from distal to

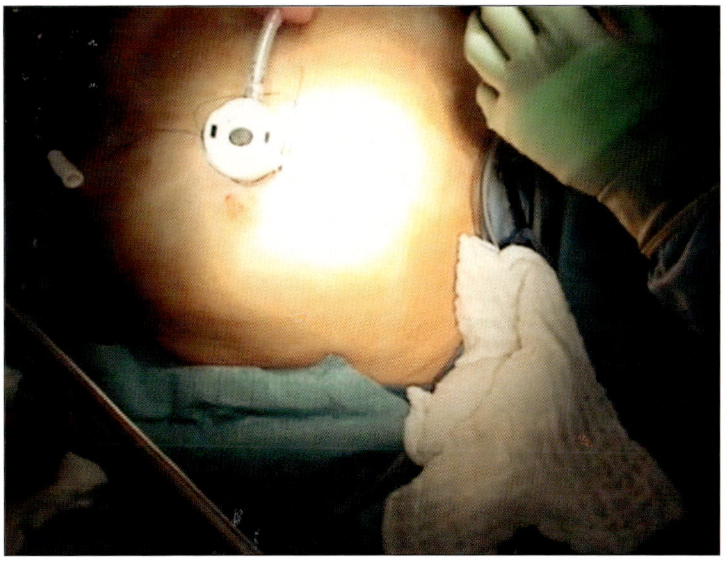

FIGURE 1. Establishment of the umbilical port.

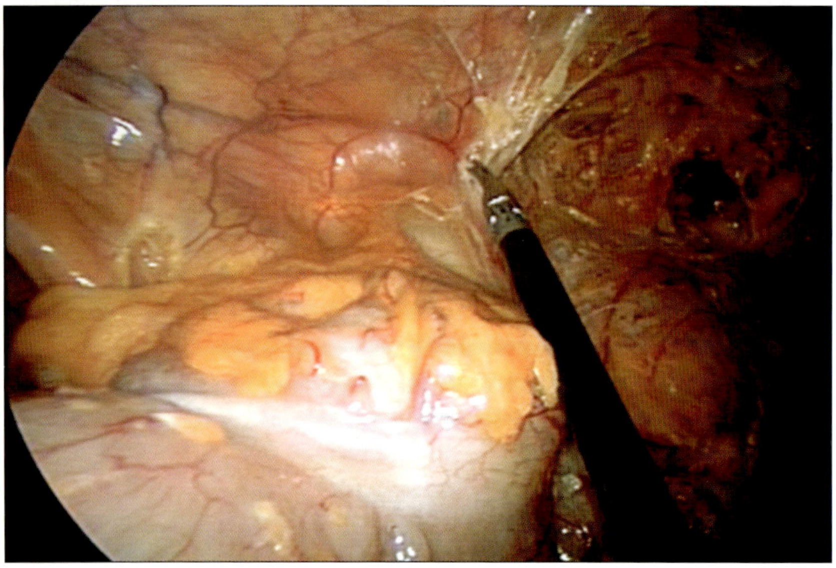

FIGURE 2. Division of the avascular plane of the line of Toldt.

cephalad it may be useful to gradually tilt the table to an anti-Trendelenburg and right side down position as the inspection proceeds towards the duodenojejunal flexure.

The actual dissection commences by the surgeon gently grasping the right colon with an "atraumatic" 10 mm diameter clamp inserted through the left iliac fossa port. The surgeon's right hand then uses the 10mm diameter ultrasonic scissors (harmonic scalpel; Ethicon Endosurgery, Inc., Cincinnati, OH) to incise the line of Toldt from the right iliac fossa up to and around the hepatic flexure (Figures 2 and 3). The gastrocolic omentum can either be taken down from the transverse colon along its avascular plane using the harmonic scalpel or by dividing it with the harmonic scalpel. Any larger vessels can be divided with the 10 mm diameter large endoscopic clips. In general the harmonic scalpel is sufficient for division of the omentum. The end points for this mobilization include the right ureter (Figures 4) along its length, the iliac vessels, the duodenum (Figure 5), head of the pancreas, and the middle colic vessels.[3,4] If the patient has had prior pelvic surgery such as a hysterectomy or appendicectomy, loops of adherent small bowel may need to be carefully and gently delivered from the pelvis using sharp dissection under direct vision.[5]

After full mobilization, the camera is exchanged to one of the left sided ports and a 10 mm diameter grasping forceps is then introduced through the paraumbilical port to gently grasp the cecum. The patient is then placed in a flat position and the midline port incision is then enlarged to a minimum length necessary to deliver the specimen in an atraumatic fashion

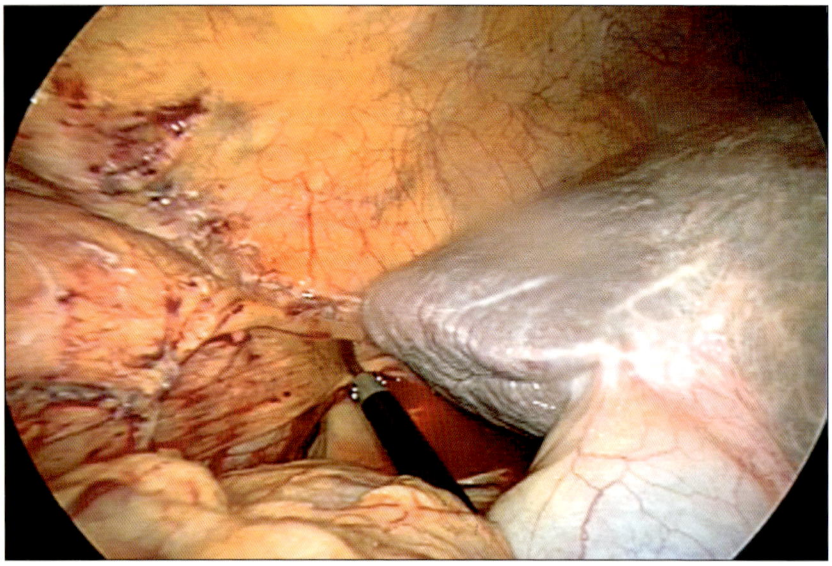

FIGURE 3. Mobilization of the hepatic flexure.

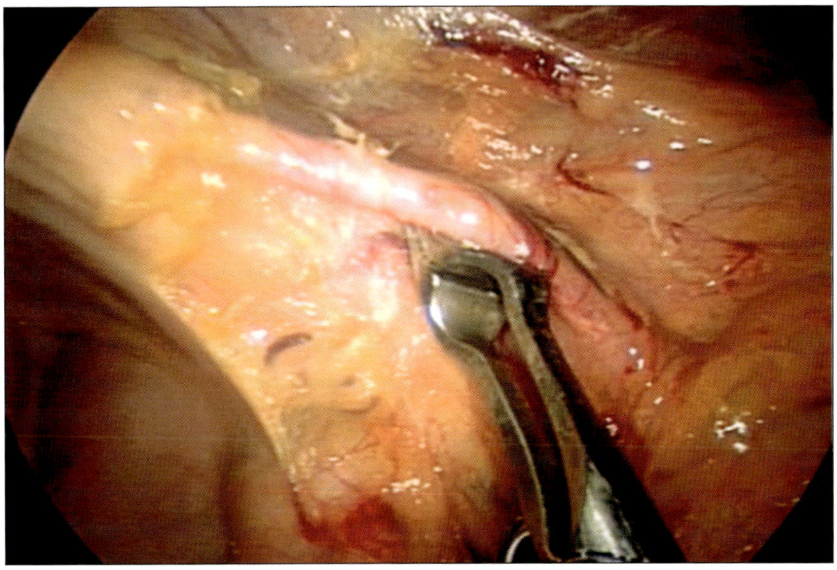

FIGURE 4. Identification of the right ureter.

(Figure 6). Thus, the patient with a 3 cm cecal polyp may be able to have a successful laparoscopic-assisted procedure with a 3cm incision length. Alternatively, the patient with a 7 cm phlegmonous mass from recurrent terminal ileal Crohn's disease may require a 7 cm incision for specimen delivery. One of the many lessons that we have learned over the last 10 years of performing laparoscopic intestinal surgery is that the incision should always be made slightly larger rather than struggling on an assisted right-sided procedure. Forcefully extracting a large specimen through a small incision can result in venous congestion and mesenteric injury with significant hemorrhage, hematoma formation, and the need to sacrifice otherwise viable bowel. Other useful points are that the incision should be made under direct vision using the insulated sheath of the instrument to divide with diathermy rather than risking internal injury. Finally, an impervious wound protector should be placed over the grasping forceps and cannula into the abdomen prior to specimen withdrawal.[6,7]

Once the specimen has been withdrawn, the mesentery is scored and all the vessels are sequentially clamped, divided, and suture ligated with 2-0 polyglactin (Viacol, Ethicon Inc., Somerville, NJ). The bowel is left in continuity. Preliminary division of the bowel can result in malrotation and anastomosis with a 360-degree twist.[8] Thus, all of the mesentery is first divided and then the mesenteric defect is repaired along most of its length, proceeding from proximal to distal, with a 3-0 polydioxane (PDS; Ethicon Inc., Somerville, NJ) suture. The ends of the bowel at the ileum and mid transverse colon (or ce-

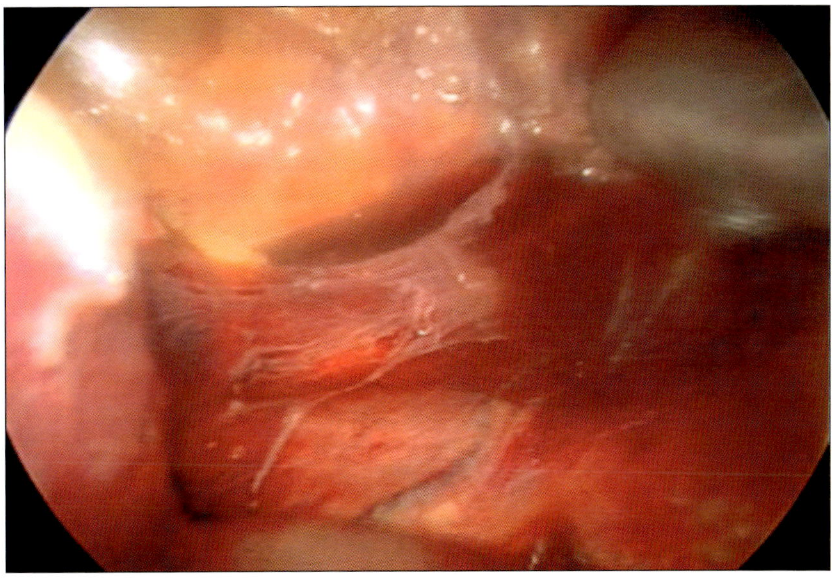

FIGURE 5. Exposure of the duodenum.

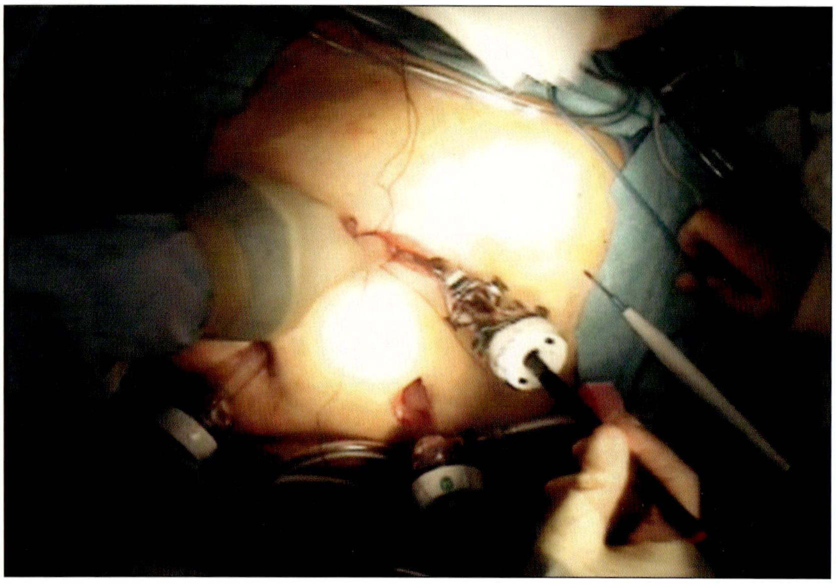

FIGURE 6. Creating the incision from which the bowel is going to be exteriorized.

cal ascending junction in the case of terminal ileal Crohn' disease) are then circumferentially cleared of fat and divided with a linear cutting device. The specimen is removed from the field and opened to ensure that the appropriate pathology has been resected (the adenoma or carcinoma in the case of neoplasia or to ensure adequate margins in patients with Crohn's disease). The antimesenteric border of each staple line is then excised and a side-to-side functional end-to-end anastomosis is then fashioned with the endoscopic linear cutter. The anastomosis is reinforced for meticulous hemostasis with 3-0 polydioxane sutures, where necessary. After verification of meticulous hemostasis, the afferent limb is secured to the efferent limb with 3-0 polydioxane sutures. The apical enterotomy is secured with a 60mm stapling device. The excess tissue is excised. The everted mucosa is then cauterized and the staple line again reinforced for hemostasis where needed with 3-0 polydioxane sutures. The mesenteric defect closure is then completed with 3-0 polydioxane sutures. After verification that the anastomosis is healthy pink, widely patent and circumferentially intact, it is returned into the peritoneal cavity. The fascia is closed at the midline site with figure of eight, 0-polydioxane sutures, and subcutaneously irrigated and verified for meticulous hemostasis. After skin closure, a dry dressing is applied. The abdomen is then re-insufflated. Through the remaining 2 or 3 ports, the abdomen is copiously irrigated, verified for meticulous hemostasis, and then desufflated. The port sites are closed with 0-polydioxane figure of eight sutures. The skin incision is closed and dressings are applied to the remaining sites.

Although this procedure can be achieved in a completely laparoscopic intracorporeal manner, such an approach becomes a triumph of technology over common sense. Specifically, the procedure is significantly prolonged and the cost significantly increased by the addition of multiple intracorporeal devices to facilitate intracorporeal vascular division, bowel transsection, anastomosis, and mesenteric defect closure. For these reasons, while we perform all of our left sided procedures in an intracorporeal manner, we have limited our right-sided procedures to a laparoscopic assisted approach.[9]

References

1. Jager RM. Laparoscopic right hemicolectomy in left lateral decubitus position. Surg Laparosc Endosc 1994;4:348.
2. Canin-Endres J, Salky B, Gattomo F, Edye M. Laparoscopically assisted intestinal resection in 88 patients with Crohn's disease. Surg Endosc 1999;13(6):595-599.
3. Young-Fadok TM, Nelson H. Laparoscopic right colectomy: five step procedure. Dis Colon Rectum 2000;43(2):267-271;
4. Fujita J, Uyama 1, Sugioka A, Komori Y, Matsui H, Hasumi A. Laparoscopic right hemicolectomy with radical lymph node dissection using the no-touch isolation technique for advanced colon cancer. Surg Today 2001;31(l):93-96.
5. Hamel CT, Pikarsky AJ, Weiss E, Nogueras J, Wexner SD. Do prior abdominal operations alter the outcome of laparoscopically assisted right hemicolectomy? Surg Endosc 2000;14(9):853-857.

6. Roe AM, Harper R, Eltringham WK, Espiner HJ. Intracorporeal laparoscopic resections for colorectal cancer: report of cases of abdominoperineal rectal excision and right hemicolectomy with 2 year follow-up. J R Soc Med 1994; 87(9): 519-521.
7. Fusco MA, Paluzzi MW. Abdominal wall recurrence after laparo-scopic-assisted colectomy for adenocarcinoma of the colon. Report of a case. Dis Colon Rectum 1993; 36(9): 858-861.
8. Bonier HJ, Lange JF. Rotation of the terminal ileum in laparo-scopic right hemicolectomy. Surg Endosc 1993; 7(6):534.
9. Bernstein MA, Dawson JW, Reissman P, Weiss EG, Nogueras JJ, Wexner SD Is complete laparoscopic colectomy superior to laparoscopic assisted colectomy? Am Surg 1996; 62(6):507-511.

CHAPTER

6

Laparoscopic left colectomy

S.D. Wexner, I.N. Oikonomakis

The patient undergoing laparoscopic left colectomy is optimally placed in a modified lithotomy position with Allen stirrups (Figure 1). Care must be taken not to flex either the knees or the hips more than 15 degrees; greater flexion impedes use of the instruments through the lower quadrant ports. The surgeon stands on the patient's right side with the camera operator on the same side while the first assistant stands opposite (Figure 2).

Port placement

The surgeon first establishes the supraumbilical port through which the camera is inserted. Under direct visualization, two subsequent ports are then created lateral to the right rectus muscle to avoid injury to the epigastric vessels. All ports should be 10-12 mm in diameter and placed at least 8 cm apart in order to avoid instrument crowding.

Sigmoid dissection from the abdominal wall

As the primary mode of retraction during laparoscopic surgery is gravity, the patient is placed in the extreme right side down and Trendelenburg position. This position helps mobilization of the sigmoid colon from the left lateral sidewall.

Dissection is carried out cephalad along the white line of Toldt using the harmonic scalpel (Figure 3). Few instrument changes are necessary due to the versatility of this instrument. Adhesions of the sig-

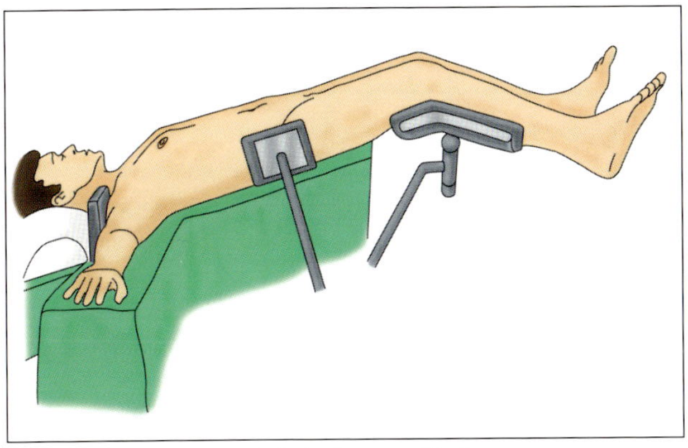

FIGURE 1. Patient positioning.

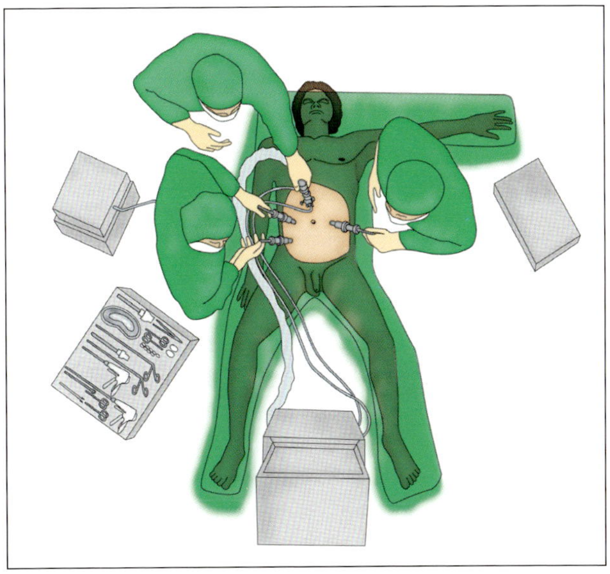

FIGURE 2. Operating room set-up.

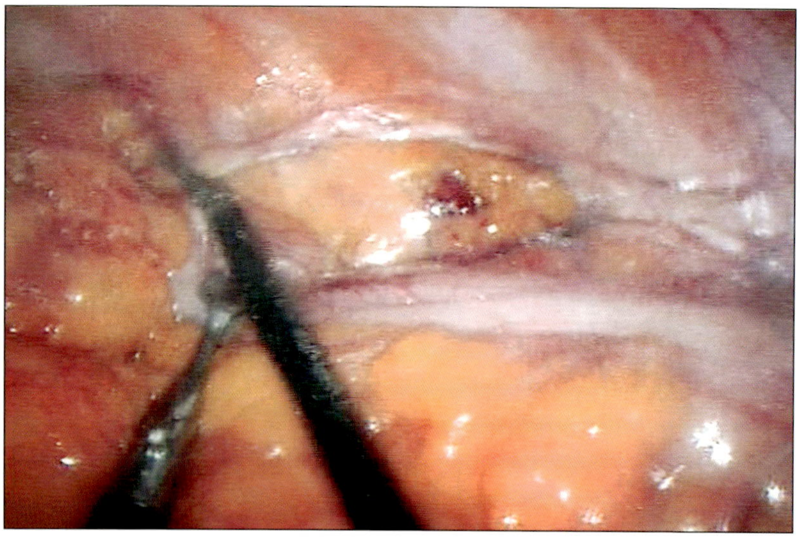

FIGURE 3. Dissection of the left colon from the left lateral sidewall.

moid colon to the left lateral sidewall are divided using gentle traction with endoscopic Babcock clamps.

After adhesiolysis is completed, attention is focused on the identification of the left ureter in the left iliac fossa (Figure 4); ureteric stents are extremely useful especially in patients with inflammatory processes.[1] The dissection then proceeds around the splenic flexure (Figure 5).

Dissection is greatly facilitated by maintaining the plane between the left colon mesentery and the retroperitoneum, which can also be challenging in patients with inflammatory conditions.

Identification and transection of the inferior mesenteric artery (IMA)

Once the sigmoid and the left colon have been completely mobilized, attention is paid to the identification and transection of the inferior mesenteric artery.[2] Using gentle traction with the endoscopic Babcock clamps, the inferior mesenteric artery is identified within the sigmoid mesentery. The harmonic scalpel efficiently dissects and thins the mesentery to expose the vessel. Windows are created within the mesentery after which a 2.5 mm vascular stapler is applied. This stapler must be applied accurately to avoid any inadverent injury to the ureters, which lie just posterolateral to the mesentery in this area (Figure 6).

Transsection of the recto-sigmoid junction

In order to insure an adequate distal resection margin, the dissection continues beyond the sacral promontory into the presacral space (Figure 7). Verification of this level of transection must be done prior to the application of the stapler by placement of an endoscopic non-crushing bowel clamp on the proximal colon and performing proctoscopy.

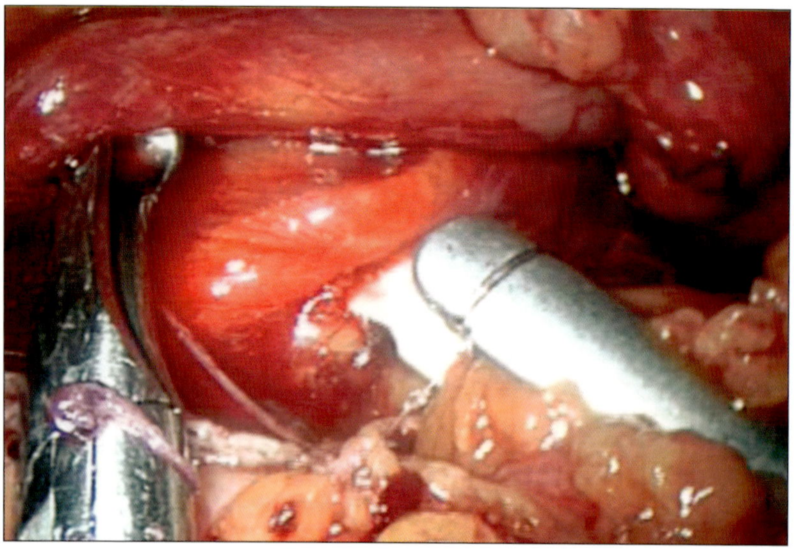

FIGURE 4. Identification of the left ureter.

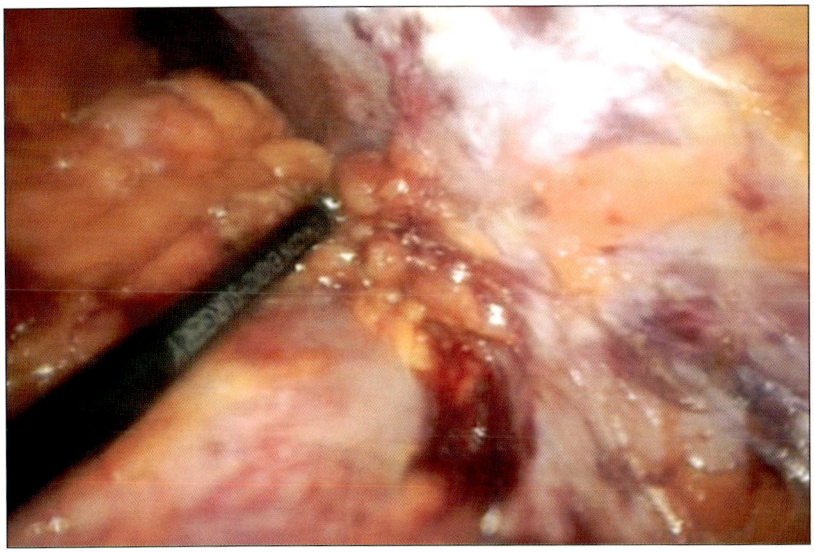

FIGURE 5. Splenic flexure dissection.

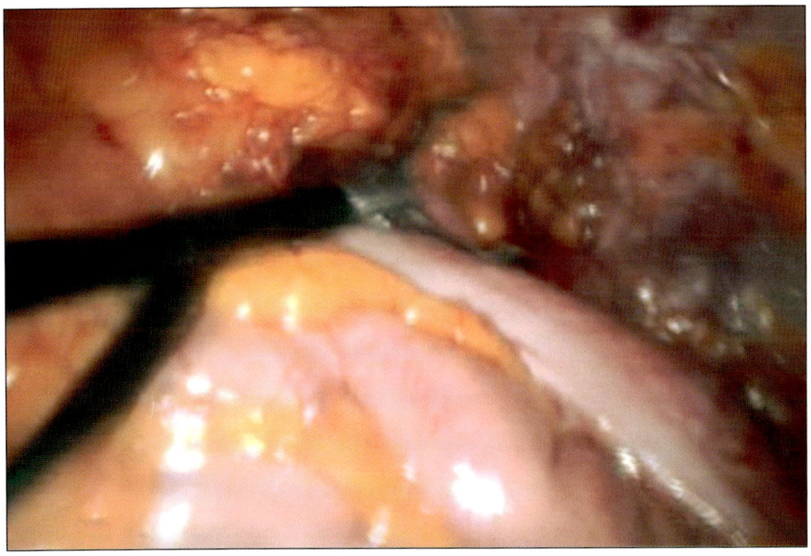

The 10-12 mm right lower quadrant port may then be exchanged with an 18 mm port over an exchange rod. The 30 mm stapler is then placed into the 18 mm port used to transect the bowel (Figure 8). More than one application of the stapler may be necessary to completely transect the bowel. Once transection has been completed, the closure of the stump may then be tested by instillation of an irrigant into the pelvis and insufflation of the rectum with air.

The pelvic anatomy should then be reconfirmed with respect to major landmarks such as the ureters, iliac

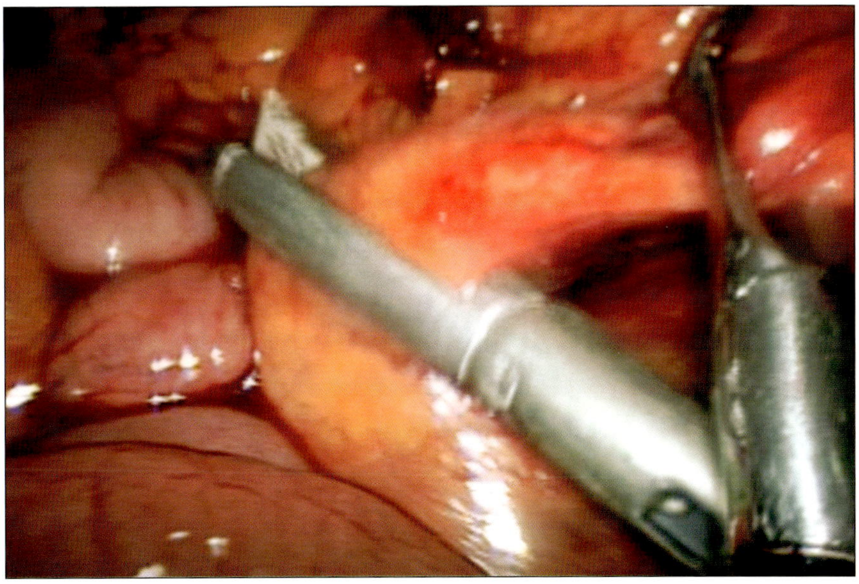

FIGURE 6. Ligation of the inferior mesenteric artery.

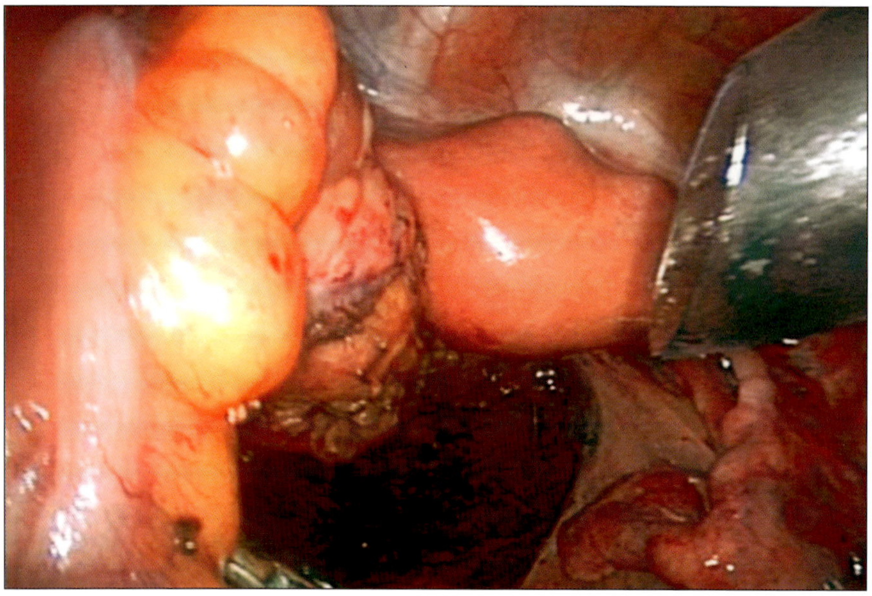

FIGURE 7. Presacral space dissection.

vessels, and the stump of the inferior mesenteric artery. Mesenteric length should be verified to ensure a tension-free anastomosis. If more length is necessary, further dissection with transection of the inferior mesenteric vein may be necessary.

Exteriorization of the sigmoid colon

Once the diseased segment has been completely mobilized, the bowel may then be exteriorized.[3] A 10-12 mm port is placed in the left lateral quadrant position under direct visualization and lateral to the left rectus muscle. The endoscopic Babcock clamp is then used to grasp the proximal resection margin in order to extracorporealize the diseased segment. The incision should be extended along the trocar length. Typically, a 5 cm incision is usually adequate for this purpose. Using a small wound protector, the diseased bowel segment can be gently removed from the abdomen (Figure 9). The wound drape may help to minimize contamination. Once the diseased segment is completely removed from the abdomen, resection may then take place extracorporeally using a standard surgical technique. A purse-string suture is placed on normal proximal bowel and the diseased segment is then transected. Removal of the purse-string suture will allow the surgeon to assess the well-vascularized margin into which the anvil of the 33 mm EEA stapler is placed. The purse-string suture is then secured and the edge of the bowel is trimmed to remove any interfering excess of fat. The bowel with the anvil is then placed back into the abdominal cavity and replaced with a 33 mm port.

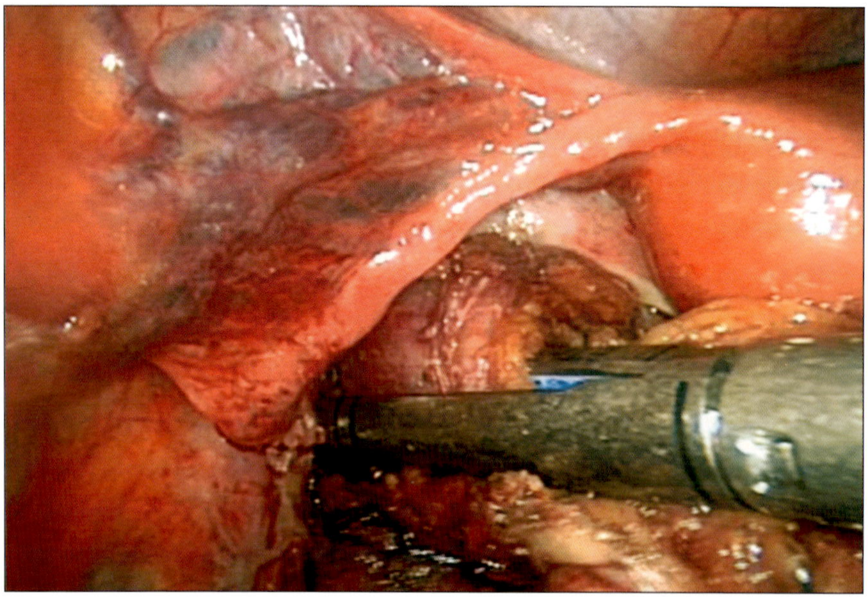

FIGURE 8. Transection of the bowel.

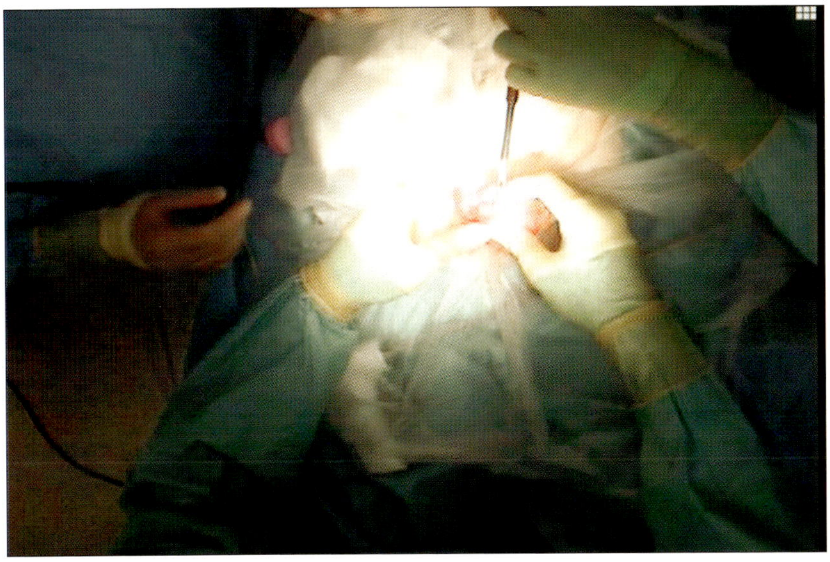

FIGURE 9. Extracorporealization of the diseased bowel.

Performing descending colorectal anastomosis

The laparoscopic phase is resumed as the 33 mm EEA stapler is placed into the rectum. The spike is discharged as close to the staple line as possible and attached to the anvil (Figure 10). Visualization is facilitated by placing the camera into the right lower quadrant port. The stapler is then closed bringing the ends of the bowel together; prior to firing the mesentery is assessed to exclude any tension and to insure proper alignment. The stapler may then be fired assuring complete mucosa to mucosa apposition. A non-crushing clamp is once again placed on the

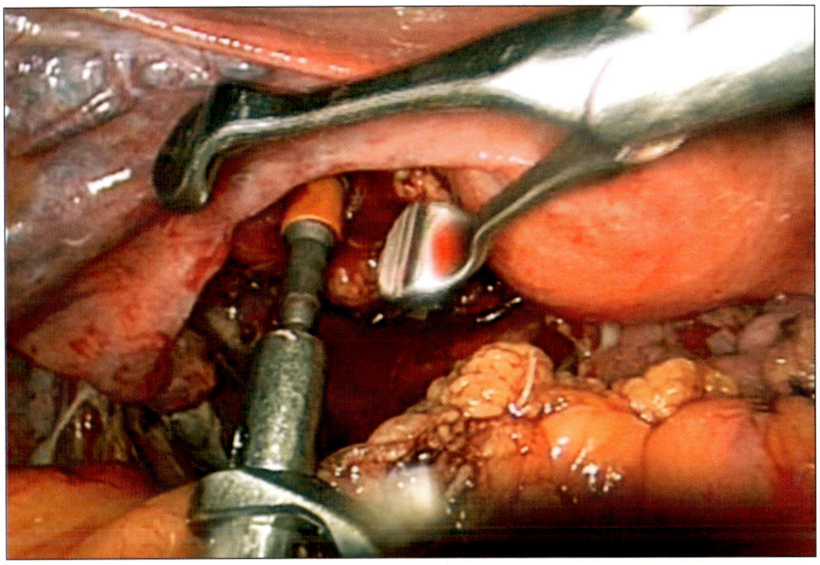

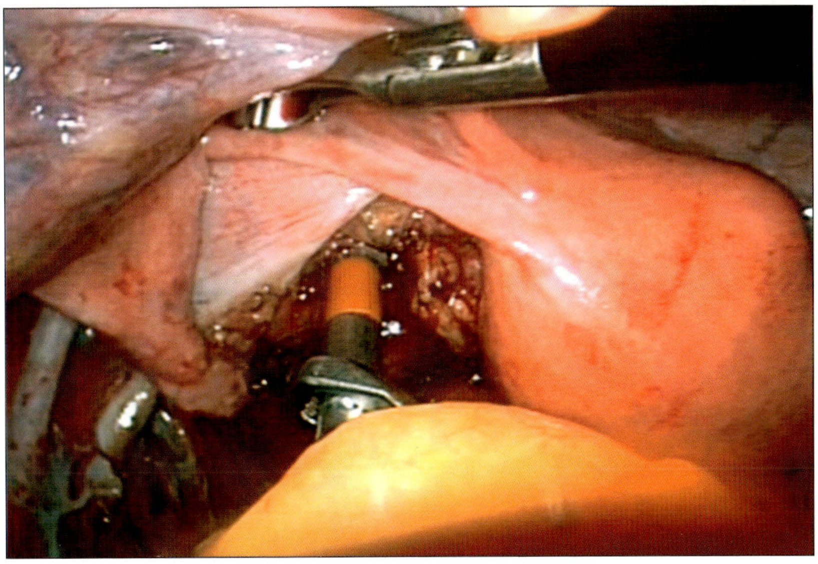

FIGURE 10. Attachment of the anvil to the stapler spike.

bowel proximal to the anastomosis, to ensure the integrity of the anastomosis. Viability of the anastomosis can be directly verified by endoscopy and indirectly by insufflation of air into a water-filled pelvis. Hyaluronic acid membrane (Seprafilm®) can be placed through the left lateral quadrant wound to minimize postoperative adhesions.[4-7] After irrigation, wounds are closed by re-approximating the fascia and then using the skin staples.

References

1. Cohen SM, Wexner SD. Laparoscopic colorectal resection for cancer: the Cleveland Clinic Florida experience. Surg Oncol 1993;2:35-42.
2. Sartori CA, Franzato B. The standardization of a technic for laparoscopic left hemicolectomy with radical lymphadenectomy. Chirltal 1999;51(4):329-334.
3. Darzi A, Hill AD, Henry MM, Guillou PJ, Monson JR. Laparoscopic assisted surgery of the colon. Operative technique. Endosc Surg Allied Technol 1993;1(1):13-15.
4. Becker JM, Dayton MT, Fazio VW, Beck DE, Stryker SJ, Wexner SD, Wolff BG, Roberts PL, Smith LE, Sweeney SA, Moore M. Prevention of postoperative abdominal adhesions by a sodium hyaluronate-based bioresorbable membrane: a prospective, randomized, double-blind, multicenter study. J Am Coll Surg 1996;183(4).297-306.
5. Moreira H Jr, Wexner SD, Yamaguchi T, Pikarsky AJ, Choi JS, Weiss EG, Nogueras JJ, Sardinha TC, Billotti VL. Use of bioresorbable membrane (sodium Hyaluronate + carboxymethylcellulose) after controlled bowel injuries in a rabbit model. Dis Colon Rectum 2000; 43(2):182-187.
6. Bums JW, Colt MJ, Burgees LS, Skinner KC. Preclinical evaluation of Seprafilm bioresorbable membrane. Eur J Surg Suppl 1997;(577):40-8.
7. Oikonomakis I. Wexner SD, Gervaz P, You, S-Y, Secic M. Giamundo P. Seprafilm®: A retrospective preliminary evaluation of the impact on short-term oncologic outcome in colorectal cancer. Dis Colon Rectum 2002; 1376-80.

Laparoscopic low anterior resection and abdominoperineal resection for rectal cancer

CHAPTER **7**

M. Sailer, K.H. Fuchs

Introduction

Treatment modalities of rectal tumours have changed considerably in the past decades. While previously abdominoperineal resection (APR) was considered the standard operation for the majority of rectal cancers, the frequency of this operation has dropped to well below 20% or even 10% in most institutions. Sphincter saving low or ultralow, i.e. intersphincteric rectal resection (LAR) can be performed for virtually all tumours situated in the mid rectum as well as for many cancers located in the lower third. Due to the introduction of new reconstruction techniques, for instance the coloanal J-pouch, postoperative functional results have also improved notably, although some patients will continue to suffer from the so called "anterior resection syndrome". Endoluminal techniques, e.g. transanal endoscopic microsurgical excision have also gained widespread acceptance in the treatment of large adenomas or well selected early rectal cancers. Furthermore, new concepts of pre- and post-operative adjuvant treatment such as radio-/chemotherapy have evolved in recent years.

The introduction of minimally invasive techniques has added yet another facet to the treatment options of gastrointestinal malignancies. However, laparoscopic colorectal resections for cancer remain a controversial issue. Opponents of this method will continue to question whether oncologic principles, including no-touch-technique, radical lymphadenectomy and the avoidance of tumour cell spillage (port site metastases), etc. can be upheld safely, while proponents of laparoscopy will publish their data which - in the majority of studies - compare favourable with the conventional open approach. To date no large randomised trials have been published to support either view, although various studies in different countries are under way to answer these questions. New insights are expected within the next two to five years.[1]

Until more evidence has accrued the general recommendation ought still be that all laparoscopic colorectal work for cancer with curative intent should be carried out within the framework of well designed studies. Furthermore, surgeons embarking on this technique need to have sufficient experience not only with laporoscopic procedures but also with colorectal surgery, as it is widely accepted that rectal cancer surgery requires special anatomic and surgical expertise.

Laparoscopic procedures have developed rapidly in the past decade which was certainly facilitated by the introduction of new instruments and modern appliances, e.g. the ultrasonic scalpel or stapling devices, to name a few. Although different levels of experience and skills are required for the various operations, it can be stated that every conventional colorectal procedure can also be carried out using minimally invasive techniques. Needless to stress that laparoscopy *per se* does not bear any influence on indications for the type or extent of the resection (i.e. APR *versus* LAR), which should solely be dictated by the individual tumour pathology, localisation, and patient specific factors, most significantly anal sphincter function. This chapter will highlight and critically discuss the techniques and results of laparoscopic abdominoperineal resection (LAPR) and low anterior resection (LLAR) for malignant disease.

Laparoscopic Abdominoperineal Resection

Indications for LAPR include tumours of the lower rectal third (within 4 cm of the dentate line) which cannot be removed by a transanal approach or excised with a sufficient distal safety margin of at least 1 to 1.5 cm which would allow a sphincter saving operation. Other indications are advanced cancers with invasion of the anal sphincter or patients with an already incompetent or impaired sphincter function who would not profit from a coloanal anastomosis due to the anticipated poor functional result. Furthermore, LAPR is indicated as a salvage operation in patients with persistent or recurrent anal carcinoma having had radio-/chemotherapy as a first-line treatment. Preoperative proceedings in terms of investigations, marking of stoma position, mechanical bowel preparation, prophylactic antibiotics, thromboembolic prophylaxis etc. should not differ from the adopted protocol in each institution for conventional APR.

Surgical technique

The patient is positioned in the Lloyd-Davies position. It is important to have adequate shoulder and pelvic supports to allow Trendelenburg position (head down tilt of up to 40°) during the operation. One should bear in mind that this position can cause compartment syndrome of the calves, especially in younger patients and after a prolonged operating time. The bladder should be drained by a urinary catheter.

Before commencing the laporoscopic part of the operation the anus should be closed by interrupted sutures. Establishing the pneumoperitoneum and inserting the ports follow the same principles and rules as for every laparoscopic operation. The principal surgeon is standing on the right side of the table and the first assistant to the patient's left and another assistant on the right side next to the legs. Ideally, there are two experienced surgeons who can alternate during the procedure. The monitor together with the other appliances (insufflator, light source etc.) are positioned between the patient's legs. The amount of working trocars differs between surgeons ranging between three and four. Apart from the camera trocar which should be positioned in the midline above the umbilicus, all other trocars (generally 10/12 mm) should be arranged in a semicircular fashion around the pelvis.

The first step should be a thorough inspection of the abdominal cavity and its contents to assess coexisting pathology and/or metastatic disease which has evaded preoperative staging examinations. In female patients it is often useful to retract the uterus using a transabdominal heavy stitch under laparoscopic control. The small bowel should be gently swept superiorly taking advantage of the Trendelenburg position. Fundamentally, all further operative steps resemble those which are performed using an open approach.

First, the left colon is mobilised by incising the peritoneal ahaesions along the line of Toldt. Early during the procedure the left ureter should be identified usually where it crosses the common iliac artery. The mesosigmoid is then further dissected in order to be able to retract the sigmoid colon anteriorly away from the aorta towards the abdominal wall. This is followed by the identification and exposition of the inferior mesenteric artery (IMA) which should be cleared completely from any surrounding tissue before it is transsected near its aortic origin. Transsection of the vessel can be safely and rapidly executed using either a linear stapler or - less expensive - large vascular clips. A division flush with the aorta should be avoided to preserve autonomic nerve fibres which are situated in this anatomic region. Obviously this step is fundamental in defining the proximal extent of the lymphadenectomy and level of bowel transsection which is carried out consecutively, again using a linear stapler device. Further division of the mesocolon down to the point of the ligated IMA will conclude the intraperitoneal component of the operation. This can be done using either a linear stapler, an ultrasonic scalpel or by simple electrocautery in combination with clips for larger vascular structures.

The pelvic part of the procedure is evidently of paramount importance as it entails the complex oncologic mobilisation of the rectum, also well known as nerve sparing total mesorectal excision (TME). This comprises initially the mobilisation of the posterior rectum along the posterior pelvic fascia preserving the hypogastric plexus which is spread out behind the Waldeyer's fascia which should be respected. Dissection is continued well down to the tip of the coccyx. Laterally and anteriorly the pelvic peritoneum needs to be incised first before the rectum can be further mobilised strictly adhering to the principles of mesorectal clearance. This includes the separation of the bowel and its connective tissue from the Denonvilliers fascia in the rectovesical plane anteriorly avoiding injury to the prostate gland or seminal vesicles. In fact, with proficient camera assistance and ample laparoscopic experience pelvic dissection in terms of TME can at times be better visualised and performed compared with laparotomy. After identification and transsection of the middle rectal artery, perirectal clearance of the pelvis is completed down to the levator plane.

The minimally invasive part of the operation is completed by extracting the divided descending colon through an enlarged left lateral portsite to create a terminal colostomy. Alternatively, the colon can be pulled out after replacing the 12 mm-port by a larger, recovery trocar. Ideally, the site should have been marked preoperatively to ensure good stoma function. After realisation of the perineal part which includes the recovery of the complete specimen it is recommended to re-establish a low-pressure pneumoperitoneum for a final intraabdominal inspection. After lavage and final haemostasis a drain can be placed in the pelvis.

Results and Literature Review

The first reports on LAPR were published in 1992.[2,3] Since then numerous centres have presented their data concerning this operation. However, compared with other laparoscopic operations, e.g. LLAR or laparoscopic hemicolectomies for malignant tumours, it has always been stressed in the literature that LAPR does have certain oncologic advantages.[4,5] The main argument is that the tumour itself is not touched or even handled during the laparoscopic phase of the operation with therefore minimal or no risk of tumour cell spillage and/or portsite metastases. Furthermore, no anastomosis is required and the retrieval of the specimen which is carried out during the conventional, perineal part of the procedure is relatively straightforward and safe. Advocates of laparoscopy assert better short-term outcomes, lower postoperative mortality and morbidity, and better immunologic response with the possible effect of an increased survival rate compared with open surgery.[6-9] Nevertheless, as already stated, there is no evidence as yet from randomised trials that patients with low rectal cancer do profit from LAPR as opposed to open APR. For cancer patients the long-term outcome in terms of (disease-free) survival is certainly of greater importance than any short-term benefits, such as shorter hospital stay or quicker recovery with less analgesics in the early postoperative period.

Perioperative complications that are specific to the laparoscopic approach and not related to the establishment of the pneumoperitoneum or siting of the various trocars, are uncommon. There is a risk of thermal injury to the small bowel if electrocautery is used, but with due care this complication can be avoided. Ureteric lesions are not more common during LAPR compared with APR. In a retrospective review including 42 patients of three different institutions undergoing LAPR who were compared with 152 patients undergoing APR the only statistical difference in terms of morbidity was the rate of perineal infection which was significantly higher in the laparoscopic group (24 vs. 8%, P=0.004).[10] The authors hypothesised that maybe the earlier ambulation could have negatively affected perineal wound healing. Mortality rates are generally very low for this procedure ranging between 0 and 2%, although one must be aware of the fact that there might be a selection bias towards patients with less cardio-pulmonary or other co-morbidity.

To date *The Laparoscopic Colorectal Surgery Study Group* from Germany has compiled the largest set of prospective data regarding LAPR.[4] A total of 116 patients underwent LAPR of which 98 (84.5%) were operated upon with curative intent. The patients were treated in 18 different institutions. Mean operating time was 226 min. (140 - 365) with a conversion rate of only 3.4%. In contrast to this study, Fleshman and co-workers[10] report a similar operating time of 234 min. but a conversion rate of 21%. As has been mentioned in previous studies on colorectal surgery, the total hospital stay is a poor indicator for the superiority of a particular operation over another. Again, when comparing the two largest trials published so far, the mean duration of hospital stay in the German study amounts to 21.6 days[4] while Fleshman et al.[10] report a mean stay of 7.4 days. Interestingly there is not only an enormous difference on either side of the Atlantic, but also between the different American institutions ranging from 5.5 to 9.6 days.[10]

Different non-randomised trials show equivalent results with regard to oncologic data[4,8,10,11] with the caveat that follow-up is generally short, usually in the range of one to two years. The report from Germany indicates that a high transsection of the I-MA and complete dissection down to the pelvic floor could be achieved in 97% of all cases.[4] However, only a mean of 12.4 lymph nodes were harvested, which again brings up the issue whether the lymph node count is an appropriate surrogate for radicality of surgery.[10,12] As lymph node recovery depends not only on the extent of resection but also on the diligence of the counting pathologist it is not at all surprising that figures differ greatly between institutions.

In summary, LAPR can be performed safely and effectively with morbidity and mortality rates similar or lower than for conventional APR. However, a certain bias towards more favourable patients in terms of co-morbidity and/or tumour stage, cannot be ruled out in most series. With regard to oncologic parameters, studies have shown that perioperative data (e.g. radical transsection of IMA, lymph node harvest, etc.) and survival data are equivalent to those of open procedures. However, these data must be interpreted with caution as the results are derived mainly from centres with a special interest in the field and - in the majority of cases - after only short-term follow-up periods.

Laparoscopic Low Anterior Resection

The concept of total mesorectal excision for the resection of mid and low rectal cancers is now widely accepted.[13] Although these results have never been verified in larger controlled trials, there is clear evidence that no other technique can yield similarly low local recurrence rates. It is therefore imperative that the laparoscopic approach to the same disease entity does not permit for any compromise in this respect. Bearing this in mind and further acknowledging that other operative principles, such as radical transsection of the IMA, complete lymphadenectomy, and utmost attention not to perforate the tumour or even better complete no-touch technique during the entire procedure, are also essential, it is understandable that LLAR for cancer is still a matter of great debate.

Surgical technique

The initial part of the operation corresponds with the procedure outlined above for LAPR. This includes the following steps: inspection of the abdominal cavity, mobilisation of the left hemicolon beginning laterally at the rectosigmoid junction, identification of the left ureter, high ligation of the IMA and transsection of the inferior mesenteric vein at the lower border of the pancreas, followed by further mobilisation of the rectosigmoid colon down to the pelvic floor incorporating the nerve-sparing excision of the intact mesorectum. Proximal mobilisation of the large bowel has to be carried out well above the splenic flexure to allow for a tension-free pelvic anastomosis.

During the pelvic dissection, again care must be exercised not to injure the presacral venous plexus which will almost inadvertently lead to uncontrollable bleeding requiring conversion, the seminal vesicles and the prostate in men as well as the vagina in women. Of course, handling the rectum requires great caution to avoid any trauma of the tumour bearing segment. Once the pelvic floor has been identified and completely freed from any surrounding tissue, the rectum can be cross-clamped using a angular linear stapler and irrigated transanaly with a cytocidal agent. This is then followed by the division of the bowel at the required level.

The transected large bowel is then pulled out either through a small incision in the midline above the symphysis pubis or else in the left lower quadrant by enlarging a trocar site. At this stage it is important to protect the abdominal wound from potential tumour cell spillage to avoid the occurrence of port-site metastases. This can be accomplished by either using a circular plastic sheath around the incision itself or by placing the specimen, i.e. distal end of the colon which includes the cancer, in a retrieval bag which has been firmly secured proximally prior to extraction.

The next steps are performed in front of the abdominal wall. It comprises the proximal transsection of the colon between non-crushing bowel clamps and the insertion of the appropriately sized anvil of the circular stapler device. At this stage a decision needs to be made as to the preferred reconstruction technique, i.e. straight end-to-end, side-to-end or J-pouch coloanal anastomosis. As usual, the anvil placed in the proximal bowel end is secured with the aid of a pursestring suture. The colon with the tightened anvil is then returned to the abdominal cavity. At this point an assistant will advance the cartridge of the device transanaly under the tactile guidance of the operator. Once in the correct position he will perforate the stapler line of the rectal remnant with the hollow central rod which will then be connected to the anvil. Attention is paid to the correct orientation of the descending colon to avoid any rotation. Cartridge and anvil are then slowly approximated and finally fired taking care not to incorporate any additional tissue, e.g. vagina, into the anastomosis. As usual, both "doughnuts" need to be inspected for integrity. The abdominal incision is then closed and the pneumoperitoneum re-established. This allows for a final inspection of the anastomosis and the pelvic region. The soundness of the anastomosis can also be checked by either transanal irrigation with an Iodine-solution or else by submersing the anastomosis under saline and insufflating air transanaly. A drain can easily be placed into the Pouch of Douglas and all instruments are then removed.

Alternatively, the abdominal wound can also be closed straight after the repositioning of the colon in the abdominal cavity. After re-establishment of the pneumoperitoneum already at this stage the anastomosis is fashioned laparoscopically. While fixing the central rod of the cartridge with a heavy grasper the anvil rod is brought into the pelvis with another instrument (e.g. Babcock clamps) and connected to stapler. Approximation and firing of the stapler will then take place under direct visual rather then tactile control.

Results and Literature Review

Literature reports about LLAR are even scantier than for LAPR. This does certainly reflect the more complex nature of the operation. Therefore, operating times reported range from 180 min[14] to 292 min[15] and even 450 min in one study from Japan.[16] Also of note is a comparatively high conversion rate. In the study by Hartley et al.[14] a total laparoscopic excision of the mesorectum was feasible in only 50% of the patients. However, Bährlehner and colleagues[9] had to convert merely in two cases out of 52 resections. Both patients had bulky T4 tumours with invasion of the lateral abdominal wall. They report a 100% R0 resection rate for all 50 patients undergoing LLAR with curative intent. In terms of benefits various trials could demonstrate a reduction of perioperative blood transfusion requirements, an earlier return of bowel function, less analgetic requirements, and less postoperative fatigue compared with open surgery.[17-19] Generally, morbidity and mortality in the reported series compare favourably with the conventional approach which again is in part explained by patient selection. In the largest single-institution series (n = 53) of LLAR reported in the literature three (5.6%) anastomotic leakages were encountered (no mortality). An insufficiency rate of 19%, however, was noted in the study by Hartley et al.[14]

With regard to oncologic principles there are only few data available. Köckerling and contributors[12] from *The Laparoscopic Colorectal Surgery Study Group* analysed a subgroup of 90 patients with rectal cancer. Of these 53 (upper rectal third tumour n = 29; middle third n = 24) underwent a laparoscopic anterior resection while 10 patients out of 37 with low rectal cancer (<5 cm from the anal verge) had a LLAR while the remaining 27 had an LAPR. They report a complete lateral, posterior, and anterior dissection down to the pelvic floor and a proximal vessel transsection of the IMA in all but one of the 37 patients with low rectal cancer. Oncologic follow-up data following LLAR are very scarce. In a case-control-study by Schwandner et al.[17] in which 19 laparoscopic-assisted anterior resections were compared with 19 matched controls undergoing open surgery, no difference was found with regard to survival, recurrence, and cancer-related mortality after a mean follow-up of 33 months in the laparoscopic and 31 months in the open group.

Another interesting issue is the matter of immune response during and after minimal access surgery. Various reports suggest an attenuated metabolic stress response during laparoscopic surgery compared with the conventional approach.[7,20,21] In terms of oncologic outcome it has been hypothesised that a better immune status could translate into increased survival rates for patients with malignant disease.[22] Indeed, there are two randomised trials on this issue for patients with colorectal cancer. The study from Germany investigated a total 60 patients and found significantly lower interleukin-6 (IL-6) and C-reactive protein (CRP) levels after laparoscopic resection.[18] They concluded that minimal invasive surgery leads to a less intense inflammatory response due to a milder surgical trauma. However, the most recent report from Singapore including 236 patients did not detect any differences with regard to T- or B-cell function measured three days postoperatively.[23] The authors conclude that there is no difference in the systemic immune response between laparoscopic and conventional surgery for colorectal cancer.

In conclusion, LLAR is technically feasible with acceptable perioperative complication rates. Oncological short-term outcome as documented in a few trials with insufficient patient numbers does not differ from patients undergoing conventional surgery. LLAR can serve as a prime example for the requirement of both, specialised oncological knowledge and laparoscopic expertise in order not to jeopardise the patients' short- and, more importantly, long-term outcome. However, for a final and valid assessment, prospective randomised trials are mandatory to evaluate the role of laparoscopic surgery for rectal cancer.

References

1. The COLOR Study Group. COLOR: a randomized trial comparing laparoscopic and open resection for colon cancer. Dig Surg 2000;17:617-622
2. Phillips EH, Franklin M, Carroll BJ, Fallas MJ, Ramos R, Rosenthal D. Laparoscopic colectomy. Ann Surg 1992; 216: 703-707
3. Sackier JM, Berci G, Hiatt JR, Hartunian S. Laparoscopic abdominoperineal resection of the rectum. Br J Surg 1992; 79: 1207-8
4. Köckerling F, Scheidbach H, Schneider C, Bärlehner E, Köhler L, Bruch HP, Konradt J, Wittekind C, Hohenberger W. The Laparoscopic Colorectal Surgery Study Group. Laparoscopic abdominoperineal resection: early postoperative results of a prospective study involving 116 patients. Dis Colon Rectum 2000;43:1503-11
5. Seow-Choen F, Eu KW, Ho YH, Leong AF. A preliminary comparison of a consecutive series of open versus laparoscopic abdomino-perineal resection for rectal adenocarcinoma. Int J Colorect Dis 1997;12:88-90
6. Poulin EC, Mamazza J, Schlachta CM, Gregoire R, Roy N. Laparoscopic resection does not adversely affect early survival curves in patients undergoing surgery for colorectal adenocarcinoma. Ann Surg 1999;229:487-92
7. Vittimberga FJ, Foley DP, Meyers WC, Callery MP. Laparoscopic surgery and the systemic immune response. Ann Surg 1998;227:326-334
8. Schiedeck TH, Schwandner O, Baca I, Bährlehner E, Konradt J, Köckerling F, Kuthe A, Buerk C, Herold A, Bruch HP. The Laparoscopic Colorectal Surgery Study Group. Laparoscopic Surgery for the cure of colorectal cancer. Results of a German five-center study. Dis Colon Rectum 2000;43:1-8
9. Bärlehner E, Heukrodt B, Anders S. Laparoscopic surgery for rectal cancer. Zentralbl Chir 1998;123:1164-1168
10. Fleshman JW, Wexner SD, Anvari M, LaTulippe JF, Birnbaum EH, Kodner IJ, Read TE, Nogueras JJ, Weiss EG: Laparoscopic vs. open abdominoperineal resection for cancer. Dis Colon Rectum 1999;42:930-39
11. Leung KL, Kwok SP, Lau WY, Meng WC, Chung CC, Lai PB, Kwong KH. Laparoscopic-assisted abdominoperineal resection for low rectal adenocarcinoma. Surg Endosc 2000;14:67-70
12. Köckerling F, Reymond MA, Schneider C, Wittekind C, Scheidbach H, Konradt J, Köhler L, Bärlehner E, Kuthe A, Bruch HP, Hohenberger W. The Laparoscopic Colorectal Surgery Study Group. Prospective multicenter study of the quality of oncologic resections in patients undergoing laparoscopic colorectal surgery for cancer. Dis Colon Rectum 1998;41:963-970
13. Heald RJ, Karanjia ND. Results of radical surgery for rectal cancer. World J Surg 1992; 16:848-857
14. Hartley JE, Mehigan BJ, Qureshi AE, Duthie GS, Lee PW, Monson JR. Total mesorectal excision: assessment of the laparoscopic approach. Dis Colon Rectum 2001;44:315-21
15. Bruch HP, Herold A, Schiedeck TH, Schwandner O. Laparoscopic surgery for rectal cancer. Zentralbl Chir 1997; 122: 1134-41

16. Watanabe M, Teramoto T, Hasegawa H, Kitajima M. Laparoscopic ultralow anterior resection combined with per anum intersphincteric rectal dissection for lower rectal cancer. Dis Colon Rectum 2000;43(Suppl):S94-7
17. Schwandner O, Schiedeck TH, Killaitis C, Bruch HP. A case-control-study comparing laparoscopic versus open surgery for rectosigmoidal and rectal cancer. Int Colorectal Dis 1999;14:158-63
18. Schwenk W, Böhm B, Müller JM. Postoperative pain and fatigue after laparoscopic or conventional colorectal resections. A prospective randomized trial. Surg Endosc 1998; 12: 1131-36
19. Milsom JW, Böhm B, Hammerhofer KA, Fazio V, Steiger E, Elson P. A prospective, randomized trial comparing laparoscopic versus conventional techniques in colorectal cancer surgery: a preliminary report. J Am Coll Surg 1998;187:46-54
20. Stage JG, Schulze S, Moller P, Overgaard H, Anderson M, Rebsdorf-Pederson VB, Nielsen HJ. Prospective randomized study of laparoscopic versus open colonic resection for adenocarcinoma. Br J Surg 1997;84:391-6
21. Fukushima R, Kawamura Yj, Saito H, Saito Y, Hashiguchi Y, Sawada T, Muto T. Interleukin-6 and stress hormone responses after uncomplicated gasless laparoscopic-assisted and open sigmoid colectomy. Dis Colon Rectum 1996;39(Suppl):S29-34
22. Allendorf JD, Bessler M, Horvath KD, Marvin MR, Laird DA, Whelan RL. Increased tumor establishment and growth after open vs. laparoscopic surgery in mice may be related to differences in postoperative T-cell function. Surg Endosc 1999; 13: 233-5
23. Tang CL, Eu KW, Tai BC, Soh JG, Machin D, Seow-choen F. Randomized clinical trial of the effect of open versus laparoscopically assisted colectomy on systemic immunity in patients with colorectal cancer. Br J Surg 2001;88:801-7.

CHAPTER

8

Laparoscopic nephrectomy

H. Mohseni, W.D. Shingleton

Introduction

Laparoscopy in the use of surgical treatment for carcinoma of the kidney was initially reported in 1990 by Clayman.[1] During the early years of this technique relatively few procedures were performed secondary to long operative times and concerns about incomplete resection of tumor. As the operative experience with this procedure increased, a number of investigators published selected series of patients that had undergone this procedure.[2-4] In these series there was no evidence of significant morbidity associated with the procedure. Two patients had local recurrence and 8 patients have had disease progression at 28-month follow-up. In these limited series of reports, laparoscopic nephrectomies proved to be a viable surgical technique that did require a substantial learning curve. This chapter will detail the technique required for performing laparoscopic nephrectomy and the results to date.

Laparoscopic Radical Nephrectomy

Indications

Robson popularized radical nephrectomy as the gold standard treatment for localized RCC in 1961.[5] It includes en bloc removal of the kidney and adrenal gland with the perirenal fat and Gerota's fascia intact along with regional lymph nodes. The renal artery and vein are separately ligated and divided early in the course of the operation prior to manipulation of the tumor as well as to reduce the risk of bleeding. Classically the indication for laparascopic radical nephrectomy has been a solitary tumor less than 5 CM in size. Lately, this technique has been described for larger or multiple tumors as well as bilateral tumors.

Patient preparation

The informed consent should include these key points:

1. Risk of injury to adjacent organs
2. Possibility of converting to open procedure

One day prior to surgery, patients are placed on clear fluids and are NPO after midnight. A mild mechanical bowel prep in the form of Magnesium Citrate will be helpful prior to the operation.

After the induction of general anesthesia and prophylactic antibiotic administration, a urethral catheter and nasogastric tube are inserted. The patient is put in a flank position and axillary rolls are placed and all pressure points are well padded. The table is flexed with kidney rest up and the patient is secured to the table (Figure 1). Abdomen is prepped and draped from nipple line all the way down to pubic symphysis exposing the whole abdomen including the opposite side Figure 1).

Operating room set up is shown in the (Figure 2). The surgeon and his assistant stand on the opposite side with the primary surgeon facing the patient with the patient close to the edge of the table. Al-

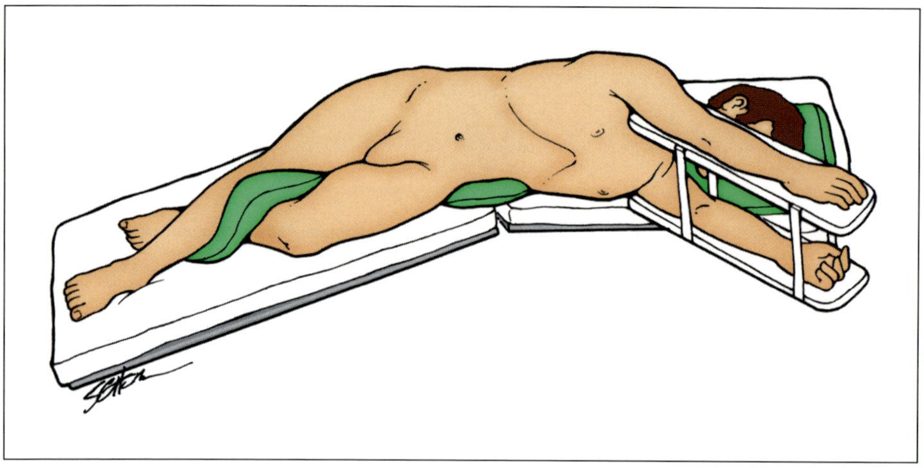

FIGURE 1. Position of the patient for right laparoscopic nephrectomy.

ternatively, the surgeon and assistant stay on the same side facing the patient, depending on the surgeon preference.

Initially pneumoperitoneum is established by inserting a Veress needle in the midline and just below the umbilicus. Alternatively, a Hasson trocar can be used under direct vision. The peritoneum is insufflated to 15 mm Hg and then the laparoscopic ports are inserted. The camera is inserted at the infraumbilical port and the under direct vision using the camera the other two ports are inserted. The first trocar, 10/12 mm in size, is placed lateral to rectus muscle

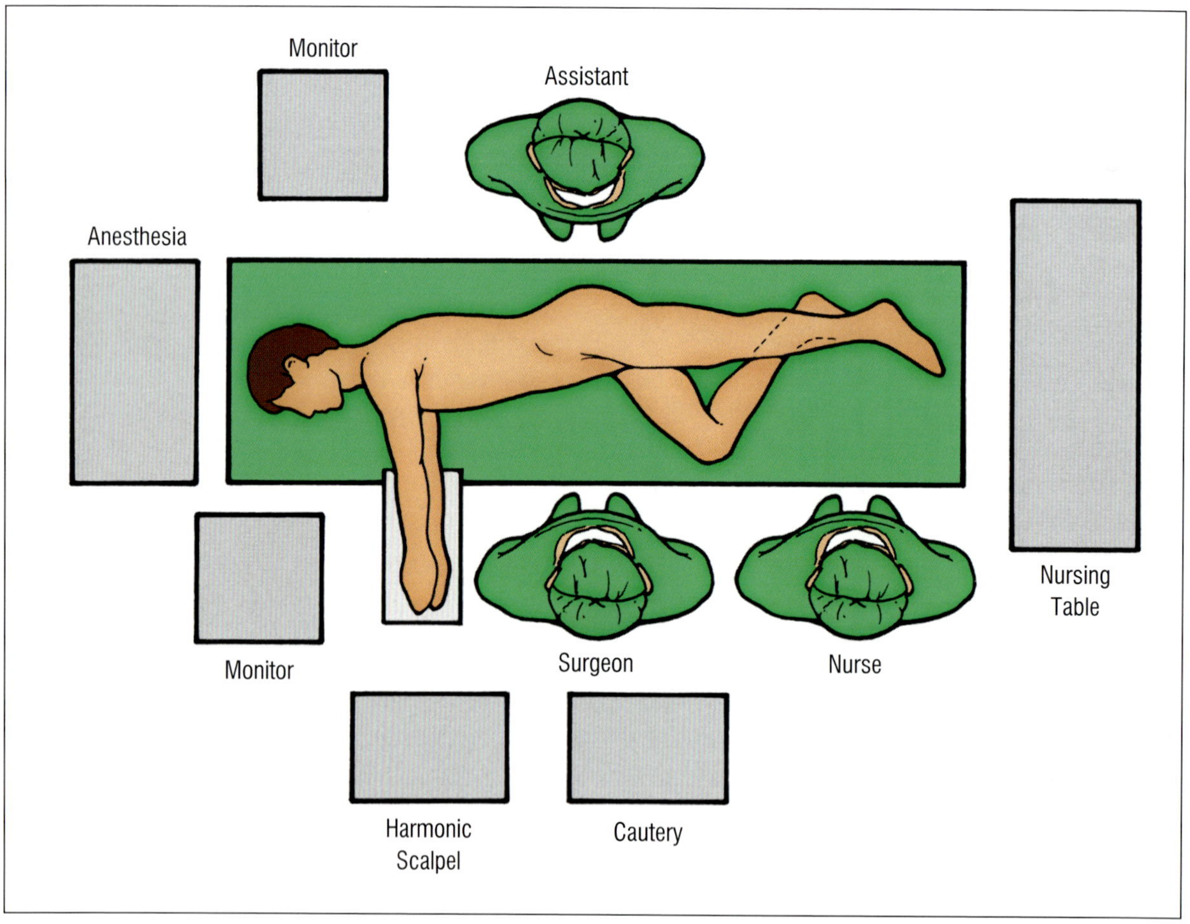

FIGURE 2. Diagram of operative room and position of surgeons and assistans.

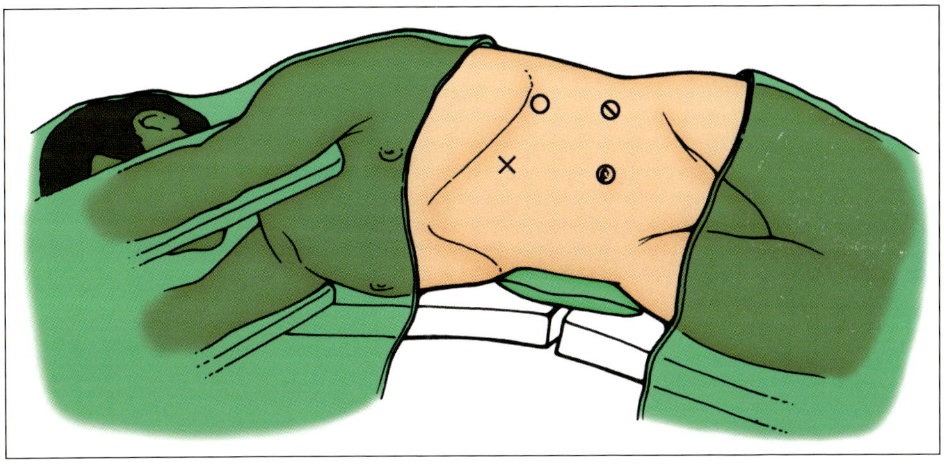

FIGURE 4. Position of ports for left radical nephrectomy.

edge midway between the umbilicus and iliac crest, while care should be taken to avoid superficial blood vessels that are visible with laparoscope. A second 5-mm trocar is inserted usually at the midline halfway between sternum and umbilicus. Usually these three ports are adequate to perform the surgery for a left sided nephrectomy, however, if more ports become necessary during the course of the operation they can be inserted in appropriate places, usually along the posterior axillary line (Figure 3). For a right nephrectomy, a fourth port is usually required to retract the liver; usually a liver retractor fan or paddle is inserted through a subcostal trocar to expose the kidney better.

Once all the ports are inserted and through inspection of the abdomen and release of the adhesion for a left nephrectomy, the descending colon is reflected and mobilized medially by sharply incising the avascular line of Toldt from splenic flexure to sigmoid colon. Using sharp dissection and electrocautery or harmonic scalpel the colon is reflected of the Gerota's fascia over the kidney medially toward the renal hilum. The dissection is carried superiorly and the attachments of the splenic flexure to the diaphragm are released. The entire colon now can be reflected medially and this will expose the s-plenorenal ligaments, which are released by electrocautery or harmonic scalpel. The spleen is further mobilized by releasing the lateral splenic attachments to the diaphragm. The spleen now can be reflected medially and the tail of the pancreas can be dissected off the kidney to expose the adrenal gland and the renal hilum. The dissection is carried at the renal hilum and the gonadal vein is dissected and is clipped and divided. The ureter is then identified inferiorly along the course of the gonadal vein and is ligated with clips at the level of the pelvic brim and divided. The kidney is dissected off the psoas muscle by incising the lateral attachments of the Gerota's fascia to the posterior abdominal wall and the kidney with the Gerota's fascia intact is mobilized inferiorly and superiorly toward the upper pole of the kidney. The kidney is freed superiorly by incising the splenorenal ligaments and the dissection is then is carried out posteriorly to free the kidney toward renal hilum. The kidney is rotated medially and this will allow dissection at the renal hilum posteriorly to identify the renal artery. The renal artery is ligated with surgical clips and divided (Figure 4). At this point a lumbar vein entering the renal

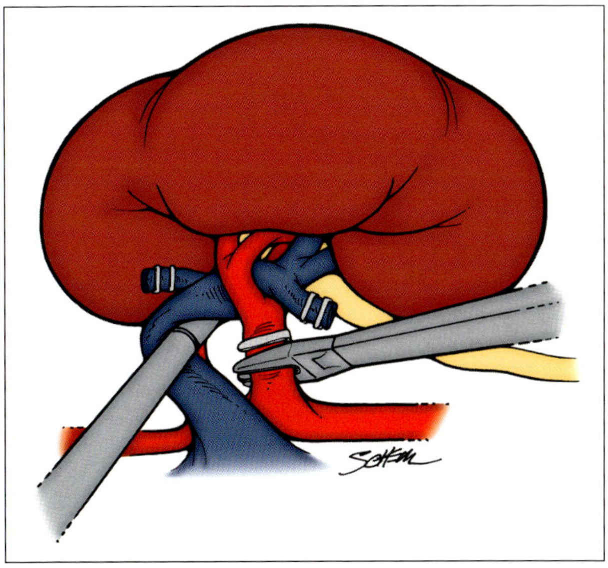

FIGURE 4. Clips being applied to left renal artery.

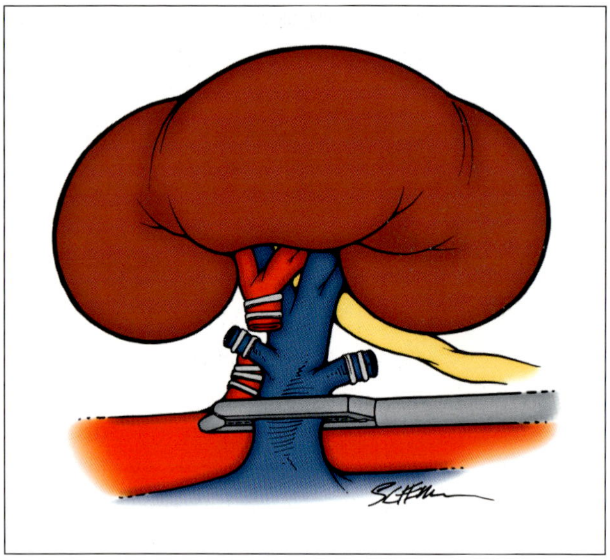

FIGURE 5. Transection of left renal vein.

vein can be ligated and divided for better exposure of the renal vein. If the adrenal gland is removed as part of the specimen the renal vein is divided with an endovascular GIA stapling device, proximal to the take off the adrenal vein (Figure 5). If the adrenal gland is spared, the renal vein is divided distal to the adrenal vein entrance. Now the kidney and the adrenal gland are only attached superiorly and superomedially. The kidney is dissected off the lateral border of the adrenal gland with the harmonic scalpel. The specimen is now free completely and is placed into an impermeable bag and delivered, in toto, outside the body, via a small muscle splitting incision through the lower port side. If the location of the tumor requires the en bloc removal of the adrenal gland, then the renal vein is divided with an endovascular GIA stapler proximal to the take off of the adrenal vein. Then the adrenal gland is dissected medially with harmonic scalpel and is included in the specimen.

The kidney can also be removed by morcellation. The advantage of this technique is that no extension of any incision is required. However, because of the risk of bag leakage and contamination of the port site with the tumor spillage, as well as lack of pathological staging, most surgeons prefer the removal of the intact specimen via an extended incision of a port site.

A right radical nephrectomy is technically more demanding because of the position of the liver over the upper pole of the kidney (Figure 6). To overcome this difficulty a fourth port is inserted subcostally to place a liver retractor and pull the liver superiorly to expose the upper pole and hilar region of the right kidney picture.

In order to expose the kidney even further the right triangular ligaments as well as the anterior and posterior coronary ligaments can be divided using electrocautery and rotate the liver medially. Next the ascending colon is mobilized by incising the line of Toldt with electrocautery and reflecting the colon medially from the cecum to hepatic flexure including the hepatic flexure. The duodenum is identified and mobilized medially with sharp dissection to expose the IVC and anterior renal hilum including the shorter right renal vein. During the dissection of the duodenum, a duodenal injury or hematoma should be avoided by careful dissection. Then the kidney with Gerota's fascia intact is dissected inferiorly and the ureter is identified, clipped and incised. The right kidney is then dissected laterally and posterior-

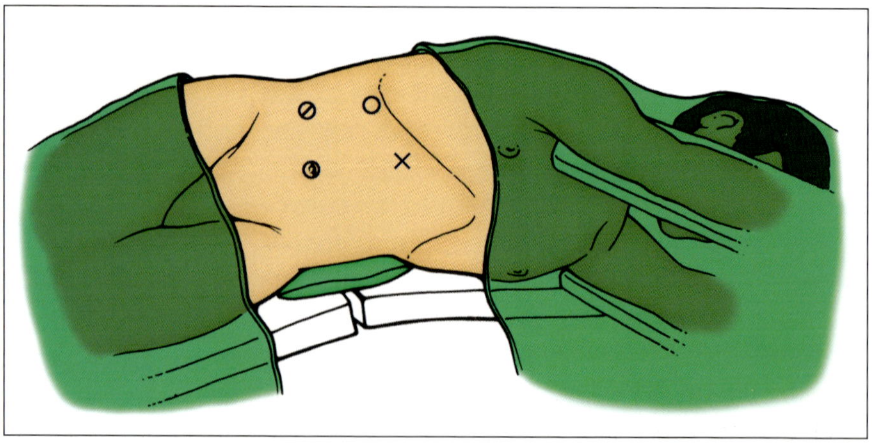

FIGURE 6. Port positioning for right laparoscopic radical nephrectomy.

ly and renal artery is identified posteriorly and is clipped and incised. The right renal vein is divided using an endovascular GIA stapler. The dissection is carried superiorly and the posterior peritoneum over the upper part of hepatorenal pouch of Morrison is incised with electrocautery and the superior part of the right kidney is freed using harmonic scalper and multiple surgical clips. If the adrenal gland is spared, the superomedial dissection is carried later to the adrenal gland. To include the adrenal in the specimen, the dissection is carried carefully medial to the adrenal gland and the adrenal vein is identified coming directly off the IVC and is double clipped and incised. The dissection is carried medially and adrenal is freed completely, included with the kidney. At this point the specimen can be removed outside the same way described for the left kidney.

Nephroureterectomy

The techniques of the nephroureterectomy are essentially the same as radical nephrectomy except that the whole length of the ureter and bladder cuff should be removed with the specimen as in a standard open nephroureterectomy. Prior to the laparoscopic nephrectomy portion of the surgery the patient is put in a modified dorsolithotomy position and cystoscoped with the ureter on the surgical side cannulated with an open ended catheter. The catheter is advanced to the kidney and then using the Collins knife, a circumferential incision is made around the ureter and ureteral orifice. This is carried deep into the perivesical fat to incorporate the bladder cuff and intramural ureter. Through this approach about 3 to 4 cm of the distal ureter and the bladder cuff should be freed. After adequate mobilization of the ureter a grasping forceps is used to pull the ureter and bladder cuff into the bladder (Figure 7). The bladder is filled with irrigation and then under direct vision an Endoloop device is inserted suprapubically to tie off the distal ureter over the ureteric catheter to prevent tumor spillage during the laparoscopic nephrectomy part of the operation. After the intramural ureter and bladder cuff has been managed endoscopically the patient is repositioned for the laparoscopic part of the operation. Alternatively, the distal ureter and the bladder cuff can be managed laparoscopically. After the kidney and proximal ureter part of the dissection is completed the ureter is not cut. Additional ports at least one or perhaps two is inserted for the dissection of the distal ureter and bladder cuff. After dissecting the bladder to the level of iliac vessels the ureter is freed distally

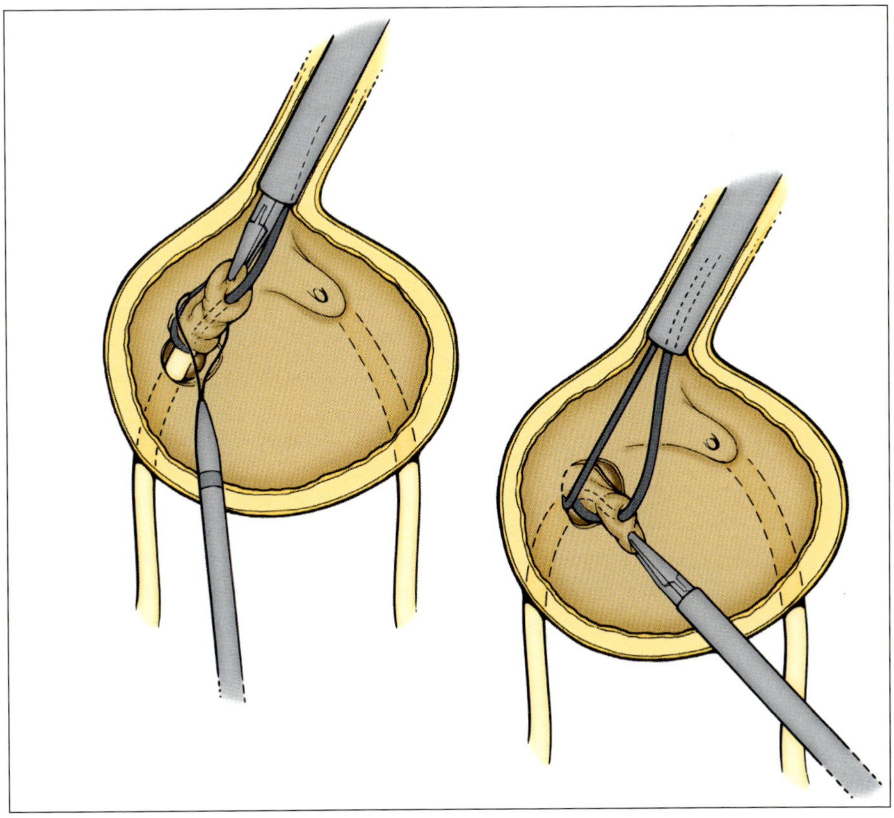

FIGURE 7. A & B - resection of distal left ureter and ureteral orifice.

toward the bladder. The vas deferens or round ligament is clipped and divided followed by the same procedure as the medial umbilical ligament. The ureter is mobilized to its entry to the bladder at the UV junction. At this point, while retracting the ureter, cephaled an absorbable stapler device, can be used to divide the distal ureter and bladder cuff from the bladder (Figure 8).

Hand-Assisted Laparoscopic Nephrectomy

Hand-assisted laparoscopic nephrectomy is becoming popular among urologic surgeons because it is easier to perform technically. In this approach the surgeon uses his nondominant hand during laparoscopy. He uses his hand to retract, dissect, and direct his instruments. Additionally, the hand port is used to bring the specimen to the outside. In this approach, after the pneumoperitoneum is achieved and the appropriate ports are inserted accordingly, the periumbilical site is extended enough to accommodate the hand port that will be used for the surgeon's nondominant hand. Once the hand and the appropriate ports are in place the surgery is performed in a similar manner as described for laparoscopic nephrectomy.

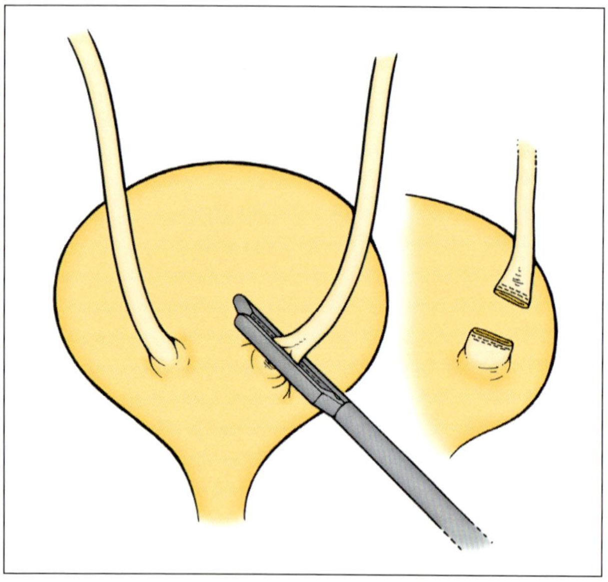

FIGURE 8. Transection of right distal ureter.

Extraperitoneal Laparoscopic Nephrectomy

In this technique the retroperitoneum is accessed through a small incision at the tip of 12th rib. The retroperitoneal space is expanded bluntly with a fingertip and then under direct vision, a special trocar with an inflatable balloon is used to dissect the kidney from the psoas muscle. This creates a space for laparoscopic work, as well as, performing a major part of the dissection posteriorly. Once the space is created two other ports are introduced and the rest of the surgery is performed.

The disadvantage of this approach is the limited space to work. However, since the peritoneal space is not violated postoperative ileus is less frequent and recovery is faster than a transperitoneal approach along with loss of postoperative pain.

Results

The published reports of laparoscopic nephrectomies have increased over the past few years as more investigators are performing the procedure and the length of follow-up has increased. The majority of the reports have been for the transperitoneal approach.

Ono et al reported the results for 60 patients with an operative time of 5.2 hours, a short recovery time (3 weeks) and lower blood loss than for an open nephrectomy.[2] Five year survival was 95.5% which is comparable to that for open radical nephrectomy. No patient developed local recurrence and only 3 patients had distant metastasis. Cadeddu et al described the results in 157 patients in a multi-institutional review.[7] Three percent of the cases required conversion to an open surgical procedure. There was one intraoperative death; however, the overall 5-year survival was 91%. Again, the rates are comparable to the open radical nephrectomy series. Dunn et al reported the Washington University experience on 61 patients.[7] The operative time was longer than in a series of open radical nephrectomies. However, the laparoscopic patients had a lower blood loss, narcotic pain medication requirement, and hospitalization stay. Barrett and associates reviewed these results in 72 patients with a mean operative time of 2.9 hours and a 12% conversion rate.[8]

The published reports in regards to retroperitoneal laparoscopic nephrectomies have been less than a transperitoneal approach. Gill et al has reported on 47 patients with a mean operative time of 2.9 hours, 1.6 hospital day stay, and a recovery period of 4 weeks.[9] The Japanese experience was described by Ono in 1997 on 14 patients noted a longer operative time (4.9 hours) and greater blood loss than Gill.[10] Abbon et al compared 29 open and 29 retroperitoneal laparoscopic cases and noted an equivalent operative time with lower blood loss and a shorter hospital stay in the laparoscopic patients.[11] In terms of hand-assisted radical nephrectomy, there have been no reports of a series of patients undergoing this approach with follow-up at this time.

Complications

There have been a variety of major and minor complication reports with laparoscopic nephrectomy. Gill reviewed four series of patients with a total of 266 patients who had 16% minor and 7% major complication rate.[12] The overall conversion rate to open procedure was 4% and there was a 1% perioperative mortality rate. Cadeddu et al in a series of 157 patients from five different institutions noted a 9.6% perioperative complication rate of which 4 patients required open conversion.[6]

Conclusion

The routine use of laparoscopic nephrectomy is being widespread in the urologic community. Although there is a definite learning curve associated with the procedure, once the surgeon is comfortable performing it, the morbidity and mortality rate is similar to that of open radical nephrectomy. Continued monitoring of patients who had the procedure performed will be necessary to ensure that the survival rate of these patients is equivalent to that of patients undergoing open surgery.

References

1. Clayman RV, Kavoussi LR, Soper NJ, et al. Laparoscopic nephrectomy: initial report. J Urol.1991 Aug;146(2):278-82.
2. Ono Y, Katoh N, Kinukawa T, et al. Laparoscopic nephrectomy, radical nephrectomy, and adrenalectomy. Nagoya experience. J Urol.1994 Dec;152(6 Pt1):1962-6.
3. Ono Y, Kinukawa T, Hattori R, et al. Laparoscopic radical nephrectomy for renal cell carcinoma: a five-year experience. Urology. 1999 Feb;53:280-6.
4. Robson, CJ: Radical nephrectomy for renal cell carcinoma. J Urol. 1963 Jan;89:37-42.
5. Barrett, PH, Fentie, DD. Longer follow-up for laparoscopic radical nephrectomy with morcellation for renal cell carcinoma. J Endourol. 1999 Feb;13:A62.
6. Cadeddu JA, Ono Y, Clayman RV, et al. Laparoscopic nephrectomy for renal cell cancer: evaluation of efficacy and safety: a multicenter experience. Urology. 1998 Nov;52(5):773-7.
7. Barrett PH, Fentie DD, Taranger LA. Laparoscopic radical nephrectomy with morcellation for renal cell carcinoma: the Saskatoon experience. Urology. 1998 Jul;52(1)23-8.
8. Dunn MD, Portis AHJ, Shalhav AL, et al: Laparoscopic versus open radical nephrectomy for renal tumor: The Washington University experience (abstract). J Urol. 1999 161:166.
9. Ono Y, Katoh N, Kinukawa T, et al: Laparoscopic radical nephrectomy: The Nagoya experience. J Urol. 1997 Sept; 158(3) 719.
10. Abbou CC, Cicco A, Gasman D, Hoznek A, Antiphon P, Chopin DK, Salomon L. Retroperitoneal laparoscopic versus open radical nephrectomy. J Urol. 1999 Jun;161(6):1776-80.
11. Gill IS. Laparoscopic radical nephrectomy for cancer. Urol Clin North Am. 2000 Nov;27(4):707-19.

CHAPTER

Laparoscopic management of prostatic cancer

9

W.B. Shingleton, H.F. Mohseni

Introduction

Carcinoma of the prostate is the most common urologic malignancy in men. In the United States, it was estimated that over 180,000 new cases were diagnosed in the year 2000.[1] Thirty-one thousand men in the United States will die during the year from this disease. This chapter will discuss the role of laparoscopy in the treatment of prostate cancer. While carcinoma of the prostate is the most common genitourinary malignancy, laparoscopy has had minimal impact on this disease to date. The initial laparoscopic procedure in urological surgery was the laparoscopic pelvic lymphadenectomy and since that time radical prostatectomy is being performed laparoscopically.

Laparoscopic Pelvic Lymphadenectomy

The initial procedure to be performed in urology with the laparoscope was the pelvic lymphadenectomy. Schussler reported their experience in performing laparoscopic pelvic lymph node dissection as a staging procedure in patients with prostate cancer in 1992.[2] The main indication for performing this procedure is to determine the stage of the disease. This will allow the patient to be offered different treatment options based on the stage of the disease determined by the pathologic results of the node dissection. Initially, laparoscopic pelvic lymph node dissection became widespread as a staging procedure regardless of the patient's initial prostate specific antigen (PSA). It provided information regarding lymph node status that was inaccessible by radiographic imaging modality such computerized tomography. It was therefore applicable to any patient who was a candidate for local curative treatment.

Partin in 1993 reported that the incidence of pathological positive lymph nodes was lower than previously expected in terms of a patient's age, Gleason score, and PSA level.[3] This information, along with the development of normograms, would enable one to determine the probability of having positive lymph node metastases in relation to age, clinical staging Gleason's score, and PSA level led to a decrease in the use of laparoscopic pelvic lymphadenectomy. While the use of this technique for the staging of prostate cancer has declined, it still remains a valuable staging modality for use in bladder cancer and penile cancer.

Technique

The patient is placed under general anesthesia for this procedure, as the abdominal distention that occurs with inflation is too uncomfortable for the patient to tolerate under intravenous sedation. The use of nitrous oxide as an anesthesia agent should be avoided, as this will cause intestinal distention. A nasogastric tube and urethral catheter is placed to decompress bowel and bladder. The patient is in a supine position with slight Trendelenburg to aid in visualization of the pelvis. The intraabdominal approach proceeds with inflation of the abdominal cavity utilizing either a Veress needle (closed) or Hassan cannula (open). Either method is acceptable and depends on the surgeon's preference. After the abdominal cavity is inflated to a pressure of 15-20 cc Hg, the laparoscope is placed and the intestinal contents inspected. At this time, any evidence of intestinal injury may be detected and the decision made for repair by either a laparoscopic or open method. In no injury has occurred, the placement of the remaining trocars may take place under direct vision. Figure 1 illustrates recommended location of the trocar placement.[4] Either a 5-mm or 10 mm trocar can be utilized depending on the surgeon's preference. The two lateral trocars should be positioned lateral to the rectus muscle in order to avoid injury to the epigastric vessels. The lower midline trocar is positioned 4-cm above the pubis.

The patient is then placed in a steep Trendelenburg position with the right side of the table elevated in order to visualize the obturator fossa. Figure 2 illustrates the important structures the surgeon should identify prior to beginning the dissection. The iliac artery and vein are the lateral aspect of the dissection with the medial umbilical ligament constituting the medial aspect. The vas deferens will be a whitish appearing structure transversing the obturator fossa originating at the internal ring and proceeding medially in a horizontal fashion to cross the medial umbilical ligament. Although the ureter is shown in Figure 2, it is usually not visualized during the procedure. The initial step requires grasping the perineum and incising it to gain access to the retroperitoneum. The incision should be made parallel to the iliac vessels and extended in a vertical manner. Utilizing blunt dissection, the incision site is enlarged and the vas deferens identified. The vas is then ligated by use of the electric cautery and the laparoscopic scissors (Figure 3). The nodal package is mobilized after starting at the inferior portion (Figure 4). As the dissection begins to enter the obturator fossa, the surgeon should be careful as to identifying the obturator nerve that will be present along with the obturator artery and vein that lies deeper than the nerve. Care should be taken to mobilize the lymph node as an intact package. After the lymph nodes have been re-

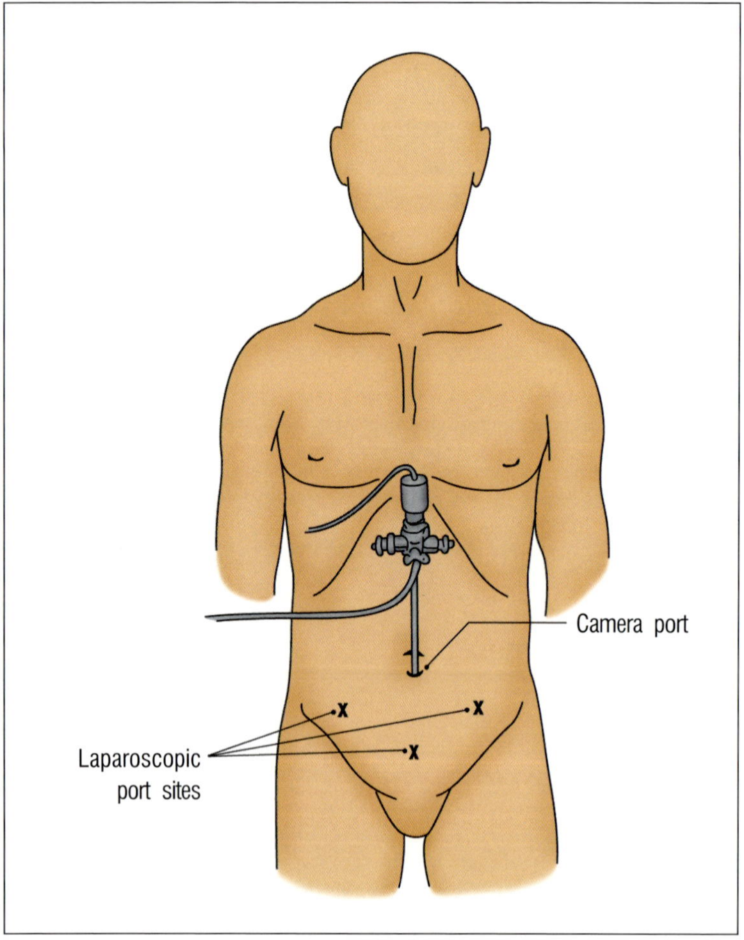

FIGURE 1. The two 5-mm trocars are placed lateral to the rectus muscle in a line approximately level with the superior aspect of the iliac crest.

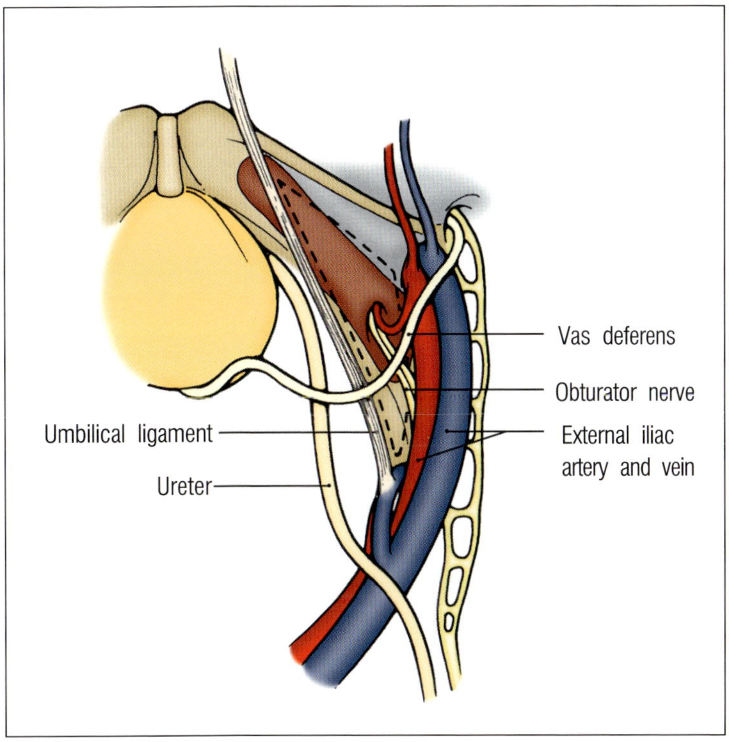

FIGURE 2. The surgeon should be certain to identify all the important anatomic landmarks.

moved from the obturator fossa, they are placed in a laparoscopic sac and removed in toto through one of the 10-mm trocar sites. After removal of the nodal package, the obturator fossa is then irrigated with normal saline and the intra-abdominal pressure lowered to allow visualization of any venous bleeding. Figure 5 illustrates how the obturator fossa should look after removal of the lymph node. If no bleeding is present, the patient is then rotated so the contralateral side is now elevated and the lymph dissection proceeds in a like manner.

The extraperitoneal approach involves avoiding penetration of the abdominal cavity and remaining extraperitoneal for the entire dissection. The advantages of an extraperitoneal approach involves avoidance of bowel during placement of trocar with possible resulting injury and the lack of necessity of mobilization of bowel prior to beginning the lymph node dissection. Additionally, the peritoneal cavity acts as a retractor preventing the bowel contents from entering into the operative field. The difficulty with the extraperitoneal approach involves having a decreased amount of space to operate in and lack of easily recognized landmarks that are present with the transperitoneal approach.

The extraperitoneal approach is initiated with a 3-cm incision made inferior to the umbilicus to allow for placement of the extraperitoneal dilating balloon. Blunt mobilization is then undertaken with the surgeon's finger to create a space for placement of the balloon. A variety of balloon devices are available commercially, as well as, utilizing surgeon's latex gloves or finger cots. The key point is to have a mechanism that will allow for the develop-

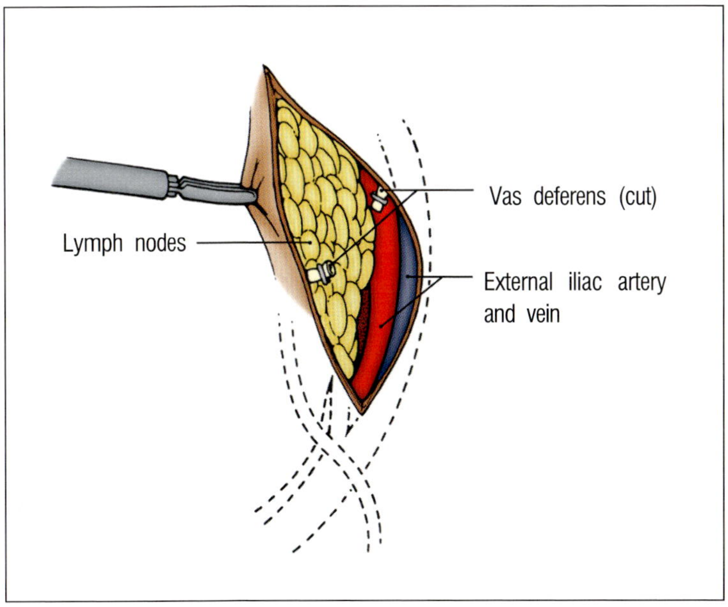

FIGURE 3. The vas deferens is grasped and mobilized from the surrounding tissue. It is divided between metal clips or with electrocautery from the scissors.

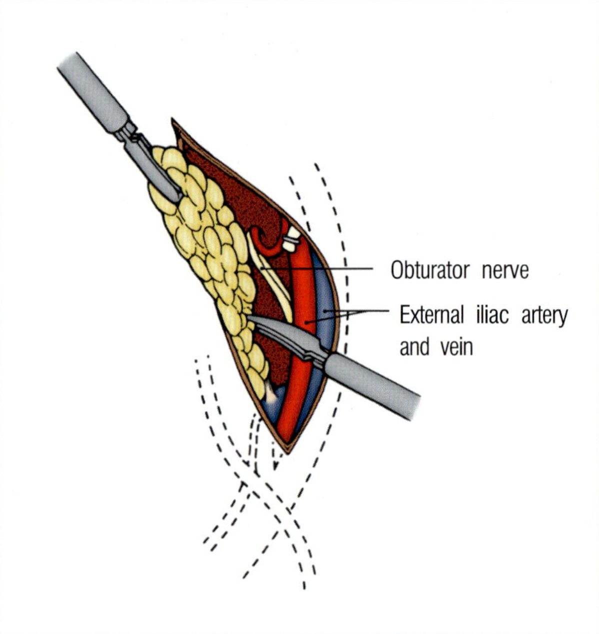

FIGURE 4. The surgeon uses a combination of blunt and sharp dissection to mobilize the lymph node package.

ment of an 800-1000 cc space in the pre-pubic space. After the space is created the Hasson cannula can be placed and further inflation achieved. The placement of the other trocars is in a manner similar as for the transperitoneal approach. The dissection can then proceed as described for the transperitoneal approach. The postoperative care for the patients having either approach consists of removing the nasogastric tube and allowing a clear liquid diet the evening after surgery. The patients are usually discharged home within 24 hours with routine wound care instituted for the trocar sites.

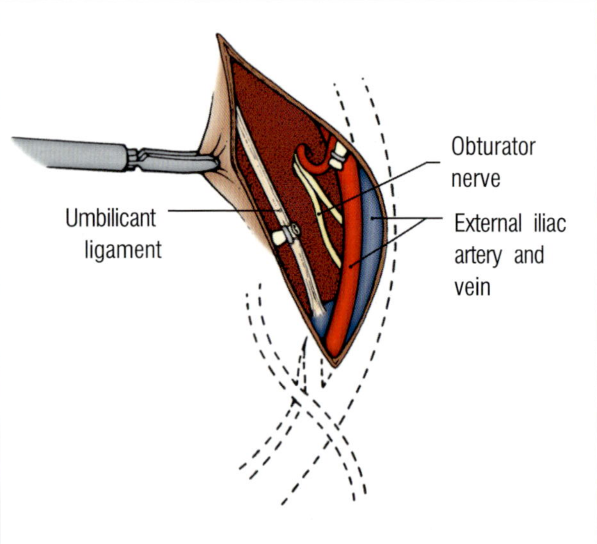

FIGURE 5. A completely dissected obturator fossa. The important structures are identified.

Results

Laparoscopic pelvic node dissection has been performed for a number of years and results have been gathered that allows an open pelvic node dissection. Kerbel et al, as well as, other investigators has shown that the 3-6 lymph node tissue yield is comparable between the laparoscopic and open technique.[5-7] Winfield reports an average yield of 4.6 and 4.5 nodes from over 200 patients treated with the laparoscopic approach.[7] The initial operation time was longer 199.4 versus 102.4 minutes than that reported by Kerbel, but as the operation experience increased the reported time as decreased.

One of the advantages of the laparoscopic technique is less morbidity that has been well documented by various investigations. Kerbel reported a decreased hospitalization, 1.7 days, lower analgesic use (1.50 mg morphine) and a faster return to normal activities (10.8 days) as compared to patients undergoing an open pelvic node dissection5.

Kavoussi has reported the overall complication at 15% in a series of 378 patients.[8] In later reports, other investigators have reported low complication rates that probably account for the increased experience by the surgeons.[9] There have been no reported complication rates for the extraperitoneal approach but the rate should be similar if not lower than the transperitoneal approach.

In regard to financial costs associated with laparoscopic pelvic lymphadenectomy, Troxel reported that the cost of the laparoscopy technique was 52% higher than the open approach.[10] The main reason for this higher cost was the use of disposable instruments as compared to reusable instruments utilized in the open technique. Conversely, the postoperative charges were estimated to be 280% higher for patients undergoing an open procedure as compared to the laparoscopic group.

Some investigators have been performing laparoscopic seminal vesicle dissection at the time of pelvic lymphadenectomy.[11] This was then followed by the radical perineal prostatectomy. Levy reported in their experiences on 37 patients and they noted an average operation time of 244 minutes with a mean hospitalization of 5.7 days.[11] Teichman reported a series of patients undergoing radical retropubic versus laparoscopic pelvic lymphadenectomy and seminal vesicle dissection followed by a radical perineal prostatectomy.[12] The mean operative time was approximately the same for the two groups. However, the laparoscopic groups had a shorter hospitalization and lower pain medication requirement.

Laparoscopic Radical Prostatectomy

The initial report of laparoscopic radical prostatectomy was by Schuessler et al in 1997.[13] He described the results of nine patients who underwent this procedure for localized prostate cancer. This technique involved placement of five trocars in a fan arrangement over the lower abdomen. This allowed the approach to be transperitoneal to the prostate. Initially, upon entering the retroperitoneum, the vas deferens was identified and cut. The vas is then followed to the point where the seminal vesicles are located and transected. The vesicle is then freed from its surrounding structures and Denovillier's fascia is then entered and the rectum bluntly dissected free from the prostate. The prostatic pedicles are then transected with a vascular stapler. The prostatic ligaments were identified and sharply transected and the dorsal vein is sharply divided without prior ligation of the vessel. The bladder neck was entered posteriorly and the incision carried around anteriorly without preservation of the bladder neck. The urethra was then sharply divided distally to the apex of the prostate. The specimen is placed into a laparoscopic bag and then removed at the end of the case through the umbilical port. The anastomosis was performed through a transverse incision placed in the bladder dome. A 20 F Foley catheter was placed and the anastomosis performed with interrupted 3-0 Vicryl sutures. The cystotomy was closed in two layers with intracorpeal suturing. A pelvic drain was placed and then removed on the second postoperative day. The urethral catheter was removed two weeks postoperatively.

The average operative time was 9.4 hours with mean hospitalization of 7.3 days. This length was mainly due to two patients who had two postoperative complications (cholecystitis and femoral vein thrombosis) and with exclusion of these patients, the hospital time was only 3.4 days. Only one surgical specimen had a positive margin and 6 of 9 patients were continent.

It was their conclusion that laparoscopic radical prostatectomy was technically feasible, however, there was no significant advantage over standard open surgery in regards to continence or potency in their small series.

Guillonneau and colleagues reported in 1999 their experience with laparoscopic radical prostatectomy in 40 patients.[14] Their operative procedure consisted of performing a transperitoneal pelvic lymphadenectomy prior to the prostatectomy. The initial steps in their procedure are similar to that described by Scheussler. The posterior vesical peritoneum is incised and the vas deferens identified and transected. The seminal vesicles are then identified and freed from surrounding tissues and cut. Denovillier's fascia is entered and dissected off the rectum from the prostate. Attention is then turned to the anterior portion of the prostate and after entering the retropubic space the dorsal vein complex is ligated times two with 3-0 Vicryl then divided. The Foley catheter is removed and replaced with a metal urethral dilator to aid in dissection of the apex of the prostate and proximal urethra. The urethra is then divided on the posterior aspect. A Hegar intrarectal bougie is placed to assist in dissection of the rectum. The bladder neck dissection is performed in such a manner as to preserve as much of the bladder neck as possible. The prostatic pedicles are coagulated with electric cautery. The anastomosis is completed utilizing 4-0 Vicryl interrupted sutures with an average of 6-9 sutures per anastomosis. A pelvic drain is placed with laparoscopic assistance and removed after 1-2 days. The urethral catheter was removed after five days. Five of 40 patients required conversion to an open surgical procedure. The mean operative time was 270 minutes. The average blood loss was 425 cc with a total of seven patients requiring blood transfusions with an average of 2.8 units transfused per patient. Eighty-two percent of the surgical specimen had negative margins. There was no report of continence or potency in their initial series of patients.

Jacob et al reported their laparoscopic experience with twenty patients in 2000.[17] Their operative time, blood loss, transfusion rate, and negative surgical margin results were similar to that reported by Guillonneau. Additionally, 75% of its patients were continent one month after surgery with 30% of the patients reported having erections. A followup report by this group of French urologists expanded their results to 43 patients[18]. There was a change in their surgical technique from performing the anastomosis with interrupted sutures to two hemicircumferential running sutures. The mean operative time had decreased to 4.3 hours with an average catheterization time of 4 days. Eighty-four percent of the patients were continent at one-month followup.

Guillonneau and Valancien described their further experience with laparoscopic radical prostatectomy in an expanded series of patients in 2000.[17] Overall, there were 120 patients reported on with a mean follow-up of 6 months. They reported their results by dividing this series of patients into three groups of 40 to assess improvements in surgical outcome, operative time, continence, and potency results with an increase in surgical experience. They had an improvement in mean operative time from 282 to 231 minutes. None of the patients in the most recent surgical group (group 3) required open surgical conversion compared to 4 in the first group of patients (group 1). There was also noted a decrease in blood loss for a mean of 574 cc to 277 cc from group 1 to group 3. The percentage of positive surgical margins remained approximately the same among the three groups. The continence rate was 72% at 6-month follow-up for the first 60 patients.

Conclusion

The initial results for laparoscopic lymphadenectomy for the staging of prostate cancer has been proved over time to yield reproducible results with minimal morbidity. Unfortunately, the procedure is being utilized less and less in urological surgery. Conversely, during the same time that procedure was decreasing in use, the performance of laparoscopic radical prostatectomy began. While there are only short-term results available now, to date this technique holds great promise. However, five-year data with well-documented outcome results will be necessary before adding this procedure to the urologists' armenterium.

References

1. M. Cancer Statistics, 2001, Ca, Greenlee RT, Hill-Haman, MB, Murray T, et al: A Cancer Journal for Clinicians 51, 15-36, 2001.
2. Laparoscopic pelvic lymphadenectomy for prostatic adenocarcinoma. Schuessler WW, Vancaille TG, Reich H, Griffith DP: Urol Clin of North America 19:407-415, 1992.
3. The use of prostate specific antigen, clinical stage, and Gleason score to predict pathological stage in men with localized prostate cancer. Partin AW, Yoo JH, Carter HB, et al: Journal of Urology 150: 110-114, 1993.
4. Laparoscopic pelvic lymphadenectomy. Shingleton WB: Surgical Clinics of North America 76, 3, 585-593, 1996.
5. Staging pelvic lymphadenectomy for prostate cancer: A comparison of laparoscopic and open techniques. Kerbel K, Clayman RV, Petro JA, et al: Journal of Urology 150: 396-399, 1993.
6. Staging pelvic lymph node dissection: Comparison of results with open pelvic lymphadenectomy. Parra RO, Andrews C, Boullier JA: Journal of Urology 147: 875-878, 1992.
7. Comparative effectiveness and safety of laparoscopic vs open pelvic lymph node dissection for cancer of the prostate (abs). Winfield HN, See WA, Donovan JF, et al: Journal of Urology 147: 244A, 1992.
8. Complications of laparoscopic pelvic lymph node dissection. Kavoussi LR, Sosa G, Chandhoke P, et al: Journal of Urology 149: 322-325, 1993.
9. Complications of first 100 laparoscopic pelvic lymph node dissections: comparative analysis of first 50 vs. second 50 (abs). Ruckle HC, Lang GS, Hutton D, et al: J. Urology 149: 417A, 1993.
10. Comparative financial analysis of laparoscopic pelvic lymph node dissection (LPCND) performed in 1990-91 vs 1993-94 (abs). Troxel SA, Winfield HN: J. Urol 153: 357A, 1995.
11. Laparoscopic pelvic lymphadenectomy and radical perineal prostatectomy: A viable alternative to radical retropubic prostatectomy. Levy DA, Resnick MI: J Urol 151: 905-908, 1994.
12. Laparoscopic pelvic lymph node dissection laparoscopically assisted seminal vesicle mobilization and total perineal

prostatectomy versus radical retropubic prostatectomy for prostate cancer. Teichman JMH, Reddy PK, Hulbert JC: Urology 45: 823-830, 1995.
13. Laparoscopic radical prostatectomy: initial short-term experience. Schuessler WW, Schulan PG, Clayman RV, et al: Urology 50: 854-857, 1997.
14. Laparoscopic radical prostatectomy: Technical and early oncological assessment of 40 operations. Guillonneau B, Cathelisseau X, Barrett E, et al: European Urology 36: 14-20, 1999.
15. Laparoscopic radical prostatectomy-preliminary results. Jacob F, Solomon L, Hoznek A, et al: Eur Urol 37: 615-620, 2000.
16. Laparoscopic radical prostatectomy: Preliminary results. Abbou CC, Solomon L, Hoznek AA, et al: Urology 55, 630-634, 2000.
17. Laparoscopic radical prostatectomy: The Montesouris technique. Guillonneau B and Vallancien G: Journal of Urology 163, 1643-1649, 2000.

CHAPTER

10

Laparoscopic adrenalectomy

G.N. Tzimas, J. Amaral

Since the introduction of laparoscopic cholecystectomy in 1987, the enthusiasm surrounding minimally invasive techniques has rapidly expanded into many areas of abdominal surgery.

The adrenal gland offers itself to laparoscopic removal because it is small, and the majority of adrenal tumors are benign. The open approach to the gland typically requires a large incision to expose a small working field, resulting substantial postoperative morbidity. According to several reports morbidity of open adrenalectomy has been as high as 40% with mortality in the range of 2% to 4%.[1,2]

That is why there are probably few operations better served by laparoscopy than adrenalectomy initially described by Gagner in 1992.[3] The advent of better instrumentation for dissection and hemostasis, improved video imaging, better familiarity with endoscopic equipment by the operating room staff and increasing patient awareness and demand for these procedures has led to the growth of these minimally invasive techniques.

The obvious advantages of this approach include: decreased intraoperative blood loss, smaller incisions, possibly shorter operative time, and shorter length of stay with decreased need for narcotics as well as increased patient satisfaction.[4,5,6,7]

The chapter that follows describes the author's experience with, and recommendations for laparoscopic adrenalectomy.

Initially basics of adrenal anatomy will be discussed; next the approaches of laparoscopic adrenalectomy will be described, followed by the current indications and contraindications to the procedure.

The operative technique of the lateral approach will be described in detail, and the other approaches will be briefly described.

At the end of the chapter we will discuss the results from large series including our own institutional experience.

Adrenal Anatomy

The pathologic adrenal gland is usually small (between 3 and 6 cm).

It is located in the upper retroperitoneum superior and posterior to the respective kidneys. Both glands are closely related to major vascular structures.

Arterial anatomy

The arterial supply to the gland classically derives from three sources:

1. Superior adrenal artery arising from the inferior phrenic artery.
2. Middle adrenal artery from the abdominal aorta.
3. Inferior adrenal by some branches coming off the renal artery.

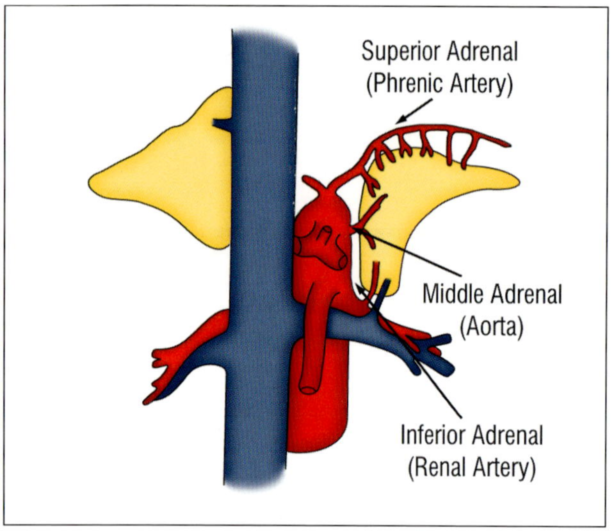

FIGURE 1. Adrenal Arterial Anatomy.

Venous anatomy

The venous drainage of the adrenal gland deffers between the two glands.

The right adrenal gland drains throught the much shorter (6 mm) right adrenal vein to the posterior wall of the inferior veca cava.

The left adrenal gland drains throught the longer (30 mm) left adrenal vein to the left renal vein, which empities to the inferior veca cava.[8]

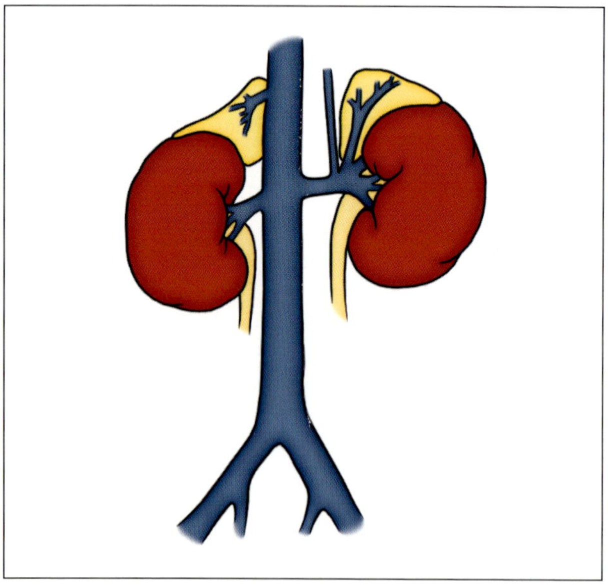

FIGURE 2. Adrenal Venous Anatomy.

Approaches to Adrenalectomy

Adrenalectomy can be performed through an open or laparoscopic approach, including:

1. Laparoscopic lateral or flank transabdominal approach for the majority of adrenal tumors.
2. Laparoscopic anterior transabdominal approach.
3. Laparoscopic posterior or retroperitoneal approach for small tumors or for bilateral adrenalectomy.
4. Open transabdominal or retroperitoneal approach for tumors > 10 cm or cancer with possible local invasion.[4,5,7,9,10,11,12]

The transperitoneal lateral approach first described by Gagner et al is the preferred method used by the authors because it provides a large working space. Also patient positioning allows visceral retraction by gravity. However if bilateral adrenalectomy is required the patient needs to be repositioned.

The anterior transabdominal approach provides a conventional view of the peritoneal cavity and allows bilateral adrenalectomy without repositioning the patient. The drawback of this approach is that it requires additional ports and has been associated with increased operative times compared to the lateral approach.[4]

The retroperitoneal approach avoids entrance in the peritoneal cavity and may be used in patients with previous abdominal surgery and in obese patients.[4] A problem with this approach is the limited working space, making it difficult to extract big tumors as well as difficulty in controlling bleeding from the inferior vena cava if it occurs.

Lastly the open transabdominal approach still may be preferred for large tumors (>10 cm) that may harbor locally invasive malignancies.

Indication for Laparoscopic Adrenalectomy

The indications for laparoscopic adrenalectomy vary little from that of open.[9]

Currently we favor laparoscopic adrenalectomy for the following indications:

1. Cushing's syndrome caused by a benign cortisol producing adenoma.

2. Cushing's disease that has not improved with other forms of therapy, mandating bilateral adrenalectomy.
3. Aldosterone-producing adenoma (Conn's syndrome).
4. Androgen producing adrenal tumors.
5. Benign adrenal pheochromocytoma.
6. Non-functioning adenomas or incidentalomas that meet the accepted criteria for adrenalectomy.
7. Benign lesions that are symptomatic.

Preoperative Evaluation

1. **Pheochromocytoma:** the classic presentation of pheochromocytoma (incidence 1-2/100.000 adults per year) occurs only in 30% of the patients. Atypical presentations include normotensive patient with episodic hypertension or hypertensive patient without symptomatic episodes.[17] Urinary metanephrines, normetanephrines, vanillylmandelic acid, and fractionated catecholamines constitute an appropriate initial evaluation. Measuring plasma catecholamines, drawn after selective adrenal vein catheterization with the patient at rest, can increase diagnostic accuracy. With confirmed the biochemical diagnosis, CT scan or MRI imaging is used to localize the tumor. Scintigraphy with 131iodobenzylguanidine may identify multiple tumors, unsuspected metastasis or extraadrenal pheochromocytoma.
2. **Aldosterone producing adenoma:** hypertensive patients with hypokalemia, not on diuretics should raise the suspicion of primary hyperaldosteronism. Patients with an aldosterone producing adenoma have an elevated plasma aldosterone level with a decrease plasma renin activity. Before testing, b-blockers and ACE inhibitors should be discontinued for 14 days. A plasma aldosterone (PA) to plasma renin activity (PRA) of more than 20 suggests primary hyperaldosteronism. Some endocrinologists prefer the saline loading test. In cases where the diagnosis is still debatable 24-hour urine aldosterone of more than 20 mcg/dl suggest primary hyperaldosteronism. Bilateral adrenal hyperplasia must always be ruled out and CT scan commonly does so. For remaining questions iodocholesterol scintigraphy or adrenal venous sampling should be performed.
3. **Non-functioning adenomas and incidentalomas:** considering the fact that 0.3% to 0.5% of all CT scans of the abdomen performed for non-adrenal reasons will demonstrate an incidental adrenal mass,[14,15,16] determination whether an incidentaloma is a functioning tumor is of paramount importance, since practically all functioning tumors should be resected.

   Evaluation of an incidentaloma includes careful history and physical examination. Biochemical work-up should focus on the findings. Serum potassium and 24-hour urine collection for metanephrines, VMA, 17-hydroxycorticosteroids and free cortisol should be obtained.

Common locations of 107 pheochromocytomas in 100 patients:

89 adults:
77 intraadrenal (2 bilateral)
12 extraadrenal (abdominal paraganglia 6, bladder1, organ of Zuckerkandl 6)

11 children:
6 intraadrenal (1 bilateral)
5 extraadrenal (1 thorax, abdominal paraganglia 6, organ of Zuckerkandl 3).[13]

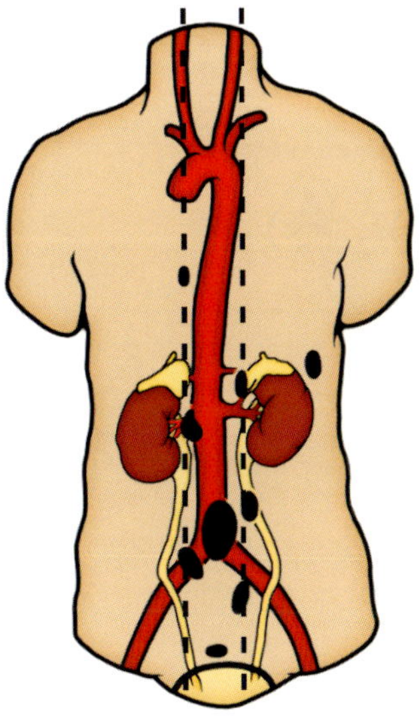

FIGURE 3. Extraadrenal Pheochromocytoma.

If the tumor is non-functional repeat CT scan is performed in 6 months. Resection is recommended for tumors bigger than 4 cm or for subsequent growth.

4. **Cushing's syndrome:** excess glucocorticoid production can be caused by Cushing's disease (pituitary adenoma), ectopic ACTH production, adrenal adenoma, adrenal carcinoma, or macronodular adrenal hyperplasia.
   Patients with adrenal adenoma and adrenal carcinoma should undergo resection, although laparoscopic resection of a carcinoma is highly debatable. Rarely bilateral adrenalectomy is required for patients with pituitary tumors or ectopic ACTH production, when pituitary or primary tumor resection fail to control excess hormone production. These tumors result elevated urinary free cortisol and 17-hydroxycorticosteroid levels. The 1 mg overnight dexamethasone suppression test can be used for equivocal cases. As soon as the diagnosis is established the patient needs to be determined if he has ACTH-dependent (pituitary pathology 70%, ectopic 15%), or ACTH-independent disease (adrenal tumor 15%). Finally CT scan differentiates adrenal tumor from adrenal hyperplasia in the majority of cases.
5. **Androgen-producing adrenal tumors:** rare tumors causing virilization.

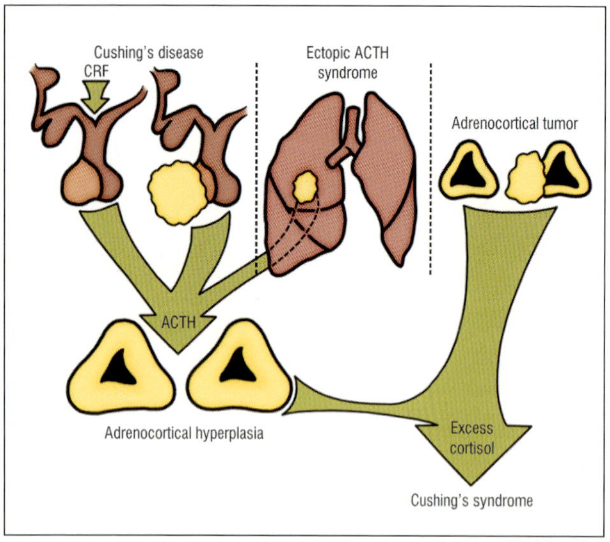

FIGURE 4. Cushing's syndrome.

These patients should have 24-hour urine collection for 17-ketosteroids and also plasma levels of testosterone and dehydroepiandrosterone.

Perioperative Considerations

All the electrolytic abnormalities should be corrected prior to surgery (e.g. hypokalemia, alkalosis, hyperglycemia).

Before the adrenalectomy hypertension should be controlled. Patients with pheochromocytoma require a-antagonists (e.g. phenoxybenzamine, prazosin, doxazosin); if despite adequate blood pressure control they remain tachycardic they require b-blockers.

Patients with aldosterone-producing adenoma should be treated with spironolactone.

Patients with Cushing's syndrome after surgery require glucocorticoid replacement to prevent postoperative adrenal insufficiency.

Finally patients with suspected adrenal malignancy should have a complete metastatic workup.

Technique

Transperitoneal Lateral Left Adrenalectomy

A. Positioning. The flank to be operated on is placed up.

Axillary pad and inflatable bag under the waist.

Open costopelvic angle with the kidney rest and by flexing the table.

The upper arm should be suspended from the anesthesia screen and the hips should be taped.

B. Trocar placement. 10 mm port 2 cm inferior to the costal margin at the anterior axillary line, additional 10 mm ports inferior to the costal margin at the midclavicular line and anterior to the 11th or 12th rib.

A 0 degree or 30 degree scope can be used.

C. Dissection. Using laparoscopic shears or the Harmonic Scalpel (Ethicon Endo-surgery, Cincinnati, OH) the spleen is mobilized by dividing the splenocolic, the splenorenal and the splenophrenic ligament.

Gravity will cause the spleen to fall medially exposing Gerota's fascia. The patient then is placed in Tredelenburg's position and dissection of the adrenal gland from lateral to medial is begun at this point by grasping the surrounding fat, avoiding tears at the delicate adrenal capsule.

Preferably the adrenal vein should be identified and ligated early during the dissection; however sometimes the size of the tumor prohibits ligation of the vein until the superior and medial dissection of the gland is completed.

The vein is usually 1 cm in diameter and can be controlled by clips.

If not already done the medial and superior portion of the dissection is completed.

The arteries are usually easy to control with the Harmonic Scalpel; however inferior phrenic branches when identified should be clipped.

When the adrenal gland has been completely dissected from its bed, it is placed into a bag and removed through the anterior port sites.

Drainage of the area is not routinely required. The fascia is closed with single absorbable suture.

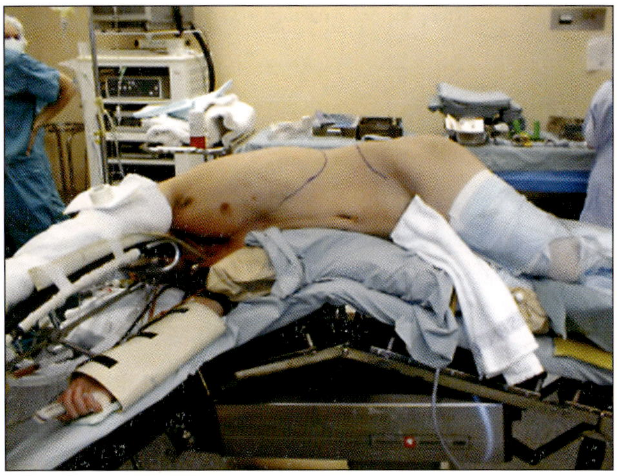

FIGURE 5. Left adrenalectomy position.

Transperitoneal Lateral Right Adrenalectomy

A. Positioning. Position the patient in the same way with the right flank up.

Flex the table and elevate the kidney rest to open the costopelvic space.

Place axillary pad and place arm on axillary rest.

B. Trocar Placement. Four trocars are usually used. They are placed 2 cm inferior to the costal margin in the anterior, midaxillary and posterior axillary lines, with the fourth in the mid-clavicular line. A fan-shaped retractor is used for the liver and the scope is placed in the second most medial port.

C. Dissection. The right triangular ligament of the liver is divided with the Harmonic Scalpel, allowing the right lobe of the liver to be retracted medially.

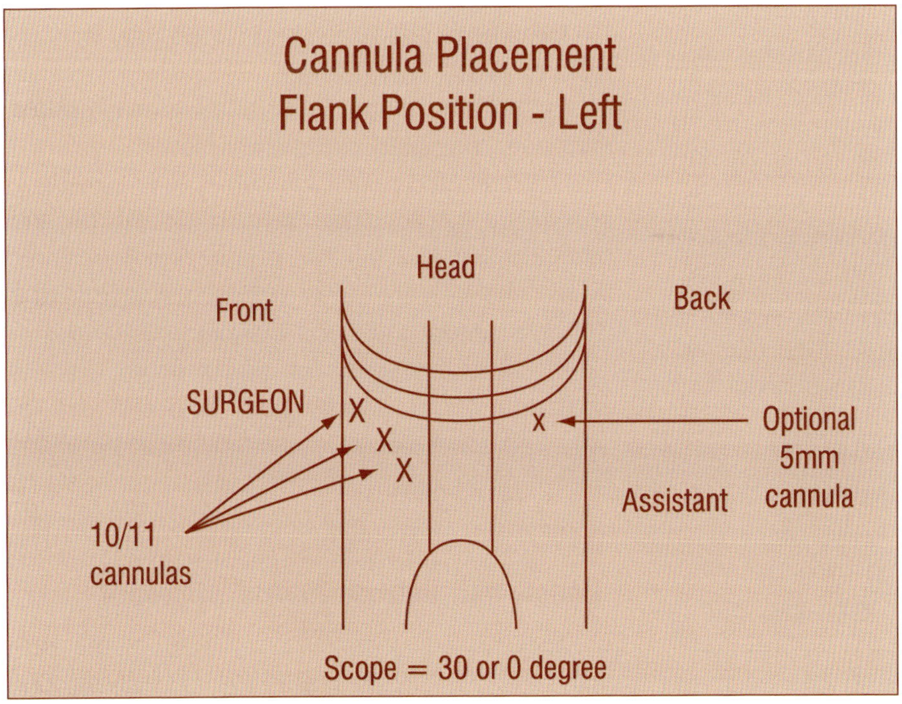

FIGURE 6.

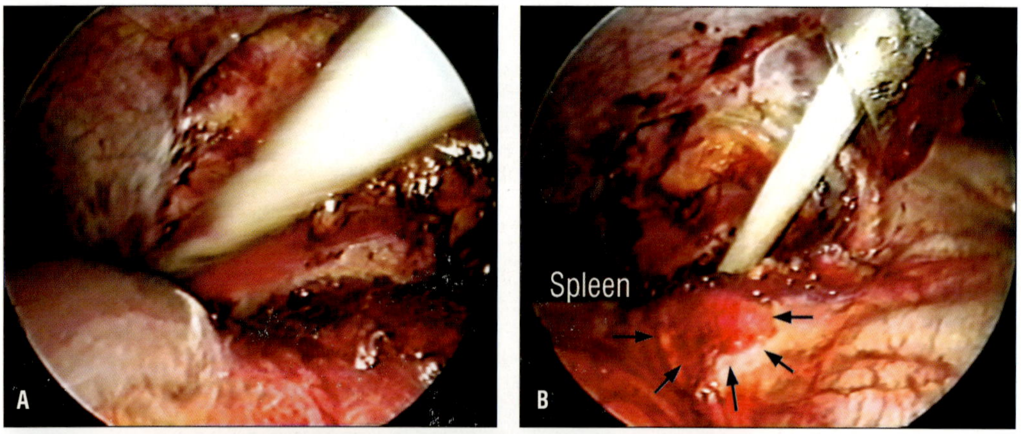

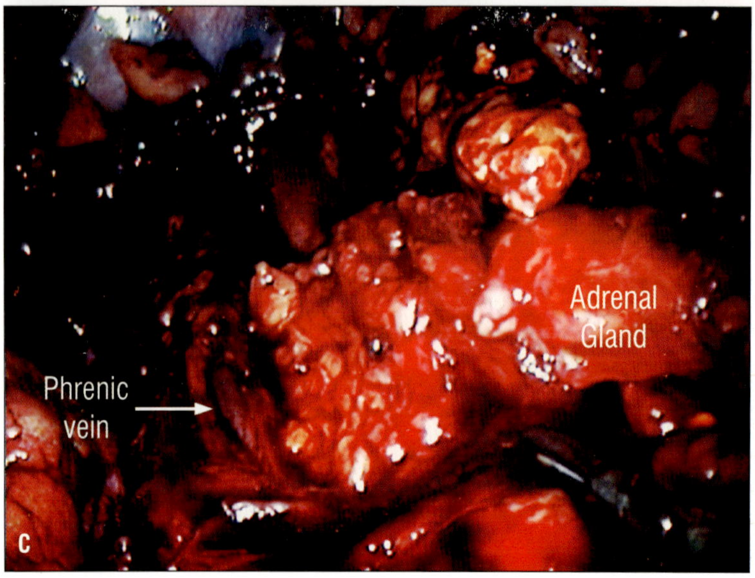

FIGURE 7. A, B, Spleed fully mobilized. **C,** Phrenic Vein.

The IVC is identified and the adrenal gland is dissected from superior and anterior, proceeding from lateral to medial.

As the dissection proceeds medially the IVC is retracted gently medially with a probe to expose its junction with the adrenal vein. The vein is clipped and divided with two or three clips left on the caval side.

The rest of the adrenal gland is dissected free, is removed and surgery is completed as described for left adrenalectomy.

Transperitoneal Anterior Adrenalectomy

The patient is positioned supine, and using the Veress needle technique or an open technique, insufflation of the abdomen is achieved.

Two 10 mm ports are placed in the midline above the umbilicus, and two additional ports are placed in the midclavicular and the anterior axillary lines 3 to 4 cm below the costal margin, on the side of the tumor.

Patient is placed in Tredelenburg position and rotated so that the operated side is up.

For left adrenalectomy the left colon is fully mobilized and retracted medially, exposing the left kidney and adrenal gland. The left renal vein is identified and its superior border is dissected all the way to the junction with the adrenal vein, which then is clipped and divided.

The adrenal gland then is dissected free, with occasional vessels being clipped.

The gland is removed with a heavy endobag, and surgery is completed in the usual fashion.

For right adrenalectomy the hepatic flexure is completely mobilized by taking down the hepatocolic ligament and the lateral peritoneal attachments exposing thus the upper pole of the right kidney, the right adrenal gland and the inferior vena cava.

The lateral border of the cava is traced until the right adrenal vein is identified, dissected and ligated. The gland then is removed by dissecting it free from the surrounding adipose tissue.

Endoscopic Retroperitoneal Approach

The patient is placed in a prone jackknife position

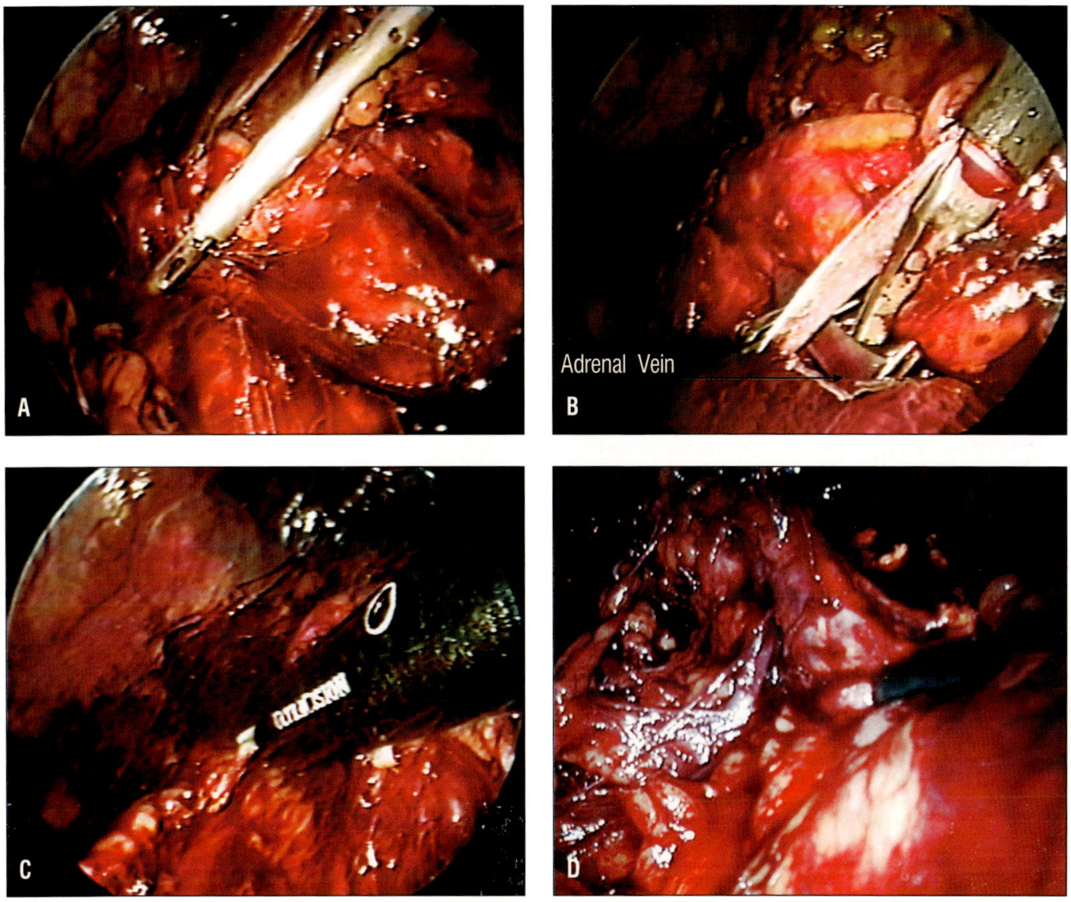

FIGURE 8. **A, B,** Ligation Adrenal Vein. **C, D,** Mobilization of Adrenal gland.

with the surgeon standing on the side from which the adrenal gland is to be removed.

Through an incision inferior to the 12th rib, balloon dissection is used to create the retroperitoneal space. A standard port can be placed by this incision. Two to three additional ports are placed under direct vision in this working space along the curve that is formed by the tips of the 11th, 12th and the subcostal margin of the 10th rib.

The ports should be separated by at least 4 cm. Retraction of the kidney downward opens up the retroperitoneal space, and dissection is performed through the most lateral ports with the camera in the medial one. Dissection is begun on the superior and lateral surfaces, proceeding medially and anteriorly by Harmonic Scalpel, or endoclips as necessary.

As the adrenal veins are encountered, they are ligated in a similar fashion as for the lateral approach.

With the adrenal gland completely dissected, it is removed and surgery is completed as earlier described.

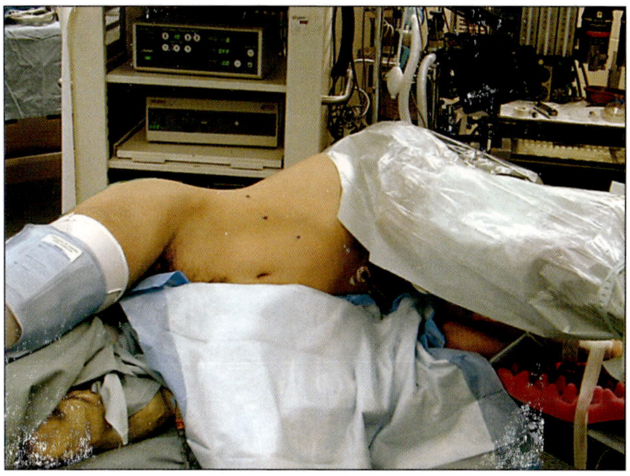

FIGURE 9. Positioning.

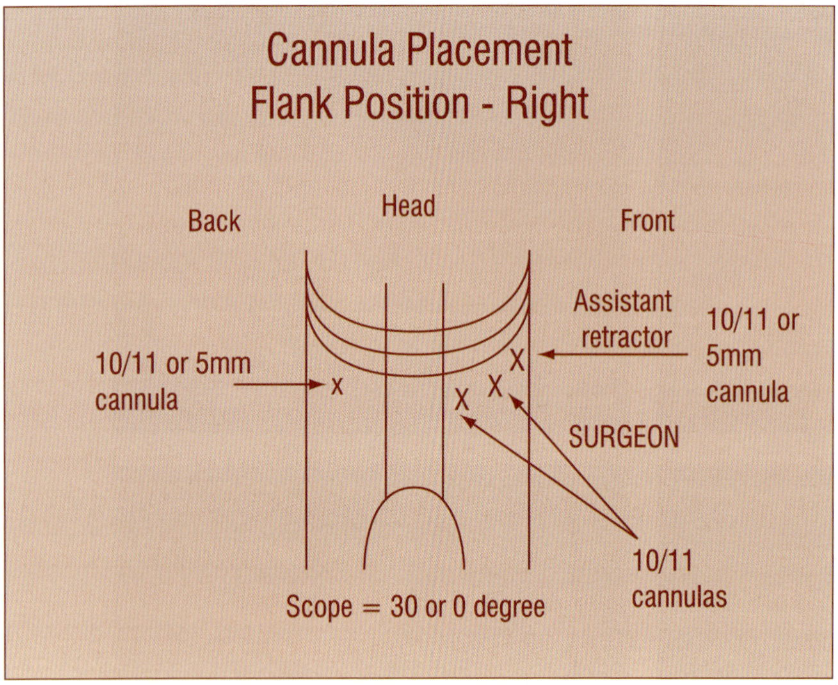

FIGURE 10.

Postoperative Care

The postoperative course for these patients is similar to that for laparoscopic cholecystectomy. Nasogastric tube and urinary catheter is removed at the completion of the surgery. Oral intake is initiated the day of surgery. Intramuscular or intravenous narcotics are usually required for the first 24 hours but after that, patients can tolerate oral narcotics and regular diet. The ma-

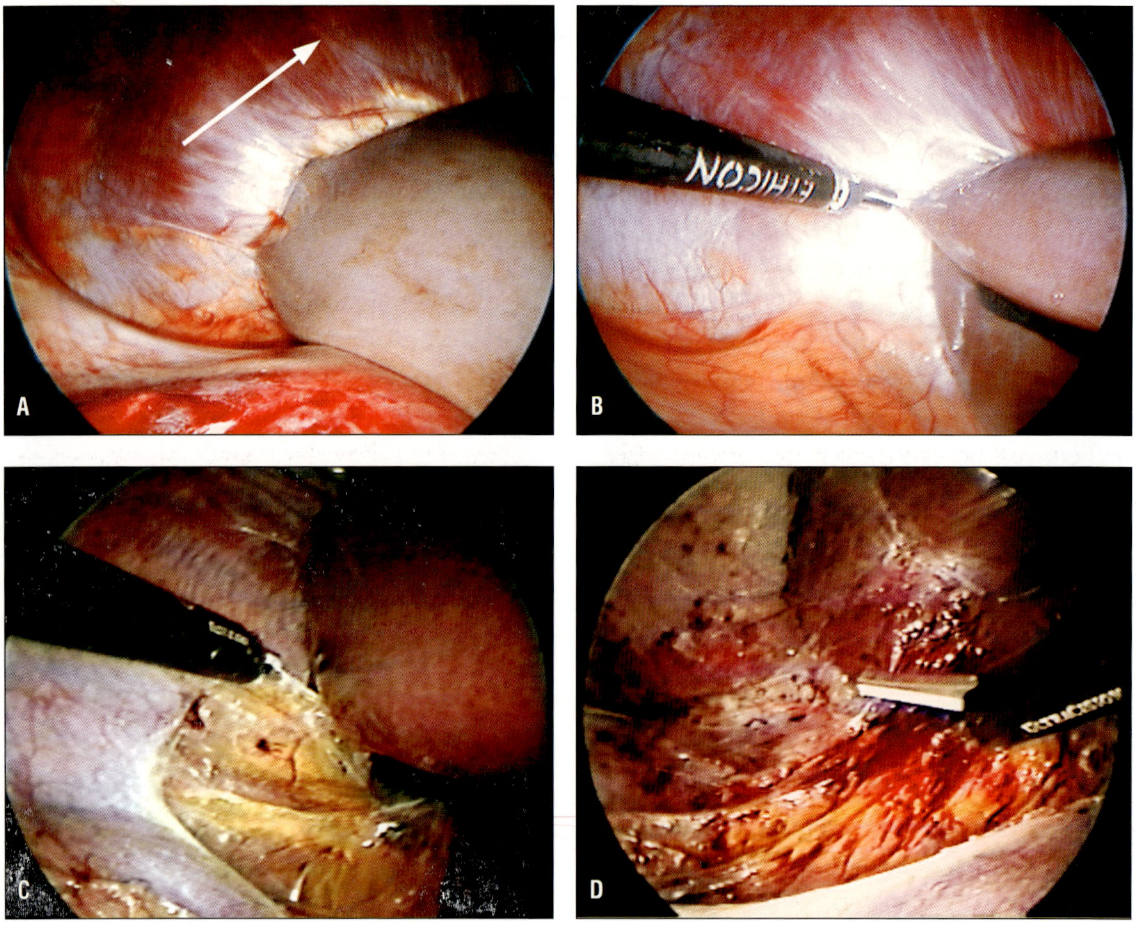

FIGURE 11. **A, B,** Right Triangular Ligament. **C, D,** Continued division of triangular ligament.

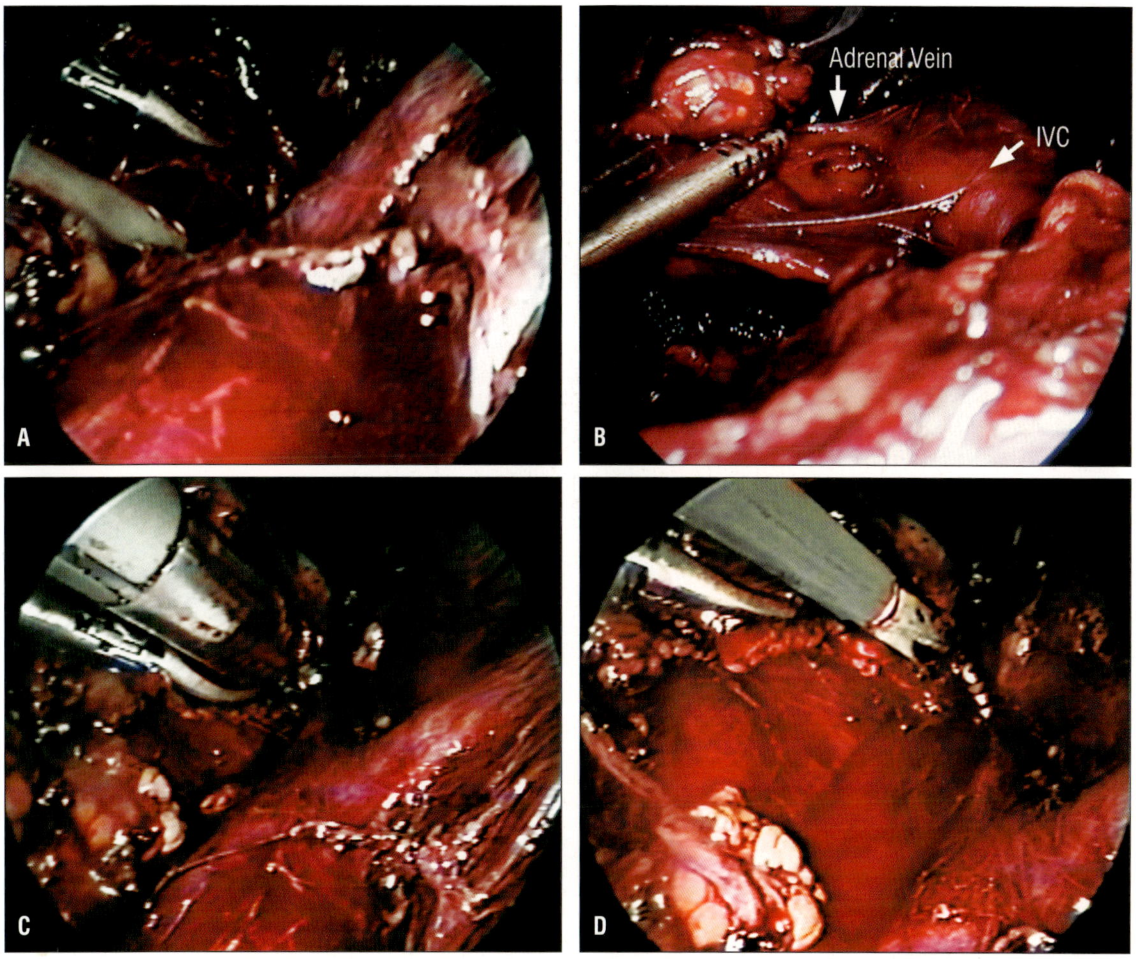

FIGURE 12. A, B, Adrenal vein identified. C, D, Adrenal vein clipped & divided.

jority of the patients can ambulate the evening after the procedure and usually they are discharged one to three days postoperatively.

Outcome Review

Currently there are no prospective randomized trials comparing the laparoscopic with the open adrenalectomy. Since the safety of the laparoscopic approach has been established, such trials would be obsolete.

However there are multiple retrospective studies comparing the two techniques.

In a study by Thompson et al, who compared 50 patients undergoing open adrenalectomy with 50 patients undergoing laparoscopic adrenalectomy in a matched, case-controlled study, they found that as for the majority of laparoscopic procedures there was a steep learning curve, leading to an increased operative time for the laparoscopic technique (167 min vs 127 min), but a significantly decreased hospital stay (3.1 days vs 5.7 days), postoperative pain and long term morbidity.

These results were reproduced by multiple studies.

Overall the reported mean operative time is between 116 minutes and 297 minutes compared with that for the open approach that ranges between 79 and 174 minutes.

The overall conversion rate is in the range of 0% to 14% but definitely these numbers improve with surgeon's experience.

The estimated blood loss is uniformly less with the laparoscopic approach, as well as the postoperative narcotic requirement and the length of stay.

Our Institutional experience as was reported by Soares, Amaral et al[18] demonstrated decreased operative time of the laparoscopic technique compared with the open (116 min vs 166 min), de-

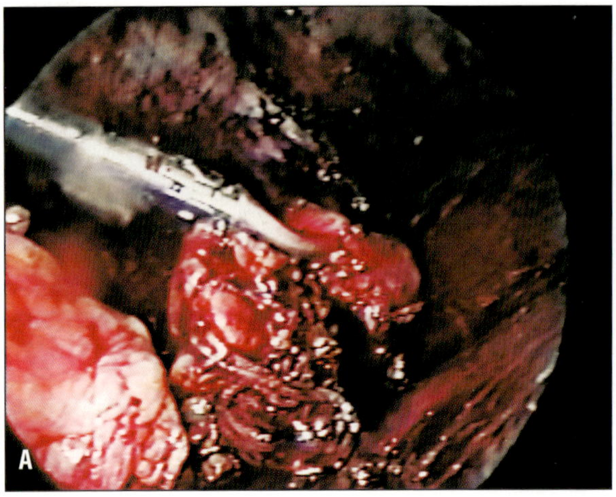

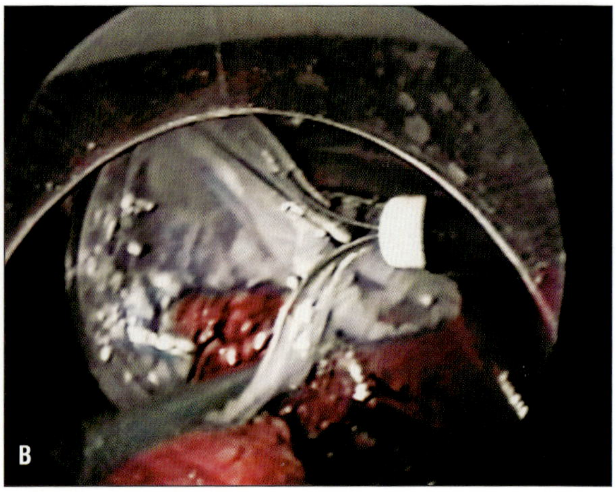

FIGURE 13. **A**, Gland free. **B**, Gland placed in endobag.

creased blood loss (132 cc vs 278 cc), decreased length of stay (2.1 days vs 5.4 days), and finally earlier resumption of regular diet, with an average of 1.7 days vs 4.7 days for the open technique. The mean operative charges were comparable in the two groups (4,084$ for the laparoscopic approach vs 4,538$ for the open approach).

Concluding we can safely say that laparoscopic adrenalectomy is associated with usually minor complications, such as port site bleeding, hematomas, subcutaneous emphysema, urinary tract infections and deep vein thrombosis. More severe complications occur less frequently secondary to vena cava injury or to solid organ injury.[19]

Overall the rate of intraoperative and early complications seem to be similar among the two techniques, but the laparoscopic approach avoids many long term complications making it thus the standard of care in North America for benign adrenal neoplasms.

References

1. McLeod MK: Complications following adrenal surgery. J Natl Med Assoc 83: 161, 1991
2. Sarkar R, Thompson NW, McLeod MK: The role of adrenalectomy in Cushing's syndrome. Surgery 108: 1079, 1990
3. Gagner M, Lacroix A, Bolte E: Laparoscopic adrenalectomy in Cushing's syndrome and pheochromocytoma. N Engl J Med 327:1033, 1992
4. Brunt LM, Doherty GM, Norton JA, et al: Laparoscopic adrenalectomy compared to open adrenalectomy for benign adrenal neoplasms. J Am Coll Surg 183:1-10, 1996
5. Gagner M, Pomp A, Heniford BT, et al: Laparoscopic adrenalectomy: Lessons learned from 100 consecutive procedures. Ann Surg 226: 238-247, 1997
6. Prinz RA: A comparison of laparoscopic and open adrenalectomies, Arch Surg 130: 489-494, 1995
7. Thompson GB, Grant CS, van Heerden JA, et al: Laparoscopic versus open posterior adrenalectomy: A case-control study of 100 patients. Surgery 122: 1132-1136, 1997
8. Claude A, Claude M, Martine P, et al: Surgical anatomy and embryology of the adrenal glands. Surg Clin North Am 1: 403-415, 2000
9. Barresi RV, Prinz RA: Laparoscopic adrenalectomy. Arch Surg 134: 212-217, 1999
10. Mercan S, Seven R, Ozarmagan S, et al: Endoscopic retroperitoneal adrenalectomy. Surgery 118:1071-1076, 1995
11. Prinz RA: Laparoscopic adrenalectomy. J Am Coll Surg 183: 71-73, 1996
12. Wells SA, Merke DP, Cutler GB Jr, et al: Therapeutic controversy: The role of laparoscopic surgery in adrenal disease. J Clin Endocrinol Metab 83: 3041-3049, 1998
13. Manger WM, Gifford RW, Melikow MM: Locations of 107 pheochromocytomas in 100 patients. Pheochromocytoma, New York, Springer-Verlag: 45, 1977
14. Angeli A, Osella G, Ali A, et al: Adrenal incidentaloma: An overview of clinical and epidemiological data from the National Italian Study Group. Horm Res 47: 279-283, 1997
15. Barry MK, van Heerden JA, Farley DR, et al: Can adrenal incidentalomas be safely observed? World J Surg 22: 599-604, 1998
16. Barzon L, Scaroni C, Sonino N, et al: Risk factors and long-term follow-up of adrenal incidentalomas. J Clin Endocrinol Metab 84: 520-526, 1999
17. Casola G, NicoletV, vanSonnenberg E, et al: Unsuspected pheochromocytoma: Risk of blood pressure alterations during percutaneous adrenal biopsy. Radiology 159: 733-735, 1986
18. Soares R., Amaral J., et al: Laparoscopic adrenalectomy for benign adrenal neoplasms. Surgical Endoscopy 13: 40-42, 1999
19. Raeburn C. and McIntyre Jr R.: Laparoscopic approach to adrenal and endocrine pancreatic tumors. Surg Clin North Am 5: 1427-1441, 2000

Chapter

11

Laparoscopic staging of pancreatic cancer

N. Alexakis, E. Leandros, J. Bramis

Pancreas cancer is the forth and sixth leading cause of cancer related death in the USA and UK respectively after lung, colorectal, and breast cancer[1]. The late presentation is responsible in part for the overall median survival of less than 6 months and 5-year survival rate of 0.4 to 5%[2-4]. Between 2.6% and 9% of patients undergo pancreatic head resection with a median survival of 11-20 months and a 5-year survival rate of 7-25%[2-7]. Cancer of the body and tail of the pancreas is rarely resectable due to the extended local invasion[4].

The natural history of pancreatic adenocarcinoma is such that only a minority of patients is candidate for potentially curative resection, so appropriate treatment depends on accurate staging of the disease. Ductal adenocarcinoma of the head of the pancreas spreads to regional lymph nodes, the liver and the peritoneum and locally invades vascular structures (postal vein and its tributaries)[4]. In the majority of patients with cancer of the body and tail, the disease at diagnosis has already spread to regional nodes, major vascular structures or metastasizes into the liver, peritoneum, omentum, at the time of diagnosis.

The gold standard method for clinical staging is *contrast-enhanced computed tomography (CT)* using multi-slice scanners with arterial and portal venous phases of contrast enhancement with an accurately in the prediction of resectability in 80-90% of cases and with 95% accuracy in predicting unresectability[4,8-10]. The assessment of local tumour extension with contiguous organ invasion, vascular involvement, hepatic metastases and lymph node metastases, correlate well with surgical findings in large tumours. The lesions that are mostly missed are small implants on the peritoneal surfaces. *Magnetic resonance imaging* has similar diagnostic and staging accuracies to that of CT and may have an advantage over CT in the detection of liver metastases[11,12].

Despite the multiple modalities available for preoperative evaluation, many patients continue to undergo celiotomy for staging and palliative purposes. This is associated with significant morbidity, mortality and diminishing quality of life for patients with limited survival. Thus, there is a strong need to identify patients with unresectable disease who might avoid unnecessary laparotomy, taking into account the availability of endoscopic biliary stents and the development of laparoscopic and duodenal biliary bypass.

In principle the surgeon in order to optimize strategic decisions, is interested whether the patient has potentially resectable disease, locally advanced disease or metastatic disease.

In patients with suspected pancreatic malignancy the identification of those with metastatic disease prior to laparotomy is important as it allows early institution of non-surgical palliation. Patients who present with metastatic disease are best palliated without surgery as their median survival is 2-6 months[4] and the same applies to unfit patients. The major symptom of advanced disease requiring intervention is obstructive jaundice. Randomized trials comparing operative bypass procedures with biliary stenting had shown that complications such as cholangitis and bile leaks are more common in bypass procedures, whilst recurrent jaundice is a feature of stenting because of stent occlusion or migration[13,14]. No significant difference was seen in median survival or procedure related deaths. Self-expanding metal stents have greatly reduced the risk of obstruction and acute cholangitis[15].

Thus the primary objective of preoperative staging is to assess distant spread or local invasion of the tumor, factors precluding curative resection. Microscopic lymph node metastases are common, but they usually do not prevent resection, although they may be associated with poorer prognosis[4,16]. It should be emphasized that the accuracy of preoperative staging in pancreatic carcinoma is worth improving, despite the effort needed and the cost incurred, because it greatly influences the therapeutic approach and spares the patients of unnecessary laparotomies. The yield from laparoscopic assessment in identifying these patients will be dependant on both the quality of the radiological imaging and patient selection.

The role of laparoscopic assessment (laparoscopy with or without intra-operative ultrasound) in the pre-operative staging of suspected pancreatic malignancy is controversial[17-20]. *Laparoscopy,* including *laparoscopic ultrasound,* can detect occult metastatic lesions in the liver and peritoneal cavity in 10-35% of cases not identified by other imaging modalities[21-24], but the true value of laparoscopy remains in dispute[4,21,25,26]. Early reports[27] suggested that laparoscopy could alter the management in up to 35% of patients by the detection of occult metastatic disease. Recent series have reported resection rates in patients considered resectable on radiological assessment (number of patients actually resected/ number of patients resectable on radiological assessment) of over 70%[28,29]; correspondingly the yield from laparoscopy has decreased to 4-15%[29] and its usefulness has been questioned[17,18,20,28]. This has led to suggestions for the selective use of laparoscopic assessment in those who are at higher risk of unresectable disease. A recent study has demonstrated for the first time that serum CA19-9 levels can reliably select those patients who are unlikely to benefit from staging laparoscopy in the preoperative assessment of suspected pancreatic malignancy[30]. Adopting a threshold of 150 KU/l would have resulted in 40% fewer laparoscopies and would have increased the yield from laparoscopy to 22%[30]. Another important aspect is that laparoscopy can also accurately stage patients who are CT unresectable but without distant metastases. These patients benefit from the new chemotherapy regiments and the results from these treatments would not be falsely lowered. A recent study of this patient group found unsuspected metastases in 34%[31].

Laparoscopy can accurately detect more than 96% of intra-abdominal metastases and 90% of liver metastases. This results from the ability of laparoscopy to detect small (1-2mm) surface metastases. Overall, the morbidity and mortality of a diagnostic laparoscopy are small. The reported incidence of major complications is 0,006%, while that of minor complications is less than 5%. With the addition of laparoscopic ultrasound (LUS), which is the most sensitive method of detecting occult liver metastases, the operator can detect small lesions, identify vascular invasion, assess the lymphatic basins and perform fine needle aspiration biopsy, with a sensitivity of 95%, specificity of 88%, positive predictive value of 95%, and negative predictive value of 88%. LUS has a steep learning curve, lesions on the surface of the liver can be missed, several factors can lead to false negative results (pancreatic edema, chronic pancreatitis, excessive fat), but with experience all these difficulties are reduced.

For patients who are relatively young with locally advanced disease, there is still benefit to undergo a surgical bypass as it may allow most of their remaining time to be spent at home without re-admissions to treat recurrent jaundice. In a series of 56 patients with unresectable or metastatic disease, using single loop biliary and gastric bypass, only four needed subsequent biliary stenting and no re-operations were required before death[32]. A recent study from the Amsterdam Medical Centre randomly allocated patients with histologically-proven unresectable tumours (using both CT and laparoscopic ultrasound) to either endoscopic or surgical palliation. The mean survival in 14 patients allocated to endoscopic palliation was 116 days, with a mean hospital-free survival of 94 days compared to 192 days and 164 days respectively in the 13 patients that had surgical palliation. These data suggest that patients who are free of major co-morbidity have better palliation by surgery rather than by endoscopy[25].

Technique

This is performed either as a separate procedure to allow for the assessment of cytologic/ histologic results and better prepare for a major resection, or in conjunction with planned exploration. Patients with small tumors (<2 cm) generally are excluded, because they are unlikely to have unsuspected metastases.

Contraindications for laparoscopy are extensive previous surgery, comorbidity that would have prevented further surgical intervention, or the presence of gastric outlet obstruction necessitating surgical bypass, even if the tumour was unresectable. Patients still undergo a trial dissection if, on the basis of intra-operative ultrasound assessment, there is equivocal vascular encasement of the hepatic portal/superior mesenteric veins or superior mesenteric artery in the absence of metastatic disease. Patients with histologically proven metastatic disease are excluded from a trial dissection.

Laparoscopy is performed under general anesthesia. The patient is placed supine on the operating table. A 1cm sub-umbilical incision is made to expose the abdominal fascia. The peritoneum is opened under direct vision and a 10mm trocar is inserted. Carbon dioxide insufflation is commenced through this trocar to an intra - abdominal pressure of 12-14mmHg. A 0 and 30-degree scope.

Examination begins with visualization of the lower abdomen and pelvis, because it is a frequent site of peritoneal metastasis. Then the attention is directed towards the upper abdomen. Inspection is carried out of the omentum, subdiaphragmatic spaces and of the anterior and posterior surfaces of the right and left lobe of the liver. With the introduction of the LUS probe from a second 10mm port at the RUQ (or from the umbilical port), the surgeon examines the liver from anterior to posterior in all directions. Any suspicious lesion is biopsied with a tru-cut needle under guidance. The bile duct is inspected. The assessment of the pancreas is carried out by placing the probe directly over it, or by pressing the stomach wall against it. The tumor characteristics are assessed. With the color doppler mode the surgeon can assess portal, SMV, SMA or hepatic /celiac artery involvement. Finally the celiac and para-aortic nodes are assessed.

Up to this stage the procedure is quite simple and effective, using two ports, providing good images of the pancreas without opening the lesser sac.

Unresectability is determined if one of the following conditions is present:

- Metastases (hepatic, serosal, peritoneal).
- Extra-pancreatic extension of the tumor i.e. mesocolic involvement
- Invasion or encasement of the celiac axis or hepatic artery
- Invasion or encasement of the portal / superior mesenteric vein and/or superior mesenteric artery

Some studies suggested that a positive peritoneal lavage cytology is an indicator of an aggressive tumor, characterized by early metastasis, and short survival[33].

In the absence of signs of unresectability at laparoscopy, the surgeon can proceed to open exploration. The operation lasts about 30 min and the patient can be discharged 24h later.

Concluding, laparoscopy is still an integral part of the staging for peri-pancreatic cancer patients as it allows optimization of therapeutic recourses and avoidance of unnecessary surgery.

References

1. Jemal A, Murray T, Samnels A, Ghafoor A, Ward E, Thun M. Cancer statistics, 2003. CA Cancer J Clin 2003; 53:5-26.
2. Bramhall SR, Allum WH, Jones AG, Allwood A, Cummins C, Neoptolemos JP. Treatment and survival in 13560 patients with pancreatic cancer and incidence of the disease. An epidemiological study. Br J Surg 1995; 82:111-115.
3. Hedberg M, Borgstrom A, Genell S, Janzon L. Survival following pancreatic carcinoma:a follow up study of all cases

recorded in Malmo, Sweden, 1977-1991. Br J Surg 1998; 85:1641-1644.
4. Alexakis N, Halloran C, Raraty M, Ghaneh P, Sutton R, Neoptolemos J. Current standards of surgery for pancreatic cancer. Br J Surg 2004; 91:1410-1427.
5. Nitecki SS, Sarr MG, Colby TV, van Heerden J. Long-term survival after resection for ductal adenocarcinoma of the pancreas. Is it really improving? Ann Surg 1995; 221:59-66.
6. Sener S, Fremgen A, Menck H, Winchester D. Pancreatic cancer: a report of treatment and survival trends for 100,313 patients diagnosed from 1985-1995, using the National Cancer database. J Am Coll Surg 1999; 189:1-7.
7. Key sites study. Pancreas report. NYCRIS. 2000.
8. McCarthy MJ, Evans J, Sagar G, Neoptolemos JP. Prediction of resectability of pancreatic malignancy by computed tomography. Br J Surg 1998; 85:320-325.
9. Chong M, Freeny P, Schmiedl U. Pancreatic arterial anatomy. Depiction with dual phase helical CT. Radiology 1998; 208: 537-542.
10. Vedantham S, Lu D, Reber H, et al. Small peripancreatic veins: improved assessment in pancreatic cancer patients using thin-section pancreatic phase helical CT. Am J Roentgenol 1998; 170:377-383.
11. Ichikawa T, Haradome H, Hachiya J, Nitatori T, Ohtomo K, Kinoshita T. Pancreatic ductal adenocarcinoma: preoperative assessment with helical CT versus dynamic gadolinium MR imaging. Radiology 1997; 202:655-662.
12. Megibow A, Zhou X, Rotterdam H, Francis I, Zerhuni E, Balfe D, et al. Pancreatic adenocarcinoma: CT versus MR imaging in the evaluation of resectability - report of the Radiology Diagnostic Oncology Group. Radiology 1995; 195:327-332.
13. Andersen JR, Sorensen SM, Kruse A, et al. Randomised trial of endoscopic endoprosthesis versus operative bypass in malignant obstructive jaundice. Gut 1989; 30:1132-1135.
14. Smith A, Dowsett J, Russell R, Hatfield A, Cotton P. Randomised trial of endoscopic stenting versus surgical bypass in malignant low bile duct obstruction. Lancet 1994; 344:1655-1660.
15. Davids P, Groen A, Rauws E, et al. Randomised trial of self-expanding metal stents versus polyethylene stents for distal malignant biliary obstruction. Lancet 1992; 340:1488-1492.
16. Connor S, Bosonnet L, Ghaneh P, Alexakis N, Hartley M, Campbell F, Sutton R, Neoptolemos J. Survival of peri-ampullary carcinoma is predicted by lymph node 8a but not by lymph node 16b1 status. Br J Surg 2004; 91:1592-1599.
17. Friess H, Kleeff J, Silva JC, Sadowski C, Baer HU, Buchler MW. The role of diagnostic laparoscopy in pancreatic and periampullary malignancies. J Am Coll Surg 1998; 186:675-682.
18. Holzman M, Reintgen K, Tyler D, Pappas T. The role of laparoscopy in the management of suspected pancreatic and peri-ampullary malignancies. J Gastrointest Surg 1997; 1:236-244.
19. Pisters PW, Lee JE, Vauthey JN, Charnsangavej C, Evans DB. Laparoscopy in the staging of pancreatic cancer. Br J Surg 2001; 88:325-337.
20. Rumstadt B, Schwab M, Schuster K, Hagmiller E, Trede M. The role of laparoscopy in the pre-operative staging of pancreatic carcinoma. J Gastrointest Surg 1997; 1:245-250.
21. Callery M, Strasberg S, Doherty G, Soper N, Norton J. Staging laparoscopy with laparoscopic ultrasonography: optimizing resectability in hepatobiliary and pancreatic malignancy. J Am Coll Surg 1997; 185:34-41.
22. Henning R, Tempia-Caliera A, Hartel M, Buchler M, Friess H. Staging laparoscopy and its indications in pancreatic cancer patients. Dig Surg 2002; 19:484-488.
23. John T, Greig JD, Carter DC, Garden OJ. Carcinoma of the pancreatic head and peri-ampullary region: tumour staging with laparoscopy and laparoscopic ultrasonography. Ann Surg 1995; 221:136-146.
24. Minnard EA, Conlon KC, Hoos A, et al. Laparoscopic ultrasound enhances standard laparoscopy in the staging of pancreatic cancer. Ann Surg 1998; 228:182-187.
25. Nieveen van Dijkum EJ, Romijn MG, Terwee CB, de Wit LT, van der Meulen JH, Lameris HS, Rauws EA, Obertop H, van Eyck CH, Bossuyt PM, Gouma DJ. Laparoscopic staging and subsequent palliation in patients with peripancreatic carcinoma. Ann Surg 2003; 237:66-73.
26. Barreiro CJ, Lillemoe KD, Koniaris LG, Sohn TA, Yeo CJ, Coleman J, Fishman EK, Cameron JL. Diagnostic laparoscopy for periampullary and pancreatic cancer: what is the true benefit? J Gastrointest Surg 2002; 6:75-81.
27. Warshaw A, Gu Z, Whittenberg J, Waltman A. Pre-operative staging and assessment of resectability of pancreatic cancer. Arch Surg 1990; 125:230-233.
28. Doran H, Bosonnet L, Connor S, Jones L, Garvey C, Hughes M, Campbell F, Hartley M, Ghaneh P, Neoptolemos J, Sutton R. Laparoscopy and laparoscopic ultrasound in the evaluation of pancreatic and periampullary tumours. Dig Surg 2004; 21:305-313.
29. Maire F, Sauvanet A, Trivin F, Hammel P, O'Toole D, Palazzo L, Vilgrain V, Belghiti J, Ruszniewski P, Levy P. Staging of pancreatic head adenocarcinoma with spiral CT and endoscopic ultrasonography: an indirect evaluation of the usefulness of laparoscopy. Pancreatology 2004; 4:436-440.
30. Connor S, Bossonet L, Alexakis N, Ghaneh P, Sutton R, Neoptolemos J. Serum CA19-9 measurement increases the effectiveness of staging laparoscopy in patients with suspected pancreatic malignancy. Dig Surg. 2005. 22;80-85.
31. Liu R, Traverso L. Laparoscopic staging of unresctable pancreatic cancer. Surg Endosc 2004; 18:S256.
32. Isla AM, Worthington T, Kakkar AK, Williamson RC. A continuing role for surgical bypass in the palliative treatment of pancreatic carcinoma. Dig Surg 2000; 17:143-146.
33. Makary M, Warshaw A, Centeno B, Willett C, Rattner D, Fernandez-del Castillo C. Implications of peritoneal cytology in pancreatic cancer management. Arch Surg 1998; 133:361-365.

CHAPTER

12

Palliative laparoscopic procedures for advanced pancreatic cancer

P. Gentileschi, M. Gagner

Introduction

The treatment of pancreatic carcinoma is almost entirely palliative. Only 10-20% of tumors are resectable at the time of diagnosis, and even in these patients survival beyond 5 years can be anticipated in no more than 10%.[1] The median survival of patients with advanced disease is 4.9 months.[2] This data underscores the importance of an optimal palliation that will guarantee the shortest possible hospital stay, and as long a survival as possible with good quality of life.

Obstructive jaundice is the most common symptom requiring palliation, occurring in 70% of patients. Duodenal obstruction, occurring in 10-25% of patients, is rarely a presenting symptom (<5%) and usually follows biliary obstruction. Most patients at presentation have some degree of pain that becomes intractable as the diseases progresses. The management of pain is difficult, especially during the terminal stage of the disease.

The palliative treatment of carcinoma of the pancreas is difficult. Careful evaluation of the patient and multi-disciplinary expertise are required to select the appropriate approach. Several risk factors are usually present: more than 50% of patients are over the age of 70 years and they often have associated medical illnesses.[3] Jaundice and poor nutritional status can further compound the problems associated with the operative treatment. Although the mortality for palliative operations has recently improved, morbidity rates have remained high.[4]

Decision-making in the palliation of carcinoma of the pancreas has become more complex in recent years. Treatment options have broadened with the advent of endoscopic and percutaneous stenting of the bile ducts, percutaneous and thoracoscopic pain relief, and laparoscopic biliary and enteric bypass.

The availability of these minimally invasive techniques has also increased the demand for accurate staging. Resectability of pancreatic lesions is determined accurately by preoperative imaging in only 47-55% of cases.[5] Diagnostic laparoscopy and laparoscopic ultrasonography are indicated in patients whose tumor is deemed resectable on preoperative imaging.[6] Using laparoscopy and laparoscopic sonography, the resectability rate can be determined correctly in 75-100% of patients.[7] In other words, 33-65% of patients can be spared a negative laparotomy for unresectable disease.[7] False-positive results-i.e., resectable lesions judged unresectable by staging laparoscopy, have not occurred in any of the reported prospectively controlled studies.[6,7,8] For these reasons, a laparoscopic approach to the palliation of advanced pancreatic cancer based on the findings of staging laparoscopy and laparoscopic ultrasonography may have the potential to replace open bypass procedures.

In this chapter the laparoscopic palliative options in advanced carcinoma of the pancreas are presented. The preferred technique is also described.

Laparoscopic Palliative Options

The surgical minimally-invasive options for palliation of biliary obstruction in patients with advanced pancreatic carcinoma range from a simple loop cholecystojejunostomy to a hepatico-jejunostomy (either using a simple loop or a Roux-en-Y loop).[9-16] Hepaticogastrostomy, allowing for hepatic segment II or III drainage into the lesser curvature of the stomach, has also been reported.[17,18] Duodenal obstruction is usually treated by gastrojejunostomy.[19-21]

Cholecystojejunostomy is simple and has particular appeal in the high-risk patient, when previous endoscopic or percutaneous attempts have failed. Before selecting the gallbladder for biliary decompression, the surgeon must ensure that the cystic duct is patent and will remain so for a reasonable length of time. The level of entry of the cystic duct and its relationship to the obstructing lesion is the most important factor in determining whether to perform a durable cholecystojejunostomy. In other words, the cystic duct must be patent and its common bile duct junction has to be at an adequate distance from the level of obstruction. Preoperative endoscopic cholangiography, percutaneous transhepatic cholangiography or intraoperative cholangiography via the gallbladder are generally used to resolve the dilemma. A 3 cm gap between the tumor and the junction of the cystic duct with the common bile duct is considered a safe distance.[22]

Laparoscopic cholecystojejunostomy was first performed in 1992.[9] Since then, many single cases and initial series have been reported.[10-14] It has the potential to fulfill the dual goals of palliation, namely the low risk of minimal access (as provided by endoscopic stenting), while affording a prospect of durable drainage through a surgical stoma.

Laparoscopic cholecystojejunostomy is a relatively easy and fast procedure. Diagnostic laparoscopy and laparoscopic ultrasonography are carried out either to confirm preoperative findings or to evaluate resectability of pancreatic carcinoma (Figure 1,2). Once a decision to perform a laparoscopic cholecystojejunostomy has been made, a loop of jejunum is brought up to the distended gallbladder. The most mobile proximal loop of jejunum is selected for the antecolic anastomosis. One or two stay sutures between the gallbladder and the jejunal loop may be applied, according to the preference of the operating surgeon. A small enterotomy is created by either cautery scissors or harmonic scalpel on the intestinal loop. A small opening is made also on the gallbladder wall in the same fashion. The gallbladder is emptied by suction to facilitate construction of the anastomosis. While maintaining traction on the stay sutures, the jaws of a 30-mm Endo-GIA stapler (US Surgical Corporation, Norwalk, USA) are inserted into the openings. The anastomosis is created with one or two subsequent firings of the stapler, to ensure a sufficiently wide diameter of the bilioenteric anastomosis. The two openings are then closed with an intra-corporeal running suture. A drain may be left close to the anastomosis.

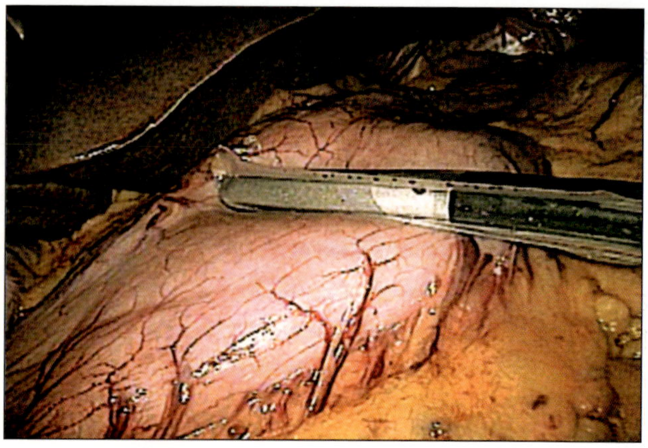

FIGURE 1. Laparoscopic ultrasonography.

While laparoscopic cholecystojejunostomy has been reported by many authors, few authors have described laparoscopic hepatico-jejunostomy for

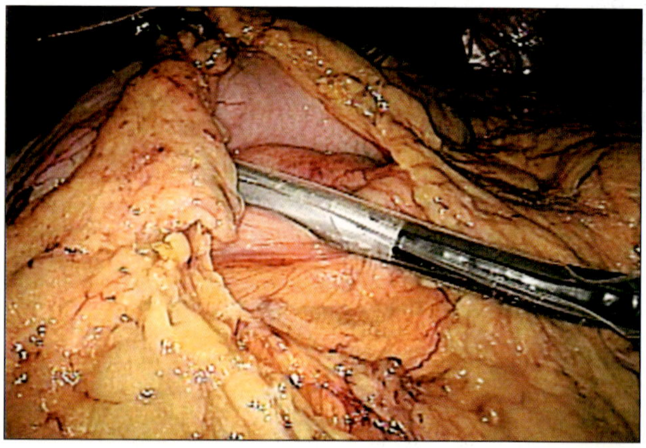

FIGURE 2. Laparoscopic ultrasonography.

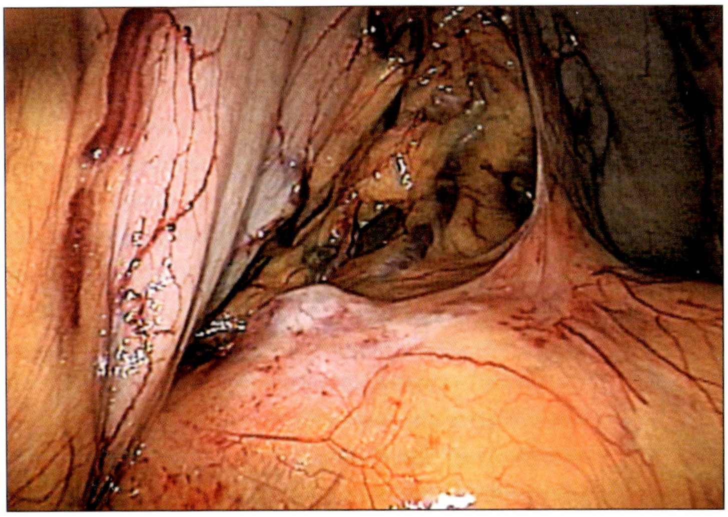

FIGURE 3. The opening of the gastrocolic ligament allows access to the anterior surface of the pancreas and the tumor is identified.

advanced pancreatic cancer.[15,16] Laparoscopic hepatico-jejunostomy is a difficult procedure, requiring expertise in advanced laparoscopy. Palliation of duodenal obstruction by laparoscopic gastrojejunostomy has also been widely described.[19-21] The following is a description of our surgical technique for laparoscopic double bypass in patients with unresectable pancreatic cancer.

When dealing with tumors deemed resectable on preoperative imaging, a complete laparoscopic evaluation of resectability, which includes laparoscopic ultrasonography, is performed. First, the liver is examined. The probe is positioned on the ventral surface of the liver with gentle pressure. The entire hepatic tissue is carefully searched for secondary lesions. The extrahepatic bile ducts and the vessels of the hepatoduodenal ligament are then scanned. Involvement of lymph nodes, hepatic artery, and portal vein are noted. This is a crucial step of the intraoperative assessment of resectability. The presence or absence of tumor invasion into the major vessels, especially the portal vein, must be ruled out. Using the stomach as an acoustic window, the pancreas is then examined (Figure 1). The size and location of the tumor may be documented at this point of the procedure. Involvement of the mesenteric vessels and the celiac trunc is ruled out. The gastrocolic ligament is then opened with the harmonic scalpel (Ethicon Endo-Surgery, Cincinnati, Ohio) and access to the anterior surface of the pancreas is achieved (Figure 3). The pancreatic lesion is usually identified, either by laparoscopy (Figure 3) or by laparoscopic ultrasonography (Figure 2).

Once the lesion is judged unresectable, and in the presence of an indication for palliation, laparoscopic side-to-side hepatico-jejunostomy and gastroenterostomy, using a simple jejunal loop, are performed.

An antecolic gastrojejunostomy is preferred as it lessens the possibility of subsequent infiltration by tumor. A small opening is made both into the posterior wall of the stomach and the jejunal loop with the harmonic scalpel (Figure 4). The jaws of an Endo-GIA stapler (U.S. Surgical Corporation, Norwalk, Usa) are inserted into the enterotomies and a wide gastrojejunostomy is created by three firings of the

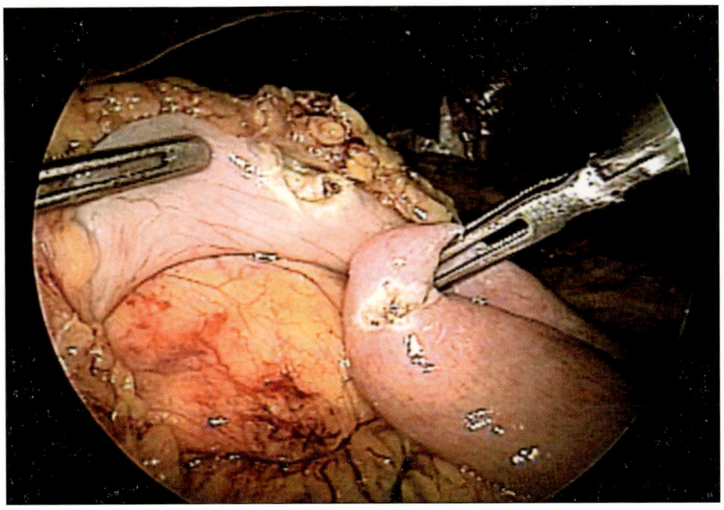

FIGURE 4. A small opening is made into the posterior wall of the stomach and the jejunal loop.

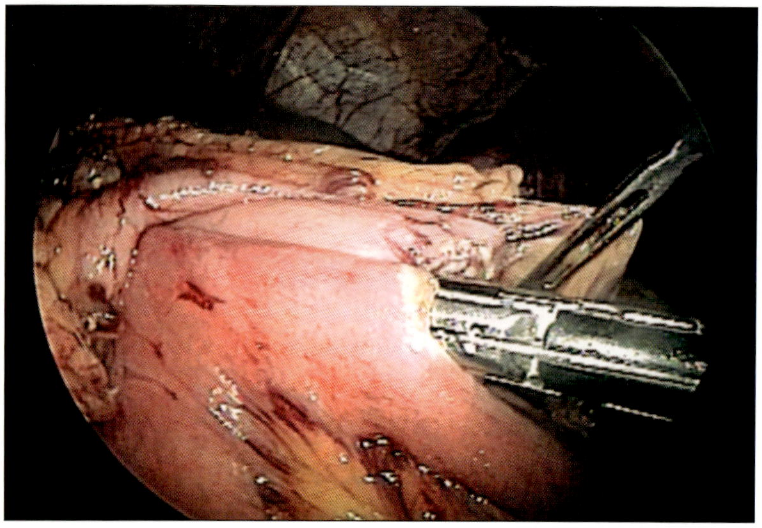

FIGURE 5. The jaws of an Endo-GIA are inserted into the enterotomies.

stapler (Figure 5). The staple line is carefully inspected for bleeding and the enterotomies are closed with a running suture (Figure 6, 7).

The hepatoduodenal ligament is further dissected and the common bile duct, cystic duct, and cystic artery are isolated. The cystic duct is divided as well as the cystic artery, and cholecystectomy is performed. The gallbladder is removed to facilitate construction of the common hepatic duct anastomosis, and to prevent the possible later complication of cystic duct obstruction and cholecystitis. An incision of approximately 1 cm is performed on the common hepatic duct (Figure 8). An eventual hepatic duct drain is therefore removed under direct vision (Figure 9). Using the same loop of jejunum that was selected for the gastrojejunostomy, a hepatico-jejunostomy is performed. Two stay sutures are applied in order to fix the loop of jejunum to the common hepatic duct. A small enterotomy is performed on the intestinal wall (Figure 10). The jaws of an Endo-GIA stapler (30 mm., US Surgical Corporation, Norwalk, USA) are inserted into the common hepatic duct and the jejunal loop (Figure 11). Using a single firing of the stapler the side-to-side anastomosis is created (Figure 12). The two openings are then closed with a running suture (Figure 13). A drain is usually left in situ.

In 1994, a new technique to palliate malignant biliary obstruction was reported.[17] Peripheral biliary diversion was obtained by hepaticogastrostomy, in which a bile duct in segment II or III of the liver was anastomosed to the lesser curvature of the stomach under combined fluoroscopic, endoscopic, and laparoscopic guidance. Before the operation, a transhepatic external biliary drainage catheter was inserted, under fluoroscopic guidance, into a bile duct of segment III (preferably) or II of the liver. Diagnostic laparoscopy was then performed to assess tumoral spread. In cases of unresectable cancer, hepaticogastrostomy was performed. The radiologist perforated the left lobe of the liver under fluoroscopic guidance, using a flexible needle, introduced through a 5-F catheter, along the external

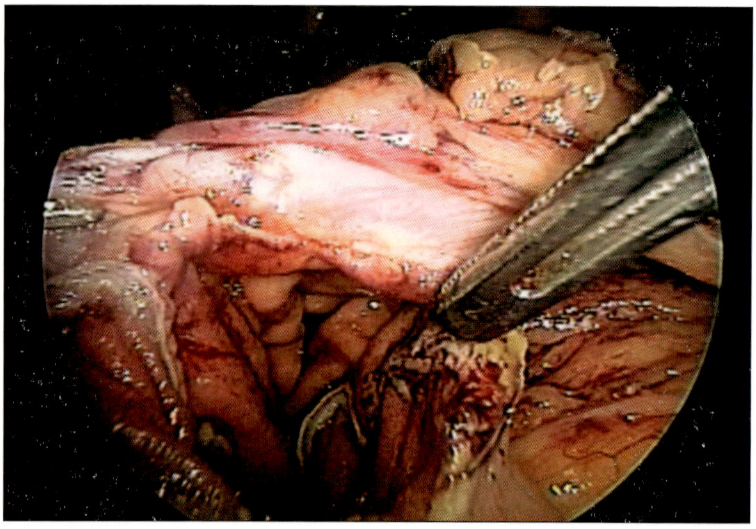

FIGURE 6. The staple line is inspected for bleeding and the enterotomies are closed with a running suture.

FIGURE 7. The staple line is inspected for bleeding and the enterotomies are closed with a running suture.

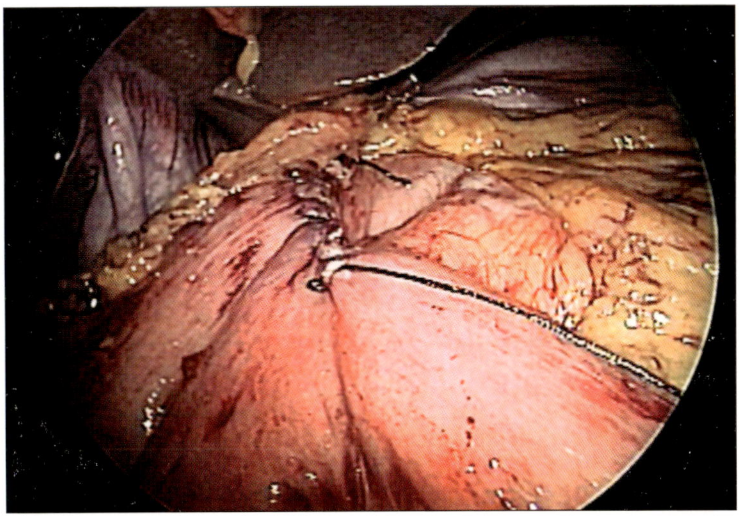

drainage catheter pathway. The needle exited the liver capsule at the inferior face of the left lobe and needle-tip positioning was assessed under laparoscopic control. The surgeon held the gastric pouch with forceps while the radiologist perforated the stomach. A snare was then introduced into the stomach through the needle and grasped by the endoscopist, who pulled it out through the patient's mouth and bound it to a 15-F percutaneous endoscopic gastrostomy tube. Side holes were added to the tube, according to the length of the intrabiliary tract. The snare was pulled by the radiologist and the gastrostomy tube was gently drawn into the stomach across the transhepatic tract. Fibrin glue was applied by the surgeon on both surfaces (liver and stomach) at the hepatico-gastric anastomosis. Slight traction was applied to the tube, which was fixed to the skin to prevent leakage. The gastrostomy tube was left in place for internal-external drainage for 15 days. At this point the tube was removed and long-term patency of the tract was preserved with a metallic stent.

Laparoscopic side-to-side gastrojejunostomy has been widely reported.[19-21] Earlier in this chapter, we have described our surgical technique. Few variations can be made. An antecolic anastomosis can be created either on the posterior wall of the stomach, as described before, or on the anterior wall of the stomach. Laparoscopic gastrojejunostomy can also be performed as a retrocolic anastomosis.[10] The transverse colon and omentum are mobilized cephalic with the use of graspers and the duodeno-jejunal junction is identified. The posterior wall of the stomach is exposed by incising the mesocolon near the ligament of Treitz. The postero-inferior margin of the greater curvature of the stomach is brought through the mesocolon and apposed to a loop of jejunum. A side-to-side stapled anastomosis is therefore created.

Pain Control

Currently, a number of options are available to manage pain in patients with unresectable pancreatic cancer. Intraoperative chemical splanchnicectomy

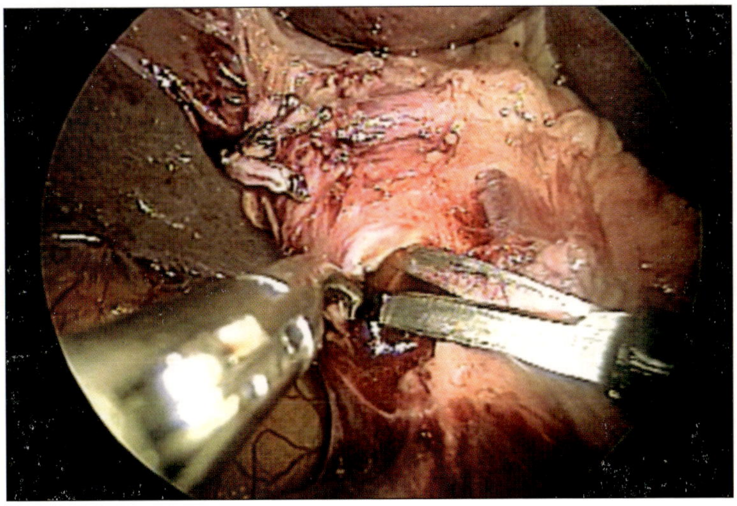

FIGURE 8. A small incision is performed on the common hepatic duct.

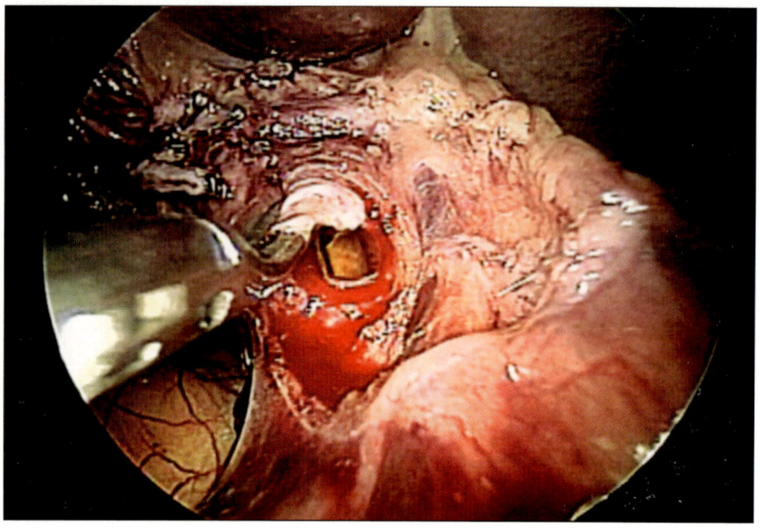

FIGURE 9. An eventual hepatic duct drain is removed under visualization.

as a method of long-term pain control was introduced in 1969.[23] The procedure is usually performed by injecting 20 mL of 50% alcohol via a spinal needle on either side of the aorta at the level of the celiac axis. A laparoscopic approach to neurolytic celiac plexus block has been developed in a porcine model.[24] The esophageal hiatus was dissected to expose the aorta at the level of the right diaphragmatic crus. The aorta was visualized with a 10-mm laparoscopic ultrasound probe. Under combined endoscopic and sonographic guidance, the celiac plexus was labeled using a mixture of 95% ethanol and India ink injected into either side of the para-aortic soft tissue via a percutaneously placed 18-gauge spinal needle. At necropsy, there were no injuries to the aorta or esophagus, and histopathologic analysis demonstrated good placement of dye-labeled sclerosant with no compromise of aortic structural integrity.

Another minimally-invasive option for pain control in patients with advanced pancreatic cancer is offered by thoracoscopic splanchnicectomy.[25,26] The procedure is usually performed unilaterally (left side), although bilateral splanchnicectomy seems to be associated with a higher rate of success than unilateral splanchnicectomy.[26] For each side, the patient is placed in the lateral decubitus position, with double-lumen endotracheal intubation allowing single-lung ventilation. The greater splanchnic nerve is visualized through the parietal pleura from its first root, along the descending aorta, to the diaphragmatic recess. A pleural incision is made in the region between the sympathetic chain and the descending aorta to expose the first root and the trunk of the greater splanchnic nerve. Care must be taken when exposing the trunk in order to avoid any vascular injury to the left hemi-azygos vein and/or intercostal vessels. Pleurotomy from the fifth intercostals space to the diaphragmatic recess is performed, and all roots of the greater and lesser splanchnic nerves and all small lateral branches are divided. A single pleural catheter drain is usually left in situ for 24 hours.

Discussion

Optimal palliation should alleviate symptoms effectively, thereby improving the

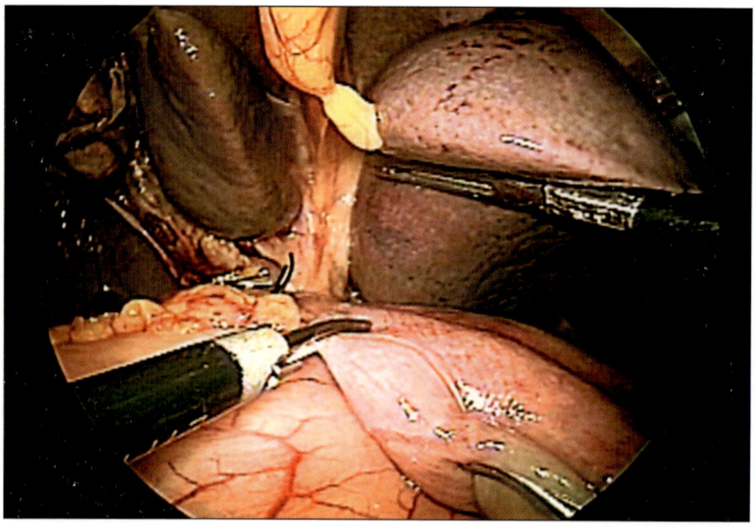

FIGURE 10. A small enterotomy is performed on the intestinal wall.

FIGURE 11. Insertion of the jaws of an Endo-GIA stapler into the hepatic duct and jejunum.

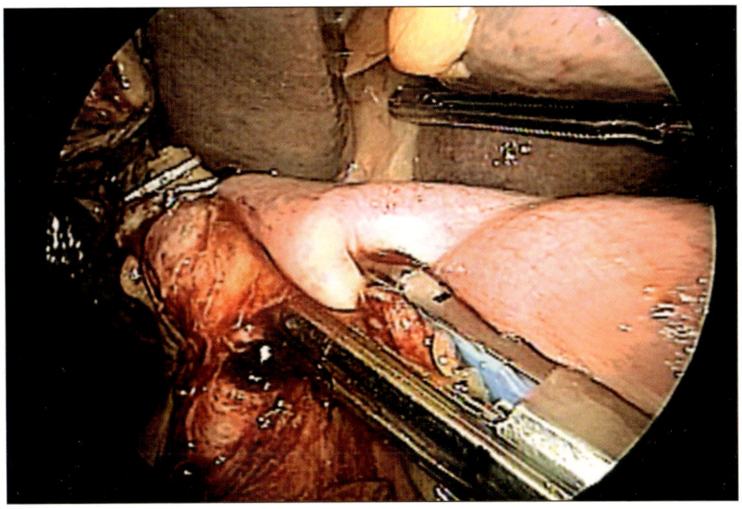

quality of life while reducing the duration of hospital stay. Palliation of patients with unresectable pancreatic cancer is aimed at three major symptoms: obstructive jaundice, duodenal/gastric outlet obstruction, and tumor-associated pain.

In a review of 8,000 patients in the English literature from 1965 to 1980,[27] the relief of biliary obstruction with surgical biliary bypass was associated with longer and more comfortable survival (5.4 months) when compared with diagnostic laparotomy alone (3.5 months). For these reasons, an attempt to palliate biliary obstruction is indicated in all but the most terminal patients.

Open palliative surgery has been associated with high mortality and morbidity rates (8-33% and 20-60%, respectively).[4,11] The introduction of endoscopic and percutaneous stenting of the bile ducts has changed the management of these patients. Several randomized studies compared biliary stenting with open bypass procedures.[28,29,30] Morbidity, mortality, and primary hospital stay were found to be lower after stenting. In particular, an excellent randomized comparative trial (surgical vs. endoscopic palliation of jaundice) was conducted at the Middlesex Hospital in London.[31] In the study, 204 patients were randomized to either surgery (n=103) or endoscopic stent placement (n=101). Technical success was achieved in 94% and 95% of surgical and stent patients, respectively. Stented patients experienced a lower procedure-related mortality (3% vs. 14%; P=0.01), major complication rate (11% vs. 29%; P=0.02), and median total hospital stay (20 vs. 26 days; P=0.001). However, recurrent jaundice occurred in 36 stented patients and only two surgical patients. Median survival was similar in the two groups (surgical = 26 weeks, stent = 21 weeks; P=0.065). The authors concluded that endoscopic stenting is easier and safer but surgical bypass provides more durable relief of jaundice. The endoscopic approach, also when compared to percutaneous stenting, demonstrated significant higher successful rate and lower mortality.[32] As for unilateral versus bilateral endoscopic hepatic duct drainage in patients with malignant biliary obstruction, the results of a prospective, randomized study demonstrated that the insertion of more than one endoprosthesis is not justified routinely.[33] Single stent insertion proved to be effective, while avoiding the risk of further procedure-related complication and

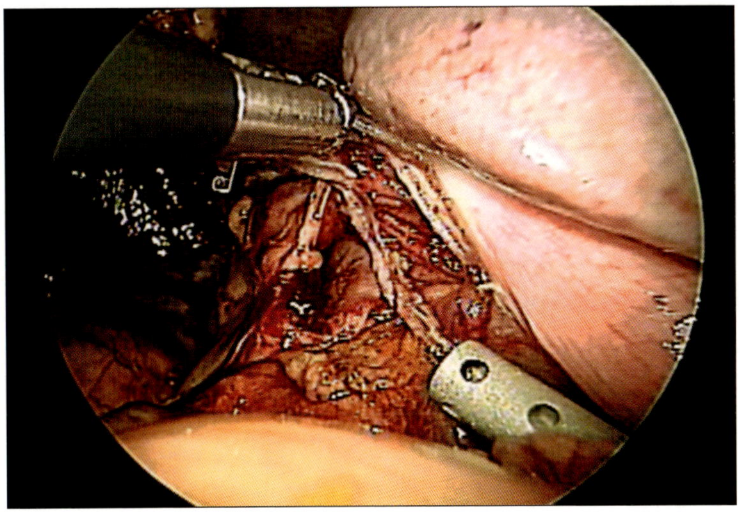

FIGURE 12. Firing the stapler, a side-to-side hepaticojejunostomy is created.

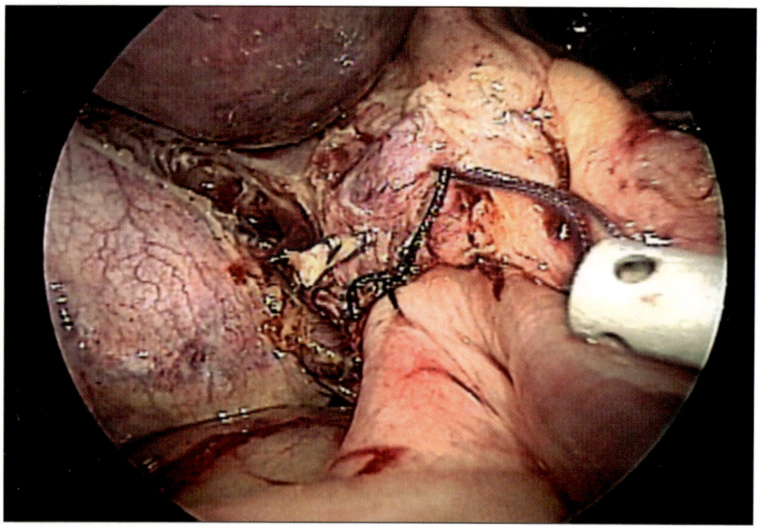

FIGURE 13. The two openings are closed with a running suture.

mortality. The major disadvantage of endoscopic stents is their short life patency. The recurrent jaundice rate ranges from 5% to 24%.[34]

These data suggest that fit jaundiced patients with unresectable pancreatic cancer benefit from surgery, whereas poor operative risk patients should be treated with endoscopic or percutaneous stenting.

Current opinion is divided regarding the preferred surgical procedure for biliary-enteric bypass. In an analysis of 600 patients who underwent open biliary bypass in 8 reported series,[35] 93 of 400 patients (23%) developed recurrent jaundice after cholecystojejunostomy compared to 14 of 200 patients (7%) after hepatico-jejunostomy. In a prospective controlled trial assessing the efficacy of biliary enteric bypass,[36] 31 patients were randomized to cholecystojejunostomy and hepatico-jejunostomy. Seven bypasses failed after use of the gallbladder and only two after using the bile duct ($p<0.04$). Prior to death, 47% of cholecystojejunostomies failed. The authors concluded that hepatico-jejunostomy is a significantly more effective palliative procedure. A meta-analysis by Watanapa and Williamson[37] found that cholecystojejunostomy carried an 89% success rate, whereas the success rate for hepatico-jejunostomy was 97%. More importantly, recurrent jaundice or cholangitis occurred in 20% of patients undergoing cholecystojejunostomy. On the basis of these data, most authors have preferred the routine use of the common bile duct for palliative biliary drainage. The described technique of minimally-invasive hepaticogastrostomy was performed in 35 patients with biliary obstruction.[18] Technical success was achieved in all patients. Two (6%) patients had anastomotic obstruction. The actuarial survival rate was 91%, 80%, 59%, and 26% at 1, 3, 6, and 12 months. The mean patency was 234 days 252. The jaundice-free rate among surviving patients was 100%, 96%, 93%, and 80% at 1, 3, 6, and 12 months. The reintervention rate was 14%. Late cholangitis occurred in seven (20%) patients. These results proved that the technique was safe and associated with good long-term patency.

Three meta-analyses have addressed the issue of duodenal obstruction, its management and treatment in patients with advanced pancreatic cancer.[22,27,37] Sarr and Cameron reviewed more than 8,000 surgically managed patients with unresectable pancreatic cancer.[27] Thirteen percent of those who did not undergo a bypass procedure at their initial operation required gastrojejunostomy prior to death and an additional 20% died with symptoms of duodenal obstruction. Another meta-analysis included 1,600 patients and reported a 17% incidence of duodenal obstruction at a mean of 8.6 months after the initial operation, requiring gastrojejunostomy prior to death.[37] Singh and Reber[22] analyzed 950 patients with advanced pancreatic cancer. Twenty-one percent required late gastrojejunostomy. In all analyses, the addition of gastrojejunostomy at the initial operation did not increase operative mortality. Conversely, when gastrojejunostomy was performed as a second operation, the mortality rates approached 25%.

Despite these data, controversy still exists over the role of prophylactic gastrojejunostomy in these patients. Espat and colleagues analyzed 155 laparoscopically staged patients with unresectable pancreatic carcinoma.[38] They received no biliary and gastric bypass procedures and were prospectively followed to determine the frequency of subsequent gastric and/or biliary bypass required prior to death. The study revealed that 98% (152 of 155) of these patients did not require a subsequent procedure to treat biliary or gastric obstruction. However, 35% of patients in this study had tumors in the body and tail of the pancreas, which represent a group with differing needs for palliation. In a recent, prospective, randomized trial the need of prophylactic gastrojejunostomy in advanced pancreatic cancer was evaluated.[39] Eighty-seven patients with no evidence of duodenal obstruction were randomized to receive either a gastrojejunostomy (44 patients) or no gastrojejunostomy (43 patients). Gastrojejunostomy did not influence morbidity, mortality and length of hospital stay. No patients experienced late gastric outlet obstruction in the gastrojejunostomy group, whereas 19% of patients in the no-gastrojejunostomy group required bypass for gastric outlet obstruction ($p<0.01$). This study provided class I evidence confirming the need of routine gastrojejunostomy in surgically explored patients with unresectable pancreatic cancer.

The pain associated with advanced pancreatic cancer is hardly managed. Pain at presentation is often a sign of advanced disease. In a recent series [40], 64% of unresectable patients presented with abdominal pain, whereas only 36% of resectable patients presented with abdominal pain ($p<0.0001$). Moreover, back pain was rarely found in resected patients (2%), but was common in unresectable patients (26%; $p<0.0001$). The results of a prospective, randomized trial comparing intraoperative chemical splanchnicectomy to placebo were reported in 1993.[41] The mean pain scores were significantly lower in the splanchnicectomy group at all postoperative time points and prior to death ($p<0.05$). Alcohol significantly reduced pain in both patients with preoperative pain and those without preoperative pain. In addition, the subgroup with significant preoperative pain receiving chemical s-planchninectomy showed improved survival than those receiving saline placebo. These data support the use of chemical splanchnicectomy in patients receiving operative palliation for advanced pancreatic cancer. In patients with known unresectable disease, pain can be managed with long-acting analgesics, computed tomography-guided percutaneous and endoscopic celiac nerve block, or external beam radiation. Most authors currently recommend percutaneous injection of 15-50 ml of 50-100% ethanol via a bilateral posterior approach with variations of the final position of the needle (retrocrural, transcrural, or transaortic). Laparoscopic chemical splanchnicectomy was found to be feasible in a chronic porcine model.[24] Thoracoscopic splanchnicectomy has been reported by many authors for the treatment of pain due to advanced pancreatic cancer.[25,26] In all experiences, thoracoscopic splanchnicectomy was found to be safe and effective. It seems to eliminate the need for progressive doses of analgesics and allows recovery of daily activities.[25,26]

The use of minimally invasive operative techniques has been applied to the management of pancreatic cancer. The role of diagnostic laparoscopy and laparoscopic ultrasonography for the intraoperative staging of pancreatic carcinoma has been well established and is the routine at advanced centers.[7] To date, many reports have described the use of laparoscopic techniques for palliation of patients with advanced pancreatic cancer.[9-21] These include laparoscopic hepatico-jejunostomy, cholecystojejunostomy, and gastrojejunostomy. Laparoscopic chemical splanchnicectomy has been performed only experimentally.[24] Initial results demonstrate technical success, with acceptable morbidity and mortality and encouraging outcomes. In a case controlled study, laparoscopic side-to-side gastroenterostomy and end-to-side hepatico-jejunostomy (Roux-en-Y) were performed in 14 unresectable patients.[15] The results were compared with a population of 14 matched patients who had conventional palliative procedures. Postoperative morbidity was 7% and 43% for laparoscopic and open palliation, respectively ($p<0.05$). There were no deaths in the laparoscopic group, as compared to 29% in the open group ($p<0.05$). Mean postoperative hospital stay was 9 days in the laparoscopic group and 21 days in the open group ($p<0.06$). Morphine derivatives were necessary for a significantly shorter period following laparoscopic palliation ($p<0.03$). These results strongly advocate the use of a laparoscopic approach to palliation of advanced pancreatic cancer. Reduced pain and early reinstitution of normal bowel motility after laparoscopy may contribute to the lower incidence of cardiopulmonary complications leading to postoperative deaths in these high-risk patients.

Another study compared the short-term outcomes of open gastrojejunostomy (22 patients) to laparoscopic gastrojejunostomy (9 diagnosis-matched controls) for the palliation of gastric outlet obstruction caused by advanced pancreatic cancer.[20] Mortality, overall morbidity, operating time, time to oral solid food intake, nonsteroidal anti-inflammatory drug consumption, opioid consumption, and survival were not significantly different between the two groups. Estimated blood loss and hospital stay were significantly reduced in the laparoscopic group ($p<0.01$ and $p<0.05$, respectively). Delayed gastric emptying had played a major role in prolonged hospital stay after open palliation, being found in 12-67% of cases.[34] After laparoscopic palliative procedures, this complication has only rarely been reported.

Further clinical trials will be needed to demonstrate an evidence-based advantage of the laparoscopic approach to palliation of patients with advanced pancreatic cancer. To date, in patients deemed resectable on preoperative imaging, a diagnostic laparoscopic approach seems reasonable. Furthermore, using laparoscopic ultrasonography, the intraoperative staging can be extremely accurate.[6,7] Unresectable patients may be further palliated by operative laparoscopic bypass. The technique described in this chapter for laparoscopic double bypass is technically challenging but has the potential to allow for a minimally invasive and durable biliary and gastric drainage. Currently, this approach is well established in advanced laparoscopic centers. Fit patients can be spared an unnecessary laparotomy while receiving a long-lasting biliary and/or gastric drainage through a surgical stoma. Whether this minimally invasive approach will be extended to a larger number of centers and patients is yet to be determined.

References

1. Warshaw AL. Progress in pancreatic cancer. World J Surg 1984; 8: 801.
2. Conlon KC, Klimstra DS, Brennan MF. Long-term survival after curative resection for pancreatic ductal adenocarcinoma: clinico-pathologic analysis of 5-year survivors. Ann Surg 1996; 223: 273-279.
3. Fentiman IS, Tirelli U, Monfardini S, et al. Cancer in the elderly: why so badly treated? Lancet 1990; i: 1020.
4. Sarr MG, Cameron JL. Surgical palliation of unresectable carcinoma of the pancreas. World J Surg 1984; 8: 906-918.
5. Yasuda K, Mukai H, Nakajima M, Kawai K. Staging of pancreatic carcinoma by endoscopic ultrasonography. Endoscopy 1993; 25: 151-155.
6. John TG, Greig JD, Carter DC, Garden OJ. Carcinoma of the pancreatic head and periampullary region: tumor staging with laparoscopy and laparoscopic ultrasonography. Ann Surg 1995; 221: 156-164.
7. Minnard EA, Conlon KC, Hoos A, et al. Laparoscopic ultrasound enhances standard laparoscopy in the staging of pancreatic cancer. Ann Surg 1998; 228: 182-187.
8. Rothlin M, Schlumpf R, Largiader F. Laparoskopisches Staging des Pankreaskarzinoms. Swiss Surg 1996; 3(Suppl): 13.
9. Shimi S, Banting S, Cuschieri A. Laparoscopy in the management of pancreatic cancer: endoscopic cholecystojejunostomy for advanced disease. Br J Surg 1992; 79(4): 317-9.
10. Kuriansky J, Saenz A, Astudillo E, et al. Simultaneous laparoscopic biliary and retrocolic gastric bypass in patients with unresectable carcinoma of the pancreas. Surg Endosc 2000; 14: 179-181.
11. Rhodes M, Nathanson L, Fielding G. Laparoscopic biliary and gastric bypass: a useful adjunct in the treatment of carcinoma of the pancreas. Gut 1995; 36(5): 778-780.
12. Raj PK, Mahoney P, Linderman C. Laparoscopic cholecystojejunostomy: a technical application in unresectable biliary obstruction. J Laparoendosc Adv Surg Tech 1997; 7(1): 47-52.
13. Hawasli A. Laparoscopic cholecysto-jejunostomy for obstructing pancreatic cancer: technique and report of two cases. J Laparoendosc Surg 1992; 2(6): 351-5.
14. Scott-Conner CE. Laparoscopic biliary bypass for inoperable pancreatic cancer. Semin Laparosc Surg 1998; 5(3): 185-8.
15. Rothlin MA, Schob O, Weber M. Laparoscopic gastro- and hepatico-jejunostomy for palliation of pancreatic cancer: a case controlled study. Surg Endosc 1999; 13: 1065-69.
16. Machado MAC, Rocha JRM, Herman P, et al. Alternative technique of laparoscopic hepatico-jejunostomy for advanced pancreatic head cancer. Surg Laparosc Endosc Percutan Tech 2000; 10(3): 174-7.
17. Soulez G, Gagner M, Therasse E, et al. Malignant biliary obstruction: preliminary results of palliative treatment with hepaticogastrostomy under fluoroscopic, endoscopic, and laparoscopic guidance. Radiology 1994; 192(1): 241-6.
18. Soulez G, Therasse E, Oliva VL, et al. Left hepaticogastrostomy for biliary obstruction: long-term results. Radiology 1997; 204(3): 780-6.
19. Casaccia M, Diviacco P, Molinello P, et al. Laparoscopic gastrojejunostomy in the palliation of pancreatic cancer: reflec-

tions on the preliminary results. Surg Laparosc Endosc 1998; 8(5): 331-4.
20. Bergamaschi R, Marvik R, Thoresen JE, et al. Open versus laparoscopic gastrojejunostomy for palliation in advanced pancreatic cancer. Surg Laparosc Endosc 1998; 8(2): 92-6.
21. Chung RS, Li P. Palliative gastrojejunostomy. A minimally invasive approach. Surg Endosc 1997; 11(6): 676-8.
22. Singh SM, Reber HA. Surgical palliation for pancreatic cancer. Surg Clin North Am 1989; 63: 599.
23. Copping J, Willix R, Kraft R. Palliative chemical splanchnicectomy. Arch Surg 1969; 98: 418-420.
24. Underwood RA, Wu JS, Quasebarth MA, et al. Development of a laparoscopic approach to neurolytic celiac plexus block in a porcine model. Surg Endosc 2000; 14(9): 839-43.
25. Leksowski K. Thoracoscopic splanchnicectomy for control of intractable pain due to advanced pancreatic cancer. Surg Endosc 2001; 15(2): 129-31.
26. Saenz A, Kurianski J, Salvador L, et al. Thoracoscopic splanchnicectomy for pain control in patients with unresectable carcinoma of the pancreas. Surg Endosc 2000; 14: 717-720.
27. Sarr MG, Cameron JL. Surgical management of unresectable carcinoma of the pancreas. Surgery 1982; 91: 123-33.
28. Andersen JR, Sorensen SM, Kruse A, et al. Randomized trial of endoscopic endoprosthesis versus operative bypass in malignant obstructive jaundice. Gut 1989; 30: 1132-35.
29. Bornman PC, Harries-Jones EP, Tobias R, et al. Prospective controlled trial of transhepatic biliary endoprosthesis versus bypass surgery for incurable carcinoma of the head of pancreas. Lancet 1986; 1: 69-71.
30. Shepherd HA, Royle G, Ross APR, et al. Endoscopic biliary endoprosthesis in the palliation of malignant obstruction of the distal common bile duct: a randomized trial. Br J Surg 1988; 75: 1166-68.
31. Smith AC, Dowsett JF, Russell RCG, et al. Randomized trial of endoscopic stenting versus surgical bypass in malignant low bile duct obstruction. Lancet 1994; 344: 1655-60.
32. Cowling MG, Adam AN. Internal stenting in malignant biliary obstruction. World J Surg 2001; 25(3): 355-8.
33. De Palma GD, Galloro G, Siciliano S, Iovino P, Catanzano C. Unilateral versus bilateral endoscopic hepatic duct drainage in patients with malignant hilar biliary obstruction: Results of a prospective, randomized, and controlled study. Gastrointest Endosc 2001; 53(5): 547-53.
34. De Rooij PD, Rogatko A, Brennan MF. Evaluation of palliative surgical procedures in unresectable pancreatic cancer. Br J Surg 1991; 78: 1053-58.
35. Bornman PC, Krige JEJ. Surgical palliation of pancreatic and periampullary tumors. In Trede M, Carter DC, Surgery of the pancreas, Churchill Livingstone, 2nd Edition, 1997.
36. Sarfeh IJ, Rypins EB, Jakowatz JG, et al. A prospective randomized clinical investigation of cholecystoenterostomy and choledochoenterostomy. Am J Surg 1988; 155: 411.
37. Watanapa P, Williamson RCN. Surgical palliation for pancreatic cancer: developments during the past two decades. Br J Surg 1992; 79: 8-20.
38. Espat NJ, Brennan MF, Conlon KC. Patients with laparoscopically staged unresectable pancreatic adenocarcinoma do not require subsequent surgical biliary or gastric bypass. J Am Coll Surg 1999; 188: 649-55.
39. Lillemoe KD, Cameron JL, Hardacre JM, et al. Is prophylactic gastrojejunostomy indicated for unresectable periampullary cancer? A prospective randomized trial. Ann Surg 1999;230:322-30.
40. Sohn TA, Lillemoe KD, Cameron JL, et al. Surgical palliation of unresectable periampullary adenocarcinoma in the 1990s. J Am Coll Surg 1999; 188: 658-69.
41. Lillemoe KD, Cameron JL, Kaufman HS, et al. Chemical splanchnicectomy in patients with unresectable pancreatic cancer. A prospective randomized trial. Ann Surg 1993; 217: 447-57.

CHAPTER

13

Laparoscopic anatomy of the liver

S.G. de la Fuente, Th. N. Pappas

1. Introduction

The safety and success of any surgical intervention on the liver depends largely on the thorough understanding of the hepatobiliary anatomy. Laparoscopic surgery mimics open liver surgery in many aspects, making a solid knowledge of the hepatic anatomy as well as techniques in open surgery crucial for the laparoscopic surgeon.

Although laparoscopic surgery has experienced a tremendous progress in the last several years,[1] minimally invasive procedures on solid organs have somewhat been limited by anatomic, technical, and equipment restrictions. Specifically to the liver, its size, its location under the ribs, and highly vascular nature have further contributed to the reluctance of general surgeons in attempting laparoscopic liver operations. Reports in the surgical literature on hepatic laparoscopic resections are relatively scant in frequency and number of patients.[2-8] Most of these studies reported in the literature are individual experiences and the lack of controlled trials with long-term results is considerable.

Concurrently to the development of hepatic laparoscopic resective techniques, there has been an increase in the implementation of this approach for the diagnosis and stratification of hepatic malignancies, implementation of intraarterial catheters for chemotherapy infusion, and the use of other therapeutic methods laparoscopically-guided such as cryotherapy, radiofrequency and alcoholization of hepatic lesions.[9-13] Nowadays, laparoscopic liver surgery is largely performed for diagnostic purposes and treatment of cysts.[14, 15] It is imperative to emphasize the specialized nature of these procedures and the importance of extensive hands-on experience and intensive clinical training necessary before attempting such procedures by the general surgeon. Laparoscopic hepatic surgery must be done with caution and it is generally performed by hepatobiliary surgeons. It is also a highly technological surgery that employs sophisticated equipment, which few centers around the world are equipped with.

2. Surgical Anatomy of the Liver

2.1. General description

The liver lies in the upper right part of the abdomen occupying the right hypochondriac and epigastric regions, and extends into the left hypochondrium and downward into the right lumbar region. It is covered by the rib cage and extends form the fourth intercostal space down to slightly below the rib margin in the normal person. In the normal male adult, the liver weights approximately 1.4-1.8 kg and 1.2-1.4 in adult females. Newborns have a relatively larger liver because of hepatic extramedullary hematopoiesis. The anterior surface of the liver is in direct contact with the diaphragm, while the visceral surface contacts the esophagus, stomach, duodenum, colon, right kidney, and right adrenal gland.

The liver's attachments to the abdominal wall, intraperitoneal organs, and diaphragm are of importance to the surgeon, especially to the laparoscopic surgeon. The liver attaches to the body wall by the falciform ligament, and above and behind to the diaphragm by the coronary ligament which form the right and left triangular ligaments. It is also attached to the stomach and duodenum by the lesser omentum or hepatogastric and hepatoduodenal ligaments. The hepatoduodenal ligament contains the hepatic arteries, portal vein and, extrahepatic bile ducts. Most of the hepatic ligaments can be appreciated displayed in figure 1.

2.2. Blood supply

Among the fascinating anatomical characteristics of the liver, its dual irrigation system is undoubtedly of significance for the hepatobiliary surgeon. The liver receives irrigation from the portal system, which supplies blood from the splanchnic system and systemic blood from the hepatic artery. The majority of the liver supply is provided by the portal vein. Junction of the superior mesenteric vein and the s-plenic vein forms the portal vein; this junction is located dorsal to the neck of the pancreas. The portal vein travels toward the liver behind the bile duct and the hepatic artery in the hepatoduodenal ligament. The vein then gives origin to two branches at the porta hepatis: the right branch, which provides mainly blood from the superior mesentery vein, and the left, branch which consists of the *pars transversus* and the *pars umbilicus*.

The hepatic artery originates from the trifurcation of the celiac trunk. The artery travels posterior and superior to the duodenum where it gives rise to the gastroduodenal artery. Proximal to the gastroduodenal artery, the hepatic artery is known as *common* hepatic artery and the segment distal to the gastroduodenal artery is refers to as proper hepatic artery. Numerous variations of the hepatic artery have been described; the most common types are display on figure 2. The artery then divides into a right and left subdivision within the hepatoduodenal ligament and then into smaller branches. Although the extrahepatic segment of the hepatic artery does not follow the portal vein, the intrahepatic portion does.

The hepatic venous blood drains into three main veins known as the right, middle, and left hepatic veins. The right hepatic vein drains blood mainly from the right lobe of the liver. The middle vein drains the medial segment of the left lobe and a portion of the anterior segment of the right lobe, while the left hepatic vein provides drainage for the

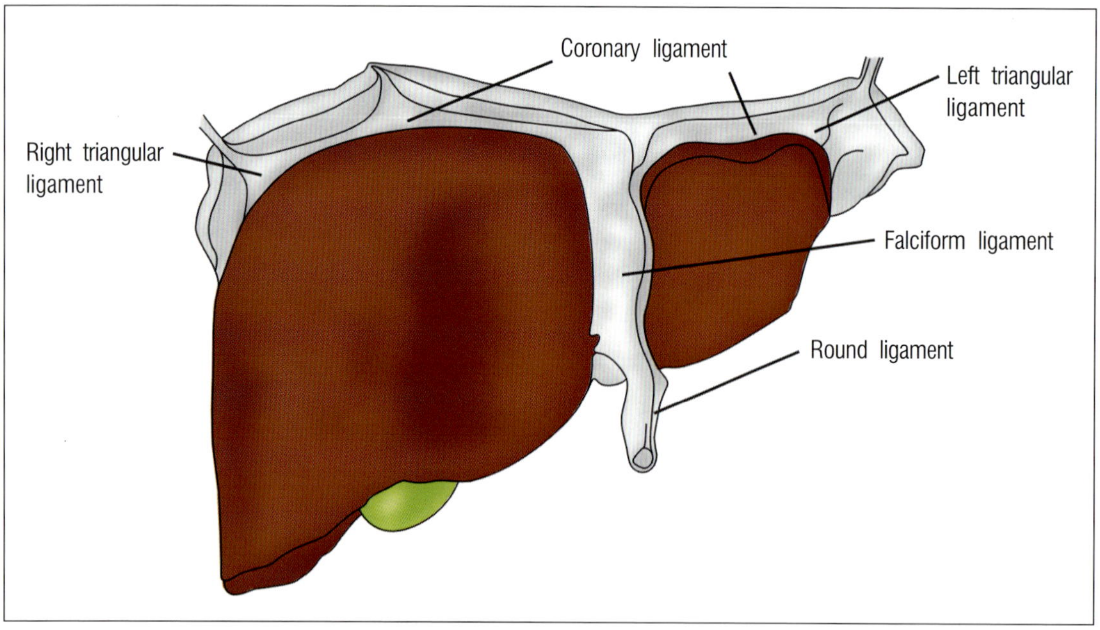

FIGURE 1. Anterior surface of the liver. Note the coronary ligament forming the left and right triangular ligaments. The falciform ligament attaches the liver to the abdominal wall; the round ligament contains the obliterated umbilical vein.

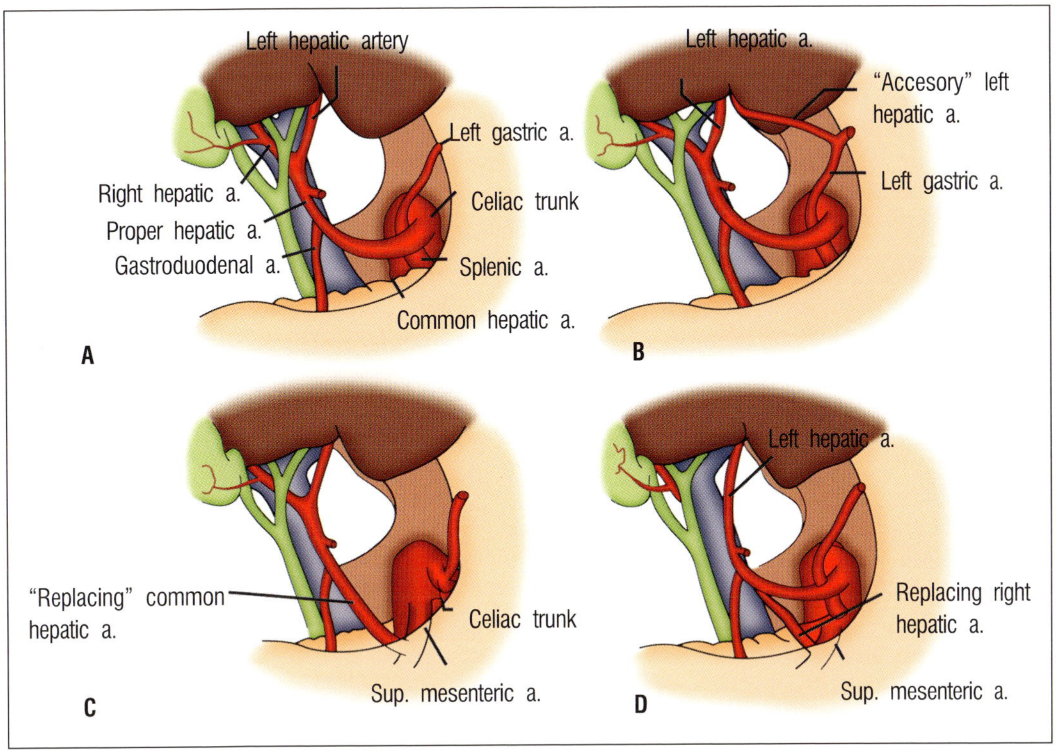

FIGURE 2. The four most common types of the hepatic arterial system variations. From Towsend CM et. al. Sabiston Textbook of Surgery, W.B.Sanders 2001; (48):1000, Fig.48-7.

left lateral segment. The hepatic veins convey blood to the inferior vena cava.

2.3. Surgical hepatic segmentation

The anatomy of the liver has been described considering its macroscopic and morphological appearance as well as its functional segmentation, which usually dictates hepatic resections. Over the years, a number of different descriptions have been published with the purposes of providing a detailed explanation of the hepatic functionality. Although such descriptions will be covered in the present chapter for clarification purposes, the authors prefer the use of the new terminology described in the year 2000 by the committee of the International Hepato-Pancreato-Biliary Association.[17]

Morphologically, the liver is divided into four lobes: right, left, quadrate and caudate (Figure 3). These lobes are divided by visible fissure but do not necessarily correspond the hepatic circulation.

When considering the functional segmentation of the liver, two different nomenclatures known as the American system and the French segmental system described by Couinaud in 1954[16] have been widely used in the past by general and hepatobiliary surgeons. The American system divides the liver in two hemilivers by a plane that starts at the left side of the gallbladder bed and extends to the left side of the inferior vena cava (Figure 4). This plane known as the Cantlie's line is based on portal and hepatic venous circulatory patterns. The left hemiliver is further divided into a medial segment, which lies to the right of the falciform ligament and a lateral segment. The right hemiliver on the other hand is subdivided into anterior and posterior segments. Couinaud's description considerers the hepatobiliary vasculature of the liver which results in eight different segments.

As mention above, to clarify and unify concepts on hepatic resection descriptions, the International Hepato-Pancreato-Biliary Association introduced a new terminology known as the "Brisbane 2000 terminology of hepatic anatomy and resections". The Brisbane terminology recognizes three subdivisions: the first-order division, the second-order division and the third-order division. Details of these divisions are displayed in figures 5, 6, 7. In addition, the committee introduced an alternative second-order division based on portal vein circulation (Figure 8). The first-order division separates the liver in two

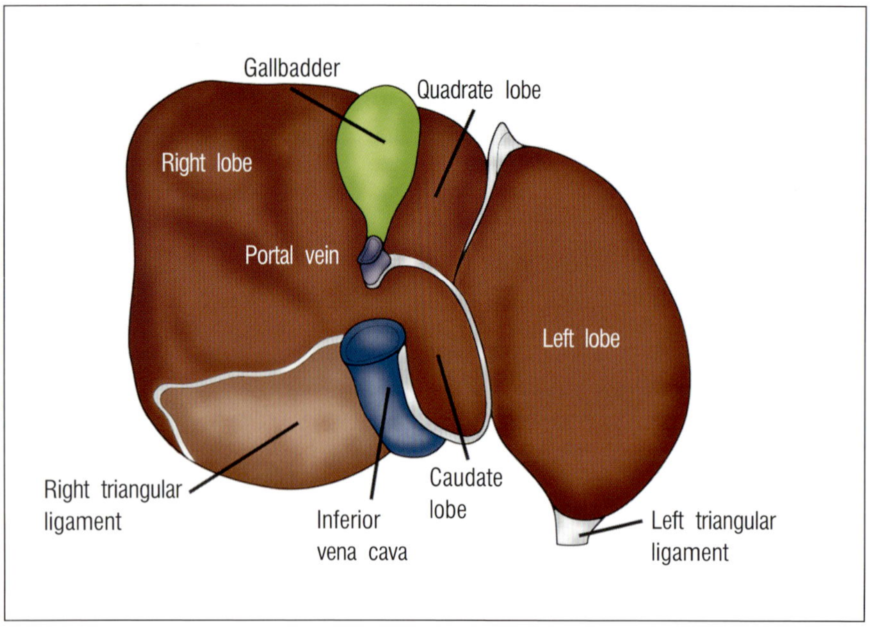

FIGURE 3. Visceral surface of the liver showing the morphological anatomy.

and hepatic artery is shown in figure 6. Figure 8 shows the alternative second-order division based on the portal vein. The anatomical term *right anterior section* corresponds to segments 5 and 8 of the old Couinaud's terminology and receives the term right anterior sectionectomy when referring to surgical resection. Resection of the *right posterior section* is known to as right posterior sectionectomy. The left hemiliver is further divided into a *left medial section* (i.e. segment 4) and a *left lateral section* (i.e. segment 2 and 3).

hemilivers (i.e. right and left hemilivers) by a plane that intersects the gallbladder fossa and the fossa of the inferior vena cava and is called the midplane of the liver (Figure 5). The term for the surgical resection of the right hemiliver is right hepatectomy while left hepatectomy refers to resection of the left hemiliver.

The second-order division based on bile ducts

Segmentectomy on the third-order division refers to resection of any of the individual segments while bidesegmentectomy refers when two contiguous segments are removed. The third-order division is displayed on figure 7.

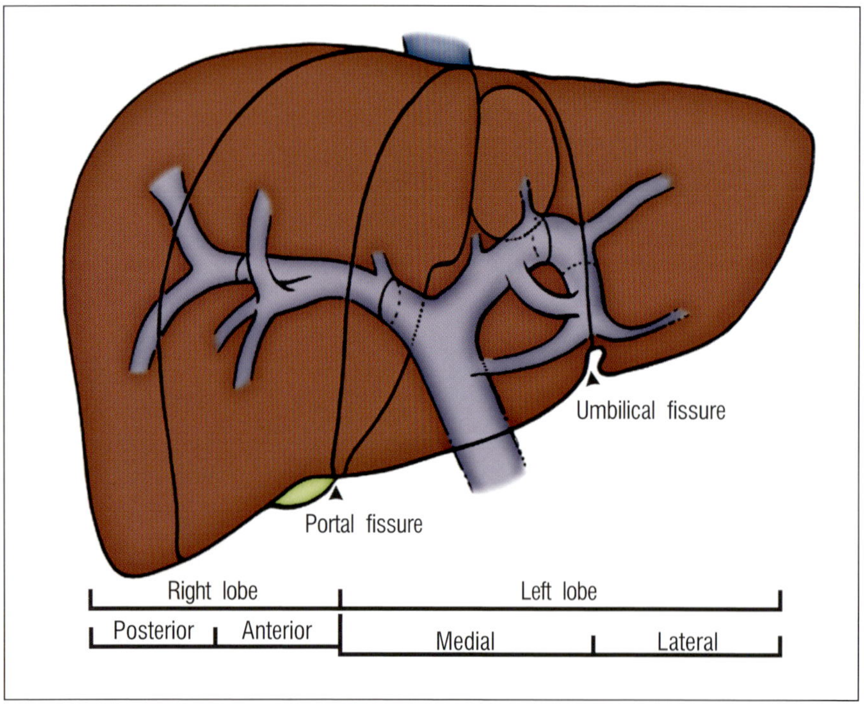

3. Special Considerations for Laparoscopic Surgeons

As mention before, the laparoscopic surgeon needs to be familiar with the hepatobiliary anatomy and open hepatic techniques to safely performed minimally invasive liver operations.

FIGURE 4. The American subdivision of the liver. From Towsend CM et. al. Sabiston Textbook of Surgery, W.B. Sanders 2001; (48): 1000, Fig 48-4.

FIGURE 5. Proposed terminology of hepatic resections introduced by the Terminology Committee of the International Hepato-Pancreato-Biliary Association in 2000. First-order division.

First-order division

Anatomical Term	*Couinaud segments referred to*	*Term for surgical resection*	*Diagram (pertinent area is shaded)*
Right Hemiliver or Right liver	Sg 5-8 (+/- Sg1)	Right Hepatectomy or Right Hemihepatectomy (stipulate +/- segment 1)	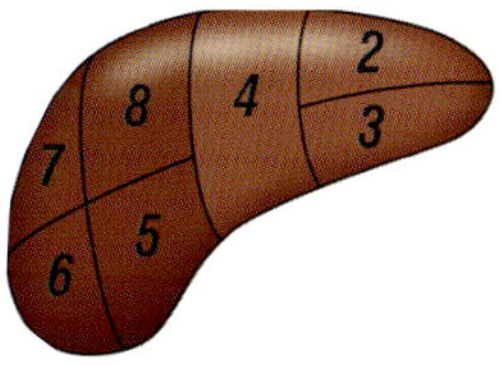
Left Hemiliver or Left liver	Sg 2-4 (+/- Sg1)	Left Hepatectomy or Left Hemihepatectomy (stipulate +/- segment 1)	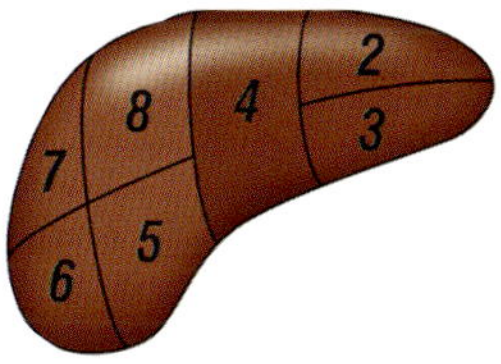

The challenges that surgeons faced when performing hepatic surgery may increase when minimally invasive approaches limit the visualization and tactic perception of the organ. However, in recent years, technologic advancements in resolution, illumination, and optical clarity have facilitated the performance of complex liver operations.

A technical advance that undoubtedly has improved and will continue to facilitate localization of hepatic lesions is laparoscopic ultrasonography.[18-21] Many surgeons advocate the use of laparoscopic ultrasonography before hepatic resections for both benign and malignant lesions are attempted.[22-24] Hepatic lesions as small as 4 mm can be detected laparo-

Second-order division

Anatomical Term	*Couinaud segments referred to*	*Term for surgical resection*	*Diagram (pertinent area is shaded)*
Right anterior Section	Sg 5,8	Add (-ectomy) to any of the anatomical terms as in right anterior sectionectomy	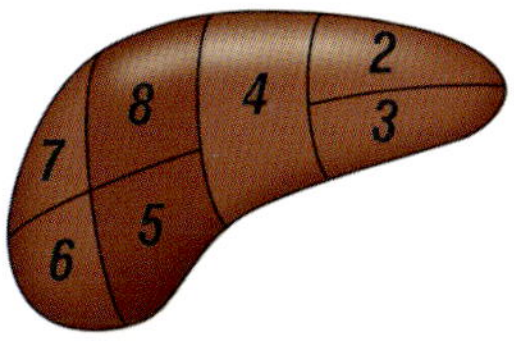
Right rosterior section	Sg 6,7	Right posterior sectionectomy	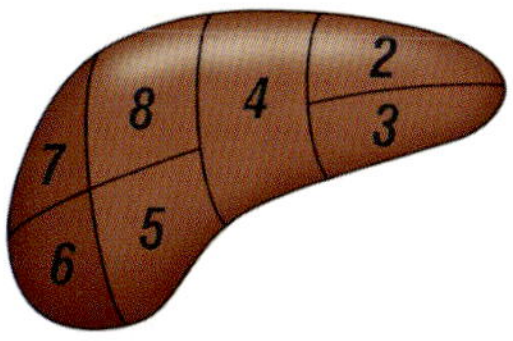
Left medial section	Sg 4	Left medial sectionectomy or resection segment 4 (also see third order) or Sectionectomy 4 (also see third order)	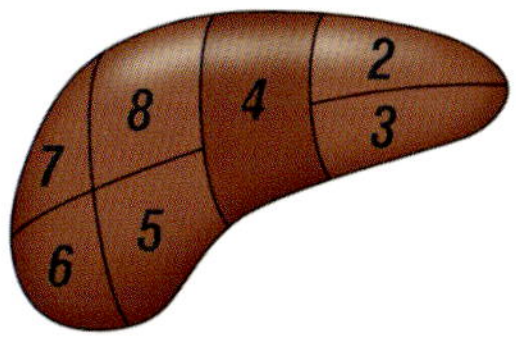
Left lateral section	Sg 2,3	Left lateral sectionectomy or Biesegmentectomy 2,3 (also see third order)	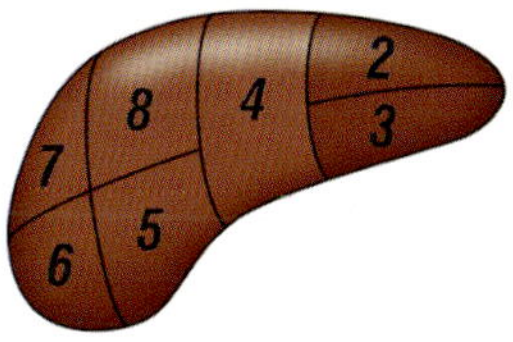

FIGURE 6. Second-order division based on bile ducts and hepatic artery.

Third-order division

Anatomical Term	*Couinaud segments referred to*	*Term for surgical resection*	*Diagram (pertinent area is shaded)*
Segments 1-9	Any one of Sg 1 to 9	Segmentectomy (e.g. segmentectomy 6)	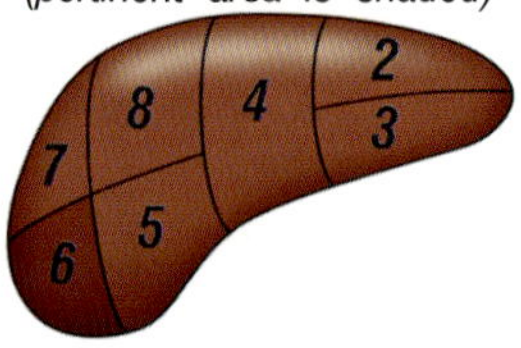
2 contiguous segments	Any two of Sg 1 to Sg 9 in continuity	Bisegmentectomy (e.g. bisegmentectomy 5,6)	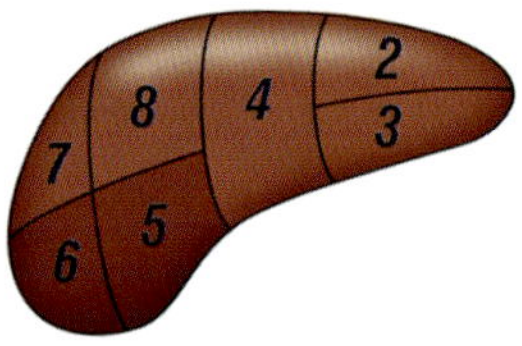

FIGURE 7.

Addendum. Alternative second-order division

Anatomical Term	*Couinaud segments referred to*	*Term for surgical resection*	*Diagram (pertinent area is shaded)*
Right anterior sector or	Sg 5,8	Add (-ectomy) to any of the anatomical terms as in right anterior sectionectomy or Right paramedial sectorectomy	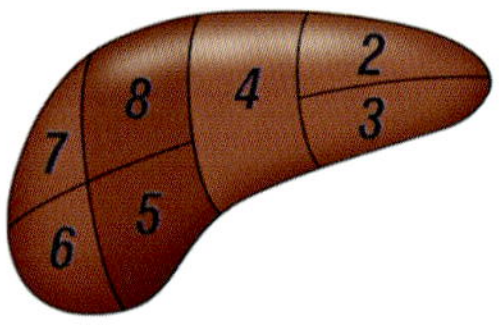
Right posterior sector or Right lateral sector	Sg 6,7	Right posterior sectorectomy or Right lateral sectorectomy	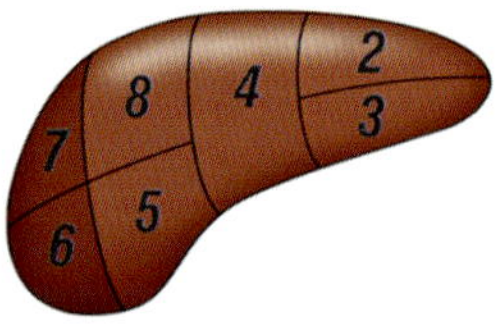
Left medial sector or Left paramedial sector	Sg 3,4	Left medial sectorectomy or Left posterior sectorectomy or Bisegmentectomy 3,4	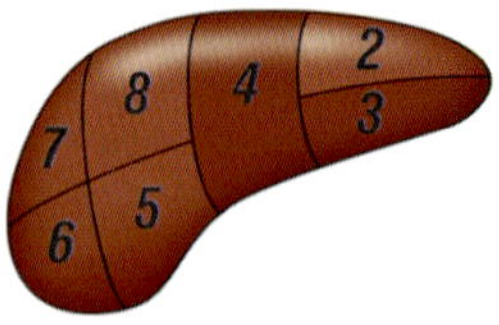
Left lateral sector or Left posterior sector	Sg 2	Left lateral sectorectomy or Left posterior sectorectomy or Segmentectomy 2	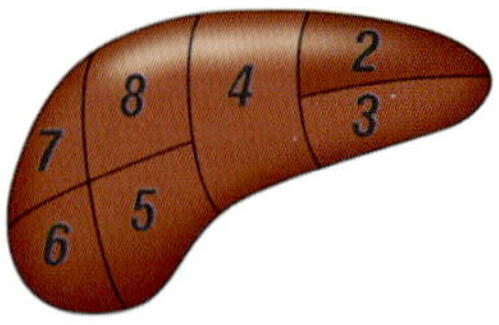

FIGURE 8. Alternative second-order division based on portal vein.

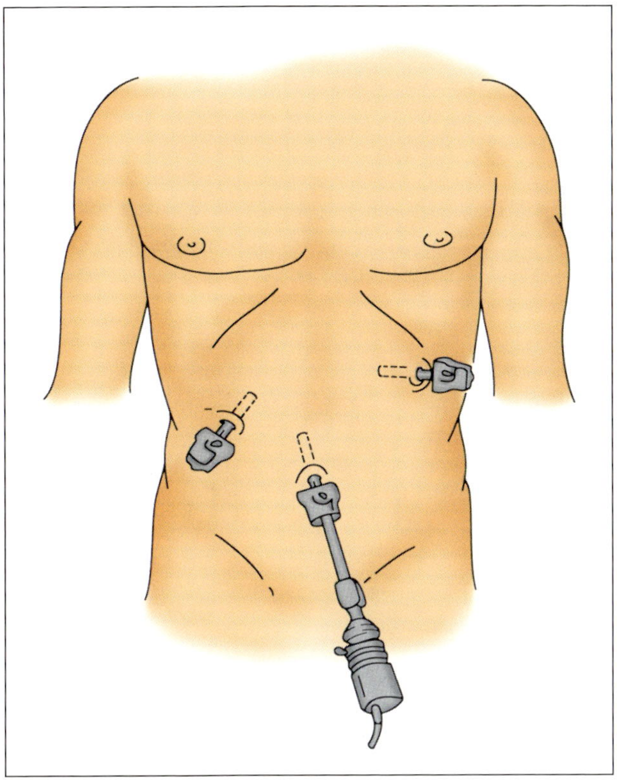

FIGURE 9. Trocar placement for hepatic biopsies. In addition to the camera port, a trocar is usually placed in a position to gain access to the area to by studied. In this example, the pathology is located in the caudate lobe; therefore, a trocar is placed in the left upper quadrant. A third trocars is used in this case to allow retraction of the liver. From Pappas TN, Schwartz LB, Eubanks WS. Atlas of Laparoscopic Surgery.1997; 11.6: Fig 11.4.

scopic ultrasonography. A comprehensive understanding of the three-dimensional anatomy of the liver is crucial for correctly interpreting the images obtained by ultrasound. It is also extremely important the adequate localization of the trocars to allow optimal evaluation of the area of interest. The ultrasound probe is generally introduced into the abdominal cavity through a 10 mm port located in the umbilicus or through a port placed in the right midclavicular line or anterior axillary line (Figure 9). The endocamera can be shifted to a different port while the ultrasound probe is in place to allow fully visualization of the liver. The flexibility of the probe's tip of commercially available ultrasounds permits exploration of the entire organ including the confluence of the hepatic veins in the inferior vena cava. The sonographic examination of the liver's parenchyma generally starts by recognizing the portal vein and the hepatic veins. A key step in the localization of intrahepatic lesion is the correct understanding of the blood vessels orientation.

The number of trocars that are employed for laparoscopic liver surgery depends largely on the type of operation being performed. If the intervention is more than a diagnostic laparoscopy, four to six -10 mm trocars are generally used. The endocamera is introduced through an umbilical port but can be shifted if further evaluation of the liver surface or abdominal cavity is required. The graspers are introduced through trocars placed on the patient's right side and, a fourth port is used on the left for irrigation and suction. For hepatic biopsies for example, two or three trocars are positioned in such way that the surgeons has access to the area in questions (Figure 8). In cases where a more extensive examination of the liver is desire such as with multifocal disease, the introduction of a laparoscopic hand port can provide additional evaluation of the hepatic parenchyma. The utilization of a hand-port also provides assessment of margins in malignant resections as well as direct digital compression should a significant hemorrhage occurs. The hand-port is usually placed along the line of a potential laparotomy ipsilateral to the tumor side. Preliminary data indicate that laparoscopic hand-assisted resection can safely be performed providing a valuable tool for the hepatobiliary surgeon.[25-26]

The preferred position of the patient for laparoscopic liver surgeries is the French position where the surgeon operates from in between the patient's legs. This position offers a symmetric view of the operating field without unnecessary bending. The surgical assistants typically stand at the patient's sides with the scrub nurse located to the right of the surgeon, which allows him or her to pass instruments to the surgeon's right hand. Two monitors are typically placed in each side of the patient's head permitting all members of the surgical team a direct visualization of the operation.

The advent of better equipment coupled with an improved understanding of the hepatobiliary anatomy has increased the number of hepatic operations that are performed daily around the world. Hepatic surgery has been shown to be amenable for minimally invasive approaches; however, proper indications, careful scrutiny of patients and adequate surgical skills will determined the progression of laparoscopic hepatic surgery in the future.

References

1. Hansen P, Ludemann R, Swanstromm LL. Minimally invasive approaches to hepatic surgery. Hepato-Gastroenterol 2001; 48:37-40.
2. Azagra JS, Goergen M, Gilbart E, Jacobs D. Laparoscopic anatomical (hepatic) left lateral segmentectomy- technical aspects. Surg Endosc 1996; 10:758-761.
3. Koneko H, Takagi S, Shiba T. Laparoscopic partial hepatectomy and left lateral segmentectomy: techniques and results of a clinical series. Surgery 1996; 120: 468-475.
4. Samana G, Chiche L, Brefort JL, Le Ropux Y. Laparoscopic anatomical hepatic resection. Report of four lobectomies for solid tumors. Surg Endosc 1998; 12: 76-78.
5. Marks J, Mouiel J, Katkhouda N, Gugenheim J, Fabiani P. laparoscopic liver surgery: a report on 28 patients. Surg Endosc 1998; 12: 331-334.
6. Mouiel J, Katkhouda N, Gugenheim J, Fabiani P. Possibilities of laparoscopic liver resection. J Hepatobiliary Pancreat Surg 2000; 7:1-8.
7. Hashizume M, Shimada M, Sugimachi K. Laparoscopic hepatectomy: new approach for hepatocellular carcinoma. J Hepato-Biliary-Pancreat Surg 2000; 7(3): 270-275.
8. Shimada M, Hashizume M, Maehara S, Tsujita E, Rikimaru T, Yamashita Y, Tanaka S, Adachi E, Sugimachi K. Laparoscopic hepatectomy for hepatocellular carcinoma. Surg Endosc. 2001; 15(6): 541-544.
9. Cuschieri A, Crosthwaite G, Shimi S, Pietrabissa A, Joypaul V, Tair I, Naziri W. Hepatic cryotherapy for liver tumors. Development and clinical evaluation of a high-efficiency insulated multineedle probe system for open and laparoscopic use. Surg Endosc 1995; 9(5): 483-489.
10. Feliciotti F, Paganini A, Guerrieri M, Chan R, Campagnacci R, Lezoche E. Laparoscopic intra-arterial catheter implantation for regional chemotherapy of liver metastasis. Surg Endosc 1996; 10(4): 449-452.
11. Yamanaka N, Tanaka T, Oriyama T, Furukawa K, Tanaka W, Okamoto E. Microwave coagulonecrotic therapy for hepatocellular carcinoma. W J Surg 1996; 20(8): 1076-1081.
12. Tait IS, Yong SM, Cuschieri SA. Laparoscopic in situ ablation of liver cancer with cryotherapy and radiofrequency ablation. Br J Surg 2002; 89(12):1613-1619.
13. Franklin ME Jr, Gonzalez JJ. Laparoscopic placement of hepatic artery catheter for regional chemotherapy infusion: technique, benefits, and complications. Surgical Laparosc Endosc Perc Tech 2002; 12(6):398-407.
14. Tsioulias GJ, Wood TF, Chung MH, Morton DL, Bilchik A. Diagnostic laparoscopy and laparoscopic ultrasonography optimize the staging and resectability of intraabdominal neoplasms. Surg Endosc 2001; 15 (9):1016-1019.
15. Katkhouda N, Mavor E. Laparoscopic management of benign liver disease. Surg Clin North Am 2000; 80(4): 1203-1211.
16. Couinaud C. Les envelopes vasculobiliares de foie ou capsule de Glisson: Leur interet dans la churgie vasiculaire, les resections hepatique et l"abord du hile du foie. Lyon Chir 1954; 49: 589.
17. Strasberg S, Belghiti J, Clavien PA, Gadzijev E, Garden JO, Lau W-Y, Makuuchi M, Strong RW. The terminology committee of the IHPBA. The Brisbane 2000 terminology of liver anatomy and resections. HPB 2000; 3: 333-339.
18. Miles WF, Paterson-Brown S, Garden OJ. Laparoscopic contact hepatic ultrasonography. Br J Surg 1992; 79(5):419-420.
19. John TG, Banting SW, Pye S, Paterson-Brown S, Garden OJ. Preliminary experience with intracorporeal laparoscopic ultrasonography using a sector scanning probe. A prospective comparison with intraoperative cholangiography in the detection of choledocholithiasis. Surg Endosc 1994; 8(10): 1176-1180.
20. John TG, Greig JD, Crosbie JL, Miles WF, Garden OJ. Superior staging of liver tumors with laparoscopy and laparoscopic ultrasound.[comment]. [Clinical Trial. Controlled Clinical Trial. Journal Article] Ann Surg 1994; 220(6): 711-719.
21. Lo CM, Lai EC, Liu CL, Fan ST, Wong J. Laparoscopy and laparoscopic ultrasonography avoid exploratory laparotomy in patients with hepatocellular carcinoma. Ann Surg 1998; 227(4): 527-532.
22. Catheline JM, Turner R, Champault G. Laparoscopic ultrasound of the liver. Eu J Ultras 2000; 12(2): 169-177.
23. Berends FJ, Meijer S, Prevoo W, Bonjer HJ, Cuesta MA. Technical considerations in laparoscopic liver surgery. Surg Endosc 2001; 15(8): 794-798.
24. Rahusen FD, Cuesta MA, Borgstein PJ, Bleichrodt RP, Barkhof F, Doesburg T, Meijer S. Selection of patients for resection of colorectal metastases to the liver using diagnostic laparoscopy and laparoscopic ultrasonography. Ann Surg 1999; 230(1):31-37.
25. Dematteo RP, Fong Y, Jamagin WR, Blumgart LH. Recent advances in hepatic resection. Sem Surg Oncol 2000; 19: 200-207.
26. Fong Y, Jamagin W, Conlon KC, Dematteo R, Dougherty E, Blumgart LH. Hand-assisted laparoscopic liver resection. Arch Surg 2000; 135: 854-859.

CHAPTER

14

Laparoscopic surgery of the liver

Namir Katkhouda, Jean Mouiel

Because of its multiple metabolic, detoxifying and filtering functions, the liver plays the role in the field of oncology. Whether it concerns primary cancer or metastases, the liver is often the seat of different tumors. Most of the intra-abdominal organs in fact have portal venous drainage toward the liver, just as other organs closer to the liver also have lymphatic drainage in the direction of this organ. The structure of the liver with different lobules constritutes an obligatory barrier to cancer cells which depending on the various conditions of number, environment and susceptibility, as well as other contributing factors, will blossom to produce hepatic metastases whether they are syncronous or metachronous. The size of the metastases varies greatly and obeys the laws of exponential tumor growth, which means that some of them cannot be detected by the conventional viewing methods because of their small dimensions.[1]

Hepatic oncological surgery is presently very advanced and the tecnology has been thorougly tested.[1-4] It is nenertheless mandatory to emphasize the specialized nature of this type of surgery. It cannot be properly done if the department has not had a long traditional involvement with the various techniques involved in hepatobiliary surgery. Unfortunately, we too often see hepatic oncological surgery which has been poorly performed or inadequately carried out, the effects of which on the survival of the patient are frequently irreversible. Laparoscopic surgery, which after several years is now out of its infancy stage, has seen its applications spread to most of the intra-abdominal organs.[5-8]

The liver remains the last taboo, the last point of resistance, due to its size, its highly vascular nature and certain mystery which surrounds liver surgery. Laparoscopic surgery of the liver in oncology will have to be performed judiciously and with caution, and only by experienced hepatobiliary surgeons.[2,9,10]

Prerequisites to Laparoscopic Surgery of the Liver

It is essential not only to have experience in open hepatobiliary surgery, but also to have an experimental laboratory in order to gain experience in laparoscopic surgery. It is indeed imperative to get used handling laparoscopic instruments for use in the liver, and to completely master techniques of hemostasis and biliostasis. This can only be achieved by carrying out experimental surgery on animals. It is also necessary to have a certain amount of specialized equipment. These requirements are more important for surgery of the liver than for surgery of other intra-abdominal organs. Unforunately, equipment for laparoscopy surgery, for example the YAG laser, can be very expensive. To alleviate this problem it is essential that the various disciplines share the equipment and thereby make it cost - effective.[3,11,12] It is, furthermore of paramount importance to provide reasonable indications and to follow these indications carefully. Finally, problems can crop up at any time during hepatic surgery and one must be able to convert immediately, for the sake of the patient' s safety. These different points will be progressively analyzed and discussed in this chapter.

Possible Complications

The major complications of laparoscopic surgery of the liver for carcinoma are the intraoperative risks of hemorrhage and possible gas emboli. These hemorrahagic risks, which at the outset appear to be under control but which suddenly arise during the operation, can take dramatic turn. One cannot stress enough the importance of making a quick decesion to convert in the event of sudden hemorrhage. As in open surgery, maintaining meticulous control of biliary radicles is also important. This can be achieved with clips or ligatures, as well as intracorporeal sutures. It is therefore essential for every surgeon embarking on this kind of surgery to be able to master the techniques of laparoscopic suturing with both intracorporeal and extracorporeal ligatures. Laparoscopic hepatic surgery is more tecnically demanding than the others types intracorporeal surgery. It is thus necessary to become familiar with the different techniques of intraoperative use the YAG laser, the ultrasonic scalpel[15] and the handling of automatic stapling devices. All of these points will be discussed in more detail in the chapter on specialized equipment. Finally, one possible problem that must be considered is the extraction of the excised specimen, once the organ has been completely separated from its attachments. There are different ways to do this, but it is necessary to emphasize the specimen must be placed in an extraction bag in order to avoid intra-abdominal spillage of neoplastic tissue. One must not hesitate to enlarge the umpilical incision or to use other means, such as a colpotomy (in female patients). An electric morcellator (Cook Medical), which preserves minimum histological features, is an important aid. This apparatus should soon be available for standard use.

Specialized Equipment

Besides the basic laparoscopic instruments, which have been described elsewhere, it is necessary to have different sets of instruments that are adapted to hepatic surgery.

High-quality scopes with a 0°, but also 30° and even 45° viewing range must be available. The 30° scope is indispensable in access to the liver, since it enables observation of the "blind" areas which cannot be seen by the traditional 0° scopes. The 30° allows visualization of the upper posterior side of the liver and the lateral regions. Moreover, the examination of the blood suply often requires a view of the base of the tumor, which can only be achieved with the 30° scope. Although it is the author's personal opinion that 30° scope is not indispensable for other intra-abdominal operations carried out laparoscopically, it is an absolute necessity for operation on the liver.

The video camera needs to be of high quality and must have descernment capacity needed to realize complete hemostasis and biliostasis. The light source must be powerful (250 W halogen or xenon). Finally, the video monitors must also have the correct dimensions (at least 51 cm) and it is necessary to have two screens, so that the surgeon and the assistants have a full comfortable veiw of the operation. There is nothing specific about the trocars, but it is noteworthy that sufficient trocars should be available, as well as sufficient instrumentation. The forceps used on the liver should be atraunatic, preferably with no teeth. The so-called "crocodile forceps", or forceps with large teeth are ineffective and increase the risc of hemorrhage. All of the forceps sould be insulated and possibly rotating. It is also desirable to have rotating coagulation scissors and an insulated hook which are entirely insulated to the tips. For laparoscopic liver surgery one cannot do without automatic clip appliers, which allow the clips to be loaded without with-drawing the instruments for reloading. Finally, stapling devices with vascular clips will be useful for certain vascular pedicles, providing complete safety. Among the more specific instruments, the Nd YAG laser and the ultrasonic dissector (CUSA-Lap, Valley-lab Inc Boulder, Colorado, Usa) should be mentioned. The Nd- YAG laser is the instument which is the most adapted to surgery of the liver. Due to its capacity of greater penetration than the CO_2 and argon lasers, it enables a correct cut to be carried out. This was demonstrated experimentally during the excision of hepatic metastases, which compared the YAG laser to conventional electrocautery. At the conclusion of this randomized prospective experimental study, the YAG laser proved to be clearly superior. This instrument is very costly, however, and acquisition is best done on a multidisciplinary basis, which will allow the different disciplines to share its utilization and costs. The ultrasonic dissector is also a valuable instrument. It enables precise dessection of the hepatic parenchyma, bearing the vasculobiliary radicles, thus allowing step-by-step dissection of these structures. The ultrasonic dissector is ideal in the field of limited tumor resection, enabling enucleation with a margin while maintaining control of the pedicles. Appropriate needle holders are also mandatory; a range of models is available.

Pretied calcut endoligatures should be available, and finer sutures should also be available for internal suturing. These should be strong and monofilament, preferably without memory. This kind of monofilament ligature is also useful for extracorporeal tying with Roeder Knot. The specimen bags must be strong and equipped with closing system.

The Tisseel fibrin glue (BAXTER, Hyland Immuno) is indispensable for hemostasis after laparoscopic hepatic resection. Its ideal application in this area is on the raw hepatic surfaces. This adhesive fibrin sealand is available in various concetrations and various setting times. It should be applied without pressure to the raw surface of the liver at the end of resection. Omentum can also be used to advantage in covering the raw surfaces of the liver, at the end of the procedure.

The four-hand technique is used to resect benign solid tumors, such as adenomas and focal nodular hyperphasia, in the event of suspected malignancy that could not be ruled out preoperatively. The resection begins with division of the round ligament and the right or left triangular ligament for lesions located in the corresponding lobe. Glisson's capsule is scored 2 cm away from the lesion using electrocautery. The Harmonic shears (LCS, Ethicon Endosurgery, Inc., Cincinnati, OH) is one of the key instruments in laparoscopic liver surgery. It can be used to mimick a Kelly fracture technique while achieving hemostasis and biliostasis of all small radicles. Its action is based on the denaturation of proteins through a heat-induced coagulation process by the oscillations of the blades at 55,000 cycles/s. Those shears are used by the first surgeon to dissect the parenchyma, while the first surgeons left hand retracts the exposed liver surface. Simultaneously, the second surgeon divides all exposed larger vascular and biliary pedicles between large hemostatic clips. Hemostasis and control of bile leak from raw liver surface are achieved by wide application of fibrin sealand (Tisseel, Baxter Healthcare Corp., Hyland/Immuno Div., Vienna Austria). Clips are used for hemostasis of large structures, and linear endovascular cutters are reserved for hepatic veins. A flexible laparoscopic sonography probe is useful in locating anatomic landmarks or vasculobiliary structures.

Position of the Patient and the Operating Team

We have opted for the so-called 'French' position: the surgeon positions himself between the patient's loweer limps, which are spread and placed in special supports. This position is very comfortable for the surgeon, who does not have to bend unnecessrily, and it provides a symmetrical view "across from" the patient. It also allows free use of the hands, while enabling the foot pedals to be maneuvered. This is also very convenient for assistants on each side. The two monitors are placed on each side of the anesthesiologist, near the head patient, so that the whole arrangement is head of the patient, so that the whole arrangement is coherent and ergonomic. The scrub nurse should be to the right of the surgeon, beside the assistant, allowing him or her to pass the instruments to the surgeon's right hand. The position of the patient will be the same as in open surgery, with a wide operating field. All of the traditional basic instruments for open surgery must be to hand in sterilized area in the operating room, in case the need for conversion arises. The usual rules of anesthesiology for hepatic surgery are followed, but it is necessary to emphasize that the anesthesiologist must be aware of the additional hazards of laparoscopic surgery. Measures must be taken to ensure that there is equipment in the room for rapid transfusion of blood: a sufficient suply of plasma and blood must also be readily available. With this preparation and equipment, laparoscopic surgery can take place in relatively comfort and safety.

Reasonable Indications

In the field of oncology, diagnostic laparoscopy can prove to be very useful in searching out small tumors of the liver which are not detectable by convertional imaging techniques (CT Scan, MRI, scintigraphy and hepatic arteriograhy). Cancer of the pancreas, for example, which is unfortunately too frequent and often fatal, is commonly accompanied by multiple hepatic metastases[8,13] which are small in size and dispersed throughout the entire liver.

Because of their size, these metastases are sometimes not detected by the usual imaging methods, but can usually be seen with the laparoscope. This makes it possible to change an indication for curative resection into palliative surgery, or even into non- entervention in advanced cases.

Another example is cancer of the gallbledder in elderly persons: preoperative imaging may indicate such a cancer, but ultrasonography will not reveal localized hepatic extension. Here too, laparoscopy introduced through the umbilicus with single trocar will allow a clear diagnosis to be made, and allow for biopsy. In the case of localized colorectal cancer (stages A and B) resection by laparoscopy should be proceeded by a thorough examination of the liver to enclude metastases. This examination can further suplemend by laparoscopic ultrasonography at the time of the attemped resection. Unfortunately this step is frequently neglected. It is also important to be able to distinguish benigh tumors to the liver at the time of lapascopy, as these tumors (adenomas and focal nodular hyperphasia) can sometimes be mistaken for hepatic metastases. After thorough evaluation of the liver by laparoscopy, one can make a completely objective decision regarding the talking of biopsies only, laparoscopic resection, or conversion to open surgery. Lymph nodes in the porta hepatis, demostrated with imaging techniques, are also an indication for diagnostic laparoscopy. In cases of cancer of the stomach, pancreas or gallblader, these lymph nodes can be involved. This changes the surgical indication from curative to palliative surgery.[14] It is often possible not only to visualize the porta hepatis but also to perform lymph node biopsies and frozen section studies, which will help in the better staging

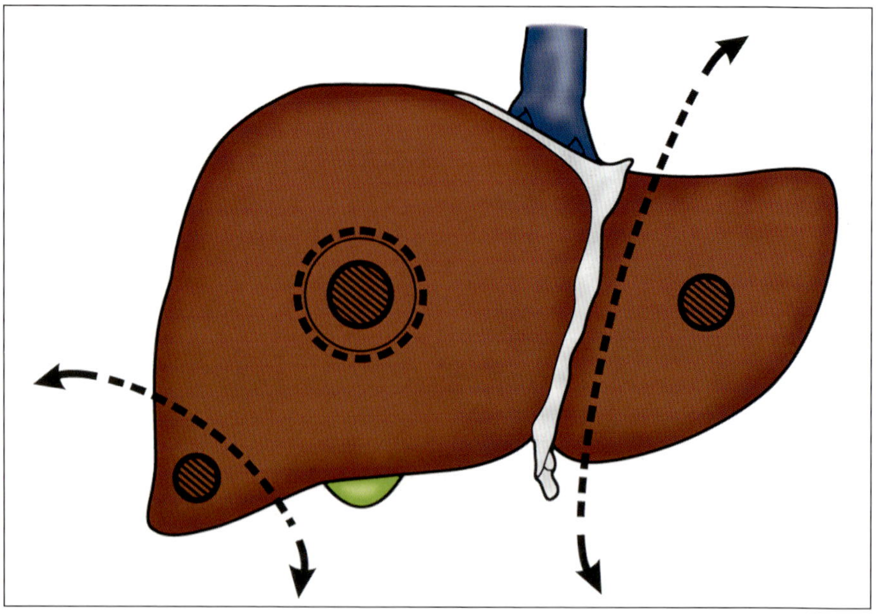

FIGURE 1. Reasonable possibilities of resection in laparoscopic liver surgery.

of the diseases. A further indication for laparoscopy is the possible laparoscopic resection of confined tumors in the liver (Figure 1) It is currently accepted that metastasectomy with a 2 cm margin is sufficient. This enucleation can be performed by laparoscopy. A segmentectomy that is limited to one, or the most two, segments can also be performed by laparoscopy. Finally, lobectomy is also possible, but this calls for considerable experience as already pointed out above. These resections mostly concern hepatic metastases, but can also be applied to non-malignant tumors for which there is a formal indication, such as a hepatocytic adenoma (in woman taking oral contraceptives) which has increased in size or been complicated by hemorrhage. Apart from from these risks of serious complications, limited resection is possible with this type of tumor, the histiologic diagnosis of which is frequently uncertain.

Unfortunately, in primary liver cancer the tumors are very often large at the time of diagnosis, and resection by laparoscopy is not a resonable procedure. Laparoscopic resection is also not recommended if the liver is cirrhotic, given the risk of hemorrhage which can occur at any time, with possible fatal consequences. For the time being laparoscopic resection in the presence of cirrhosis cannot be recommended mutinely although it has already been performed in humans.

Approach to the Liver

A minimum of four trocars and cannulas will be introduced if the planned intervention is more than diagnostic laparoscopy (Figure 2). The placement of the trocars will allow enough space between them to avoid the 'knitting needle' effect of the various instruments. The cannula for the endoscope is usually introduced in the umbilicus, with a cannula for the graspers on the left side and one for the instruments on the right side. This triangle is converted to a rectangle by placing the fourth trocal for the palpator and the irrigation/aspiration probe. This general scheme can be changed according the localization of the lesion and the working method to which the surgeon is accustomed. There is no ideal position of the trocars for this kind of surgery. All trocars must be at least 10 mm, in order to allow repositioning of the camera for visualization of the lesion and the parenchyma from different angles. Other trocars - five or six being a maximal number - will be introduced for the use of the YAG laser or the CUSA. More trocars can affect the operative ergonomy.

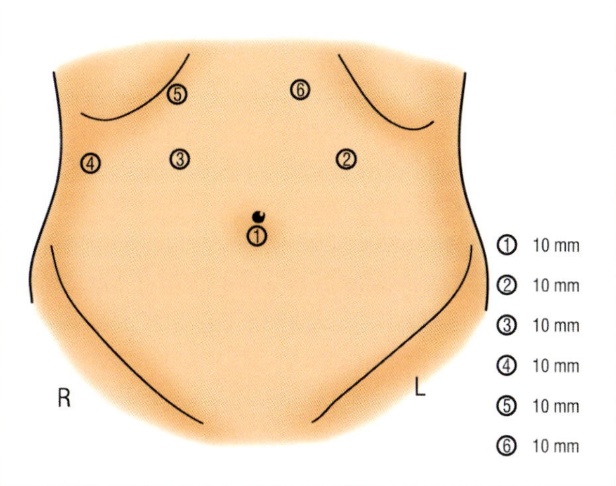

FIGURE 2. Laparoscopic approach to the liver.

Maneuvers Common to all Hepatic Laparoscopic Surgery

As in open surgery, hepatic laparoscopic surgery begins by mobilizing the liver (Figure 2). This is the key to the success of the lesion, so that there is direct and precise access. This procedure, which is familiar to all hepatobiliary surgeons, is as follows: division and ligation of the round ligament between clips; section of posterior surface of the liver can be lowered; section of the left lobe; and partial division of the right triangular ligament, which is more difficult in the case of a right posterior lesion. In the event of a major resection it is necessary to be able to approach the side of the superior vena cava and the trifurcation of the hepatic vein. A careful dissection and mobilization can prove to be extremely useful, in case a resection of the lobe becomes necessary. Once the liver is completely mobilized, an incision will be made in Glisson's capsule.

This will be done with either a coagulating hook or the YAG laser. Next, long forceps will simulate finger fracture methods. The ultrasonic dissector comes in very handy here, enabling parenchymalous pulverization while preserving the vasculobiliary elements. All these large-sized vascular and biliary radicles must be clipped and, in the case of major vessels or biliary ducts, one must not hesitate to resort to use extracorporeal ligatures (sliding Roeder knots). Finally, at the end of the operation the ablated segment must always be contained in bag which allows extraction without spillage. This extraction is usually done by enlarging the umbilical opening. The resected specimen can be partially morcellated with Kelly forceps, should an electric morcellator not be available. A specimen should never be reduced to total pulp, since this would prevent any type of postoperative histological and pathological examination. If the patien is a woman and the specimen is large, it is possible to extract it via a posterior colpotomy, which of course requires appropriate and precise reapproximation and resuturing. This type of extraction does not entail any delayed complications if the repair is done correctly.

Diagnostic Laparoscopy

As we have already specified in the discussion concerning indications, diagnostic laparoscopy of the liver is extremely important in liver malignancies, as well as in metastases. It also provides for directed biopsy to be carried out with ease, due to the magnification provided. It is also possible to examine the lesions macroscopically and to confirm or invalidate the preoperative diagnostic assessment. Laparoscopic ultrasonography is an invaluable technique in the study of the liver. Some users who already have considerable experience with it show images which are surprisingly no different from images oblained by intraoperative ultrasonography carried out during open surgery. Laparoscopic ultrasonography enables the detection of deeper-lying metaslases, as well as allowing the definition of attachment to vital structures, such as the hepatic veins. The hepatic pedicles as well as the hilum can be cleanly seen. Thanks to the intraoperative ultrasonography the biopsy can be directed without fear of causing major hemorrhage or bile leaks. These ultrasonography probes are always being improved and we can expect very effective instrumentation in the near future, which will increase the precision of laparoscopy, especially when coupled with Doppler probes.

Confined Resection of Minor Neoplastic Lesions

Metastasectomy is an example that best illustrates these techniques. A small-sized metastasis in the left lobe is the ideal example of a lesion that can safely be resected using laparoscopy. Four trocars are necessary for access: the umbilical trocar for the video laparoscope, two lateral trocars for grasping forceps and other instruments, and one subxiphoid trocar for the irrigation/aspiration probe. This same cannula can also provide access for the Nd-YAG laser fiber and the clip applier. The resection begins by incising Glisson's capsule 2 cm from the metastatic lesion. After laser incision there is less smoke than following carbonization with conventional electric cautery; this smoke must be intermittently suctioned through the xiphoid irrigation/aspiration cannula. It is then necessary to progressively dissect deeper into the hepatic parenchyma, while separating the edges of the liver with the left-handed forceps. It is sometimes necessary to add a fifth trocar for the insertion of grasping forceps to be used by the assistant in carefully moving the tumor mass. This will create a groove through which a hook or coagulating scissors can pass. Atraumatic forceps will allow the minute structures to be coagulated as they pass through this groove. In the case of larger vessels, clips must be used. It is recommended that a double-clipping technique be used to avoid inadvertent avulsion of a single clip from the vascular pedicle. It is necessary to use the irrigation/aspiration probe in the deep groove of the liver to keep the operating field dry. Maintenance of a dissection area, cannot be overemphasized. Once dissection is complete it is necessary to insert a cannula to deliver the fibrin glue (Tisseel, Baxter Healthcare Corp.,

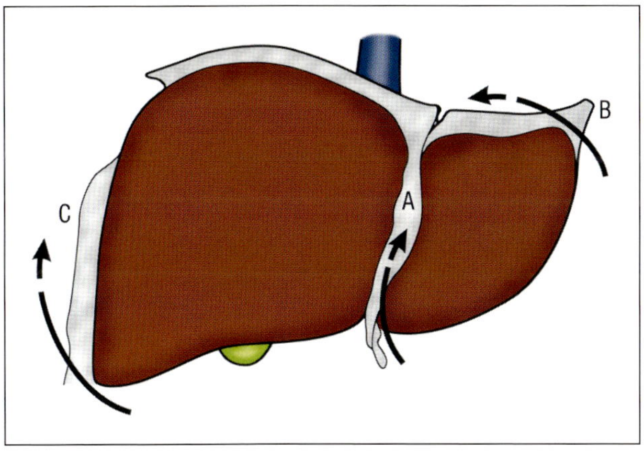

FIGURE 3. Laparoscopic mobilization of the liver. (A = falciform ligament, B= left triangular ligament, C = right triangular ligament).

Hyland/Immuno Div., Vienna, Austria). This is the last step of the operation.

In cases of small metastasectomy drainage is not necessary. In case of larger metastases we routinely perform cholangiography at the conclusion of the resection, to identify possible biliary leaks. This, of course, cannot be done without a cholecystectomy. Metastases of a maximum of 5-8 cm can be extracted without difficulty by enlarging the fascial incision at the umbilicus, so that the extracted spectmen is left intact.

Broader Resections, Left Lobectomy

This approach is aimed at larger tumors localized in the left lobe for which enucleation may prove to be incomplete and inadequate treatment. Larger lesions in the left lobe may also be best dealt with by normal lobectomy, as the enucleation procedure may actually prove to be dangerous. A left lobectomy, however, should only be considered by surgeons who have extensive experience in laparoscopy, as these maneuvers are so much easier when performed through open surgery. Laparoscopic left lobectomy nevertheless follows the same rules as in open syrgery, and must be preceded by a careful hepatic vascular isolation, which can be done with a little patience and by using extracorporeal ligatures. A dissection into the parenchyma will be done after the incision in Glisson's capsule, allowing the deep intraparenchymous dissection and encountering the different elements of segments II and III, which will be controlled with the aid of clips reinforced with ligatures, thus ensuring complete hemostasis and ligation of the biliary radicles. In general, the lobectomy specimen, which must then be placed in an extraction bag, can only be withdrawn if it undergoes some degree of morcellation or, in the case of a female patient, by posterior colpotomy. The raw hepatic surface is inspected and hemostatis completed. Here again, a cholangiographic examination for the purpose of detecting possible bile leaks proves to be very useful. The application of fibrin glue is invaluable. The greater omentum can be used to advantage in covering the raw surface of the liver at the termination of the procedure. After left lobectomy, we recommend placing two suction drains near the edge of the wound to collect any minor persistent ooze of blood or bile, and to prevent hematomas. Smaller resections, such as limited segmentectomies (wedge) are done in the same way and with the same concern for hemostasis and control to avoid CO_2 gas embolization. In general the risk in laparoscopic surgery is minimal, as the gynecological series has demonstrated. It is, however, much greater during the surgery of organs that are well vascularized, such as the spleen and the liver, since they are diredly linked to the inferior vena cava and to the heart. The risk is not insignificant and should be a constant concern. The patient must be constantly monitored by the anesthesiologist. The emboli are sometimes only detected by the recovery room staff after extubation, and staff must be aware of this possible delayed compication.

Treatment and Prevention of Intraoperative Complications

The major intraoperative complication is hemorrhage. Minimal ooze can be controlled with unipolar or bipolar forceps; a coagulating spatula enabling flat application of the coagulating current is also very useful. In the case of more serious arterial bleeding (where there is a clearly visible spurt of blood), it is necessary to grasp the artery with atraumatic forceps and immediately apply a clip or ligature. Management of venous bleeding in hepatic surgery tends to be more complicated since there is often a constant ooze, and hemostasis can be extremely difficult. Placing sutures laparoscopically is not easy, but panic should be avoided; often an appropriate temporary tamponade will stabilized the situation so that the extent of the venous injury can be assessed. Bleeding from a small lacerated vein can generally be controlled with coagulation or a clip. If the venous injury is more extensive, such as in a hepatic vein or a branch of the portal vein, one must not hesitate to convert and perform a limited subcostal incision, which will then allow precise and sufficient access and enable the operation to be concluded safely. It should be stressed that conversion is not an admission of failure, but a good surgical judgment. The safety of the patient is always the first priority. Control of biliary leaks is generally easier to accomplish, since the biliary drainage can be seen clearly with the magnification provided by the laparoscope. Another complication that can suddenly appear is that of CO_2 gas embolization. It is necessary to emphasize the importance of careful handing of large vessels inside the parenchyma and the avoidance of injury with scissors. Division of these vessels must only take place after coagulation, or control with clips or ligatures. Finally, there remains the difficulty of extracting the large specimen, which has already been mentioned.

Conclusions

It is important to approach laparoscopy liver resection with the attitude that it is a very complex operation requiring a considerable amount of experience and a high level of competence. This surgery has proved to be an attractive alternative in the field of diagnostic laparoscopy, and is very useful for the management of confined lesions. It avoids large incisions, which are painful and disabling. Laparoscopy is particularly useful in the evaluation of widespread metastases, obviating the need for laparotomy. The efficacy of this kind of surgery needs to be assessed by evaluation of the results, and therefore multicentric trials are required.

References

1. Wagner JS Adson MA, Van Heerden JA et al 1984 The natural history of hepatic metastases from colorectal cancer. A comparison with respective treatment. Ann Surg 199:502-509.
2. Katkhouda N, Mouiel J 1993 Laparoscopic applications in liver surgery. Im Zucker K (ed) Surgical laparoscopy update. QMP Inc, St. Louis, pp 395-408.
3. Katkhouda N, Nano JL, lovine L, Mouiel J 1993 An all comparative study of Nd-YAG laser versus electrocautery for liver metastatic resection in the rat. Lasers Med Sci 38:55-62.
4. Hughes k, Scheele J, Sugarbaker PH 1989 Surgery for colorectal cancer metastatic to the liver: optimizing the results of treatment. Surg Clin North Am 69:339-359.
5. Katkouda N, Mouiel J 1991 A new technique of treatment for chronic duodenal ulcer by videocoelioscopy without laparotomy. Am J Surg 161:361-364.
6. Clayman RV, Kavoussi LR, McDougall EM et at 1992 Laparoscopic nephrectomy: a review of 16 cases. Surg Laparosc Endosc 2(1):29-34.
7. Fabiani P, Katkhouda N, lovine L, Mouiel J 1991 Laparoscopic lenestration of biliary cysts. Surg Laparosc Endosc 1(3):162-165.
8. Mouiel J, Katkhouda N, White S 1992 Endolaparoscopoic palliation of pancreatic cancer. Surg Laparosc Endosc 2-3:241-243.
9. Katkhouda N, Fabiani P, Benizri E, Mouiel j 1992 Laser resection of a liver hydatid cyst under videocoelioscopy. Br J Surg 79:560-561.
10. WayL, Wetter A 1992 Laparoscopic treatment of liver cysts. Surg Endosc 6(2):89-90.
11. Dixon JA 1988 Current laser applications in general surgery. Ann Surg 207:355-72.
12. Joffe S, Brackett KA, Sanker MY 1986 Resection of the liver with the Nd-YAG laser. Surg Gynecol Obstet 163:437-442.
13. Warshaw AL, Zhuo-Yun Gu, Wittenberg J 1990 Preoperative stating and assessment of resectability of pancreatic cancer. Am J Surg 125:230-236.
14. Warshaw AL, Femandez-del Castillo C 1991 Laparoscopy in preoperative diagnosis and staging for gastrointestinal cancers. In:Zucker KA (ed) Surgical laparoscopy. Quality Medical Publishing, St. Louis, pp 101-115.
15. Tranberg KG, Rigotti P, Brackett KA et al 1985 Liver resection: a comparison using the Nd: YAG laser, ultrasonic aspirator or blunt dissection. Am J Surg 151:368-372.

CHAPTER

Laparoscopy and thoracoscopy of the esophagus

15

D.R. Urbach, L.L. Swanstrom

Introduction

The operative management of cancer of the esophagus has frustrated surgeons for many years. Patients with esophageal cancer are seldom cured by surgery, and the traditional surgical approaches to esophageal resection are associated with a high risk of operative mortality and serious complications. Transhiatal esophageal resection, by avoiding a thoracotomy, has been proposed as a less morbid procedure to the Ivor-Lewis esophagectomy. Most authorities agree that the two approaches are roughly equivalent in their oncologic effectiveness. However, open transhiatal esophagectomy is still associated with considerable operative risk, due in large part to the poor medical status of patients with esophageal cancer. Many patients have a long history of alcohol and cigarette use, and typically have comorbid chronic obstructive lung disease and poor general health. In addition, patients with symptomatic esophageal cancers are typically malnourished at the time of presentation.

The perception of poor postoperative survival and high operative risk created a sense of therapeutic nihilism among medical gastroenterologists, who referred patients for surgery less frequently, preferring instead to use palliative interventions such as endoscopic stenting of symptomatic lesions. Recently, several surgeons have reported their experience using laparoscopic techniques to achieve a minimally invasive surgical approach to esophageal cancer. Endoscopic approaches to esophageal resection offer the ability to perform an en bloc excision of the esophagus and surrounding lymph nodes, preserving the possibility of cure, while minimizing much of the perioperative risk associated with either a laparotomy or thoracotomy.

Oncologic Considerations

At the present time, there remains some controversy regarding the use of laparoscopic techniques in the management of gastrointestinal cancers. Many observers have been concerned about the ability to perform adequate oncologic resections, with surgical margins and a regional lymphadenectomy comparable to open surgery. Other concerns regarding the use of minimally invasive cancer surgery include the poorly understood phenomenon of port site metastases, as well as concerns regarding the effect of the carbon-dioxide pneumoperitoneum environment of cancer biology.[1] Because data on long term outcomes following minimally invasive esophagectomy are sparse, it is prudent to counsel prospective patients regarding the controversies surrounding the use of laparoscopic and thoracoscopic access for esophageal resection.

There are other controversies that are specific to the surgical management of esophageal cancer. Although the optimal extent of resection is debated, there is a general consensus that all tumor-bearing tissue should be removed at surgery (the "R0 resection").[2] The use of neoadjuvant therapy, typically consisting of radiation, cisplatin-based chemotherapy, or both, has been studied by a number of centers with conflicting results (see below). Some authorities recommend the use of neoadjuvant therapy to "downstage" patients with locally advanced (American Joint Committee on Cancer [AJCC] T4) lesions, to convert these cancers into resectable tumors. Controversy also surrounds the optimal operative approach to esophageal cancer (transhiatal, thoracotomy, or minimally invasive). The purpose of this chapter is to describe our technique and indications for minimally invasive esophagectomy, with the understanding that the specific operative approach must be tailored to individual patients, as well as to the experience and preferences of individual surgeons.

Minimally Invasive Resection of Esophageal Cancer

Indications

In addition to the treatment of esophageal malignancies, esophageal resection may also be indicated for some benign conditions such as end-stage esophageal disease due to achalasia, Chagas' disease, severe caustic injury, and severe cases of gastroesophageal reflux disease associated with acquired esophageal shortening and stricture that is refractory to medical treatment. The presence of pathologically well-documented high-grade dysplasia in a segment of Barrett's esophagus is considered a relative indication for esophagectomy.[3] For those who can tolerate the surgery, esophageal resection is indicated in patients with squamous-cell carcinoma or adenocarcinoma of the esophagus that has not invaded other structures (AJCC T0-T3, N0-N1 lesions), and who do not have any distant metastases at diagnosis. This recommendation is made because esophagectomy offers the possibility of cure, as well as the most durable palliation for patients who may be expected to survive more than a few months. Some authorities limit the use of minimally invasive surgery for cancer to esophageal tumors that are confined to the esophageal wall (AJCC T2 or less), and without nodal metastases (AJCC N0).[4]

Patient Preparation

All patients undergo thorough preoperative staging including computed tomographic (CT) evaluation of the thorax and abdomen. Esophagogastroduodenoscopy is performed in all patients, to confirm the pathologic diagnosis of cancer, to determine the size, location and appearance of the lesion, as well as to evaluate the suitability of the stomach and duodenum for a gastric pull-up procedure. Whenever the CT scan suggests invasion of the tracheobronchial tree, bronchoscopy must be performed to determine whether airway structures are invaded.

When permitted by the urgency of operation, pulmonary status should be improved by a combination of chest physiotherapy, smoking cessation prior to surgery, and antibiotic treatment of acute bronchopulmonary infection or heavy sputum production. If malnutrition is severe, a course of preoperative hyperalimentation may restore nutritional reserves, and improve the ability of patients to tolerate esophagectomy. Immediately prior to surgery, all patients receive a standard bowel preparation (in case a colonic interposition is required). Antibiotic wound prophylaxis and anti-embolic measures are routinely used.

Operative Procedures

Staging procedures

The current status of laparoscopic and thoracoscopic staging procedures for esophageal cancer is controversial. Our current practice is to perform a careful laparoscopic examination of the abdomen in patients immediately prior to esophageal resection. We do *not* perform a staging laparoscopy as a separate procedure to determine resectability at a later date. There are several reasons for this. The main advantage of laparoscopic and thoracoscopic staging over other staging modalities (computed tomography, bronchoscopy, endoscopic ultrasonography) is the ability to detect subtle distant metastases, such as peritoneal carcinomatosis and small liver and lung metastases, that are too small to be detected by conventional staging. The presence of distant metastases remains a contraindication to esophageal resection. Since nodal status alone does not, at the current time, affect the determination of the resectability of esophageal cancer, any advantage of laparoscopy or thoracoscopy in ascertaining nodal metastases does not affect treatment decisions.

Pre-operative staging to select patients for neoadjuvant chemotherapy or radiation is not currently recommended for two reasons. First, there is conflicting evidence on whether or not neoadjuvant therapy improves survival.[5-7] Second, even if neoadjuvant therapy is shown to be of benefit, current data suggest that it will likely be recommended either for all patients, or for all symptomatic patients (AJCC T2 lesions or higher). Neither of these criteria is determined based on minimally invasive staging. Therefore, aside from detecting occult metastases, any information obtained from laparoscopic and thoracoscopic staging procedures would not influence (1) the decision to use neoadjuvant therapy, or (2) resectability.

Our procedure for exploratory laparoscopy includes placing the first 10 mm abdominal port for a planned laparoscopic esophagectomy. The abdomen is insufflated, and careful exploration of all visible peritoneal surfaces is carried out to detect peritoneal nodules. Any suspicious lesions are biopsied and sent for histologic examination of frozen sections. If no metastases are identified, additional ports are placed and intraoperative ultrasonography is carried out with particular attention to the liver parenchyma (to detect small metastases), and the celiac and retrogastric lymph nodes. This usually requires opening a window through the gastrocolic omentum into the lesser sac, which should be created along a similar plane of dissection as that to be used for mobilizing the greater curvature of the stomach for the planned esophagectomy (see below).

Laparoscopic Resection of Esophageal Cancer

Both laparoscopic and thoracoscopic approaches use standard endoscopic surgery techniques to replicate either the open transhiatal or Ivor Lewis resections. These minimally invasive techniques require adequate experience and training in both advanced laparoscopy and open esophageal surgery. The surgeon must be able to work with both hands and suture laparoscopically. Instrumentation should include angled laparoscopes, high quality cameras, high flow insuflators and atraumatic GI graspers.

For laparoscopic esophageal surgery, the patient is positioned supine, in slight reverse Trendelenburg position. The neck is extended slightly using a shoulder roll, and the left side of the neck is prepared. Peripheral arterial and central venous access are secured for continuous blood pressure monitoring, and in case pulmonary arterial pressure monitoring is required. Many surgeons prefer endotracheal intubation with a double-lumen tube for single-lung ventilation in case a thoracotomy is required, although we routinely perform thoracoscopic surgery using only a single-lumen endotracheal tube.

Trocars are placed in a similar pattern as that for laparoscopic antireflux surgery, although each trocar should be placed as cephalad as possible to facilitate exposure and dissection in the mediastinum.(Figure 1) Our preference is to place a 10mm port in the left upper abdomen for the laparoscope. One 5 mm port placed in the right upper quadrant is used for a table-mounted self-retaining retractor. The 5 mm port for the surgeon's right-handed instrument port is placed in the left anterior axillary line below the costal margin, and the surgeon's left-handed instrument port is placed in the epigastrium, just to the left of the liver retractor (when it has been secured in place) and inferior to the left lateral segment of the liver. A final 5 mm port for an assistant's instrument is placed approximately halfway between the liver retractor and the laparoscope. During the course of the operation, additional ports may be placed as necessary, and smaller trocars are replaced with 12 mm trocars as needed to accommodate the endoscopic linear stapler.

Mobilization of the stomach is begun by reflecting the first and second portions of the duodenum off of the retroperitoneum. Mobilization of the greater curvature of the stomach begins with the

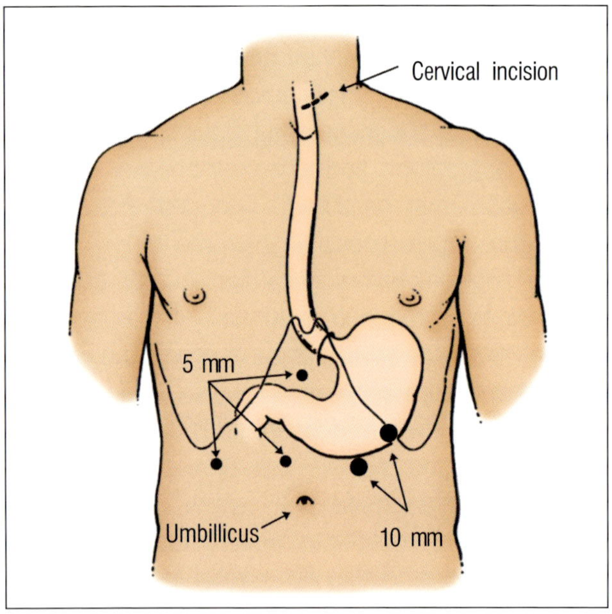

FIGURE 1. Port placement and cervical incision for laparoscopic transhiatal esophagectomy.

short gastric vessels, which are divided up to the level of the left diaphragmatic crus. The greater curvature mobilization is then carefully extended towards the duodenum by dividing the gastrocolic omentum with ultrasonic coagulating shears. Care must be taken to stay outside the right gastroepiploic vascular arcades, and extra caution must be exercised when mobilizing the distal antrum and pylorus to preserve the right gastroepiploic vessels. If communicating branches between the right gastroepiploic vein and the middle colic vein are identified, these should be divided in order to prevent shearing them when the gastric tube is drawn up to the neck. Once a wide retrogastric window has been developed, the liver retractor can be placed under the stomach to elevate it superiorly. Attachments between the posterior stomach and the pancreas, retroperitoneum and transverse mesocolon may be sharply divided with scissors.

The gastrohepatic omentum is divided from the hepatoduodenal ligament to the right crus. The celiac and perigastric lymph nodes are dissected out and removed as a separate path specimen for staging reasons. The left gastric artery may be found by following the small vessels accompanying the hepatic branch of the anterior vagus nerve proximally. This artery is divided using clips, or a linear endoscopic stapler with a vascular cartridge. Exposure and division of the left gastric artery near its origin in the celiac axis is facilitated by retracting the cardia anteriorly and superiorly. When the stomach is completely mobilized, it is divided using serial firings of a liner endoscopic stapler to create a very narrow (<3 cm) gastric tube. The line of division extends from the crow's foot to the apex of the fundus (Figure 2). The distal gastric tube is then placed in the lower abdomen and attention is turned to the esophageal mobilization.

In the case of bulky tumors of the gastroesophageal junction, a cuff of diaphragm including portions of the crura may be taken en bloc with the specimen. Otherwise, the phrenoesophageal ligament is incised circumferentially to gain exposure into the mediastinum. Wide mobilization of the mediastinal esophagus and surrounding tissue is performed by keeping the dissection on the pleural and para-aortic surfaces, sweeping all fat and nodal tissue away from these planes in continuity with the specimen. If necessary, portions of the pericardium, left pleura and right pleura can be excised en bloc with the specimen. Once the dissection has proceeded more than two centimeters above the uppermost extent of the tumor, the periesophageal

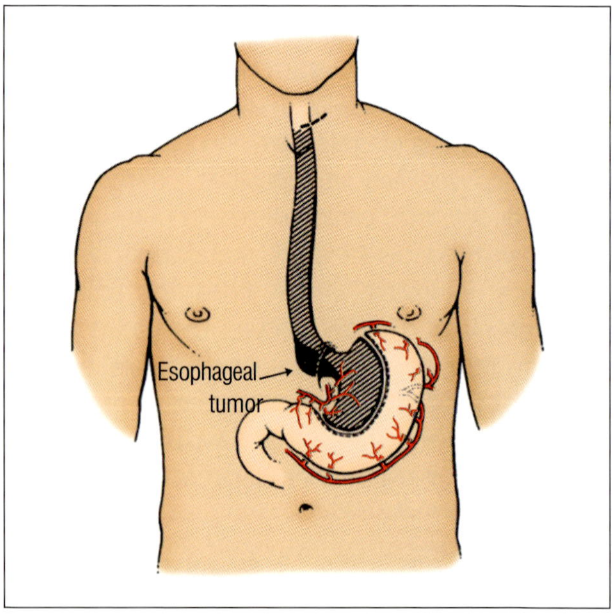

FIGURE 2. Resection lines for distal esophageal cancers should include wide margins and "tubularize" the gastric pullup.

plane may be entered for further esophageal mobilization. The dissection is extended proximally along the adventitia of the esophageal wall to the level of the carina using long (45 cm) laparoscopic instruments. Frequently, exposing the mediastinal esophagus requires one or more adjunct maneuvers, such as widening the hiatus by dividing the crura anteriorly, using a small retractor to elevate the anterior mediastinum, or using a long (or "zoom") laparoscope if available. Retrocardiac manipulation may cause the patient's hemodynamics to become labile, and the surgeon may need to stop periodically to allow the patient's blood pressure to recover. When the mediastinal dissection has been completed to the level of the tracheal bifurcation, one end of a long heavy (0) silk suture is tied securely to the gastric end of the specimen.

The cervical esophagus is exposed according the surgeon's preferred approach. Our preference is to use a 4cm left cervical collar incision. The sternocleidomastoid muscle, carotid artery, and internal jugular vein are retracted, and the omohyoid muscle is divided if necessary. The esophagus is encircled low in the neck, taking care to identify the left recurrent laryngeal nerve. Exposure of the right recurrent laryngeal nerve may be difficult, and keeping the dissection right on the esophageal adventitia will help avoid injury to this nerve. A marking suture is placed on the proximal esophagus, and the esophagus is divided as low as possible in the neck with a right-angled clamp on the distal segment. The upper mediastinal esophagus is dissected bluntly using a small sponge stick. First the posterior and anterior periesophageal planes are developed using gentle blunt dissection until the inferior mediastinal dissection is encountered. The sponge stick can then be used to retract the esophagus anteriorly, and the remaining "lateral stalks" can be divided from below under laparoscopic visualization using ultrasonic coagulating shears.

When the esophageal specimen is completely mobilized it is pulled up through the cervical incision, drawing one end of the heavy silk suture up into the neck incision. The other end of this suture is held in a "locking" grasper so it remains in the abdomen. The suture is cut, and the end is tied tightly to one end of a 24-French chest tube, which is then drawn through the cervical incision into the abdomen by pulling the silk suture from below. The apex of the tubularized stomach is then sutured securely to the chest tube, and is carefully drawn up through the mediastinum into the cervical incision by gently pulling the chest tube up from above, taking care to avoid any twisting of the gastric conduit. The stomach is sutured to the prevertebral fascia, and an esophagogastric anastomosis is performed. Our practice is to create an end-to-side esophagogastrostomy using continuous running monofilament absorbable suture. A closed suction drain is placed in the peripharyngeal space, and the neck incision is closed in layers.

Esophageal surgeons differ on the need for a gastric emptying procedure. If the surgeon's preference is to perform a pyloromyotomy or pyloroplasty, this can be done at this point, or any time after a commitment to resection has been made. Our practice is to avoid a routine gastric emptying procedure by creating a very narrow gastric tube for the conduit, with the expectation that an occasional patient may subsequently require a laparoscopic pyloroplasty as a delayed procedure. The diaphragm should be closed around the gastric tube at the hiatus using interrupted sutures. Finally, a feeding jejunostomy is placed laparoscopically in a segment of small bowel at least 40 cm distal to the ligament of Trietz. A closed suction drain is placed through the hiatus into the mediastinum. The abdomen is irrigated, and hemostasis is assured. All fascial defects 10 mm or larger are sutured closed. Even if the pleural space is entered during the dissection, we do not routinely place chest tubes unless there is evidence of a pulmonary air leak, or extensive thoracoscopic dissection has been performed (see below). Typically, a nasogastric tube is placed in the middle of the gastric pull-up, and is removed if a water-soluble contrast swallow performed on the first or second postoperative day does not demonstrate anastomotic leakage. The diet is then advanced from clear fluids to full fluids, and the cervical and abdominal drains are removed prior to the patient's discharge to home if there is no evidence of a leak.

Combined Thoracoscopic and Laparoscopic Resection of Esophageal Cancer

Some surgeons use a combined thoracoscopic and laparoscopic approach to esophageal resection. Thoracoscopy may be used routinely, in which case it is usually performed prior to the laparoscopic component of the operation. Alternatively, thoracoscopic dissection may be used selectively in difficult cases, such as when the tumor is particularly large, or closely adherent to the membranous trachea and bronchi in which case it may be performed following laparoscopic mobilization of the stomach and distal esophagus.

Thoracoscopy is performed with the patient in the left lateral decubitus position, with an axillary roll. A 10mm port for the thoracoscope is placed in the right seventh intercostal space in the mid-axillary line, and two instrument ports are "triangulated" in position superior and anterior to the telescope. Additional trocars may be added as necessary. Typically at least one additional trocar in the fifth intercostal space on the anterior axillary line will be required. If thoracoscopic esophageal mobilization is performed prior to the laparoscopic part of the procedure, exposure of the distal esophagus is improved by retracting the diaphragm inferiorly with a heavy suture in the central tendon of the right hemidiaphragm brought out through the inferior anterior chest wall.[4]

The mediastinal pleura is incised over the length of the thoracic esophagus, and the azygos vein is divided using clips or a linear endoscopic stapler with a vascular cartridge. The esophagus is mobilized, including all lymph nodes and fat surrounding the esophagus in continuity with the specimen. Once an area of the esophagus has been mobilized circumferentially, it may be encircled with a penrose drain for easier retraction. If thoracoscopic mobilization is done as the first part of a combined procedure, the entire thoracic esophagus with its surrounding lymphatic tissue is mobilized from the thoracic inlet to the diaphragmatic reflection. When the thoracoscopic dissection has been completed, the ports are removed and fascial defects 10mm or larger are closed. A chest tube is usually placed through one of the 10 mm port sites.

Complications

The immediate postoperative complications that occur following minimally invasive esophageal resection are similar to those expected after open surgery. These include cardiac complications such as myocardial infarction, ischemia, and arrhythmias (especially atrial fibrillation), and pulmonary complications such as atelectasis, pleural effusion, and pneumonia. Most of these complications are minimized by endoscopic approaches but some abnormalities are more common after laparoscopic surgery. Small asymptomatic pneumothoraces are frequently detected on routine postoperative chest radiographs, and do not require chest tube drainage if they remain stable and well tolerated. Subcutaneous emphysema may be extensive, but resolves spontaneously in all cases unless there is a persistent pulmonary air leak.

The most important serious complications specific to esophageal resection with cervical esophagogastrostomy are recurrent laryngeal nerve injury, anastomotic leak, anastomotic stricture, and chylothorax. Recurrent laryngeal nerve injuries present with postoperative hoarseness or aspiration. Half of these injuries are temporary neurapraxias, and resolve without specific therapy. Leakage at the cervical esophagogastric anastomosis is usually managed conservatively with drainage of the peripharyngeal space with the closed-suction drain, antibiotics, and enteral nutrition. Strictures can occur early, as a result of ischemia or fibrosis of the anastomosis, or late, in which case recurrent carcinoma must be suspected. Benign strictures are managed with bougienage or balloon dilatation. Most chylothoraces resolve with simple pleural drainage, and occasionally parenteral nutrition. Large-volume chyle leaks may require reoperation to ligate the thoracic duct.

Results

To date, experience with minimally invasive esophagectomy has been limited. Early reports from experienced esophageal surgeons (who are also expert minimally invasive surgeons) suggest that minimally invasive surgery is feasible. Even in the

TABLE 1 Selected "initial" series of laparoscopic and combined laparoscopic-thoracoscopic esophagectomy.

First author, year	Approach	N	Indications	OR time* (min)	ICU stay* (days)	LOS* (days)	Mortality (<30 days)	Complications	Conversion
Nguyen 2000	T+L	18	Cancer 78% Barrett's 11% Stricture 11%	364±73†	6.1±11.3†	11.3±14.2†	0	Anastomotic leak 11% Fistula 6% Respiratory failure 11%	0
Luketich 1998	L 50% T+L 37.5% MT+L 12.5%	8	Cancer 75% Barrett's 12.5% Achalasia 12.5%	460 (267-570) ‡	1.9 (0-7) ‡	13.8 (4-45) ‡	0	Anastomotic leak 12.5% Delayed gastric emptying 12.5%	25%
Swanstrom 1997	L 89% T+L 11%	9	Cancer 67% Barrett's 22% Stricture 11%	390 (285-555) ‡	0.3 (0-2) ‡	6.2 (4-9) ‡	0	Gastric conduit ischemia 11% Hoarseness T/P 67%/0%	0
DePaula 1995	L	12	Cancer 17% Stricture 8% Achalasia 75%	256 (210-370) ‡	-	7.6 (4-15) ‡	0	Anastomotic leak 8% Hoarseness T/P 25%/0 Anastomotic stricture 8%	8%

Abbreviations: ICU intensive care unit, LOS Length of hospital stay, T+L Combined thoracoscopic and laparoscopic surgery, L Laparoscopic surgery only, MT+L Combined minithoracotomy and laparoscopic surgery, T/P Temporary/Permanent
*These values are means †Plus-minus value is the standard deviation ‡Range

earliest of surgeons' experience, conversion to an open surgical approach was uncommon, and morbidity and early mortality were no worse than would be expected following open surgery (Table). Although operative times were typically long, the intensive care unit stay and total duration of hospitalization compared favorably to those seen with open esophagectomy. Data on the long-term outcomes of minimally invasive esophageal resection do not presently exist. Information on survival following minimally invasive esophagectomy for cancer should become available over the next few years.

Conclusion

Minimally invasive esophagectomy is a challenging procedure. For several reasons, we feel that at the present time it should only be performed by surgeons who are expert in difficult laparoscopic esophageal surgery, and who are also experienced in the management of patients with esophageal cancer. The technical components of laparoscopic and thoracoscopic esophageal mobilization are complex, and require the use of at least two sets of "experienced hands." We believe that the first assistant for every procedure must be another surgeon experienced in complex laparoscopic surgery. Laparoscopic esophagectomy should be viewed as an attempt to accomplish esophageal resection with less physiologic insult than open surgery. However, as in all complex minimally invasive procedures, there should be a low threshold for conversion to open surgery if required.

In some cases, thoracoscopic mobilization of the esophagus may be used as an adjunct to a conventional laparotomy for the abdominal portion of the procedure. This may be done to perform a more "precise" open transhiatal esophagectomy, or as an intermediate step to acquire competence in thoracoscopic surgery with the intention of eventually performing a combined laparoscopic-thoracoscopic procedure. It is our belief that minimally invasive esophagectomy is equivalent to open approaches in terms of the ability to perform an adequate oncologic resection. Furthermore, we believe that avoiding a laparotomy and thoracotomy in patients undergoing esophagectomy will result in less operative morbidity and mortality. Even if the oncologic results of open esophagectomy for cancer are no better with less invasive surgery, at least the reduced operative risk of these procedures will make this operation a more acceptable option for patients and referring gastroenterologists.

References

1. Ramshaw BJ. Laparoscopic surgery for cancer patients. Ca Cancer J Clin 1997;47:327-50.
2. Lerut T, Coosemans W, De Leyn P, Van Raemdonck D, Deneffe G, Decker G. Treatment of esophageal carcinoma. Chest 1999;116:463S-5S.
3. Pellegrini CA, Pohl D. High-grade dysplasia in Barrett's esophagus: Surveillance or operation? Journal of Gastrointestinal Surgery 2000;4:131-4.
4. Nguyen N, Schauer PR, Luketich JD. Combined laparoscopic and thoracoscopic approach to esophagectomy. J Am Coll Surg 1999;188:328-32.
5. Walsh TN, Noonan N, Hollywood D, Kelly A, Keeling N, Hennesy TPJ. A comparison of multimodal therapy and surgery for esophageal adenocarcinoma. N Engl J Med 1996; 335: 462-7.
6. Bosset JF, Gignoux M, Triboulet JP et al. Chemoradiotherapy followed by surgery compared with surgery alone in squamous-cell cancer of the esophagus. N Engl J Med 1997; 337: 161-7.
7. Kelsen DP, Ginsberg R, Pajak TF et al. Chemotherapy followed by surgery compared with surgery alone for localized esophageal cancer. N Engl J Med 1998;339:1979-84.
8. Nguyen N, Follette DM, Wolfe BM, Schneider PD, Roberts P, Goodnight JEJ. Comparison of minimally invasive esophagectomy with transthoracic and transhiatal esophagectomy. Arch Surg 2000;135:920-5.
9. Luketich JD, Nguyen N, Weigel T, Ferson P, Keenan R, Schauer P. Minimally invasive approach to esophagectomy. JSLS 1998;2:243-7.
10. Swanstrom LL, Hansen PD. Laparoscopic total esophagectomy. Arch Surg 1997;132:943-9.
11. DePaula AL, Hashiba K, Ferreira EAB, de Paula RA, Grecco E. Laparoscopic transhiatal esophagectomy with esophagogastroplasty. Surgical Laparoscopy and Endoscopy 1995; 5:1-5.

CHAPTER

Video-assisted thoracic surgery in staging of lung cancer

16

X. Jiao, M.J. Krasna

Staging plays a crucial role in the management of primary lung cancer. Currently, both non-invasive and invasive techniques are available for staging procedures. The initial staging of lung cancer typically involves noninvasive evaluation of the chest by chest radiographs, CT scan, or MRI. Although these noninvasive imaging techniques can provide useful information in staging of lung cancer, their sensitivity and specificity are inadequate. More recently, positron emission tomography (PET) has been shown to be highly accurate in determining the malignant or benign nature of lesions, however, it remains to be seen whether one can rely on PET alone, in the absence of histologic diagnosis of determine therapy. With the advent of neoadjuvant therapy in the treatment of locally advanced non-small cell lung cancer (NSCLC), and its apparent effect on long-term survival, preresection pathologic staging of the mediastinum has taken on new importance.[1] So far, only minimally invasive techniques can provide pathologic diagnosis, and these techniques play an important role in staging of lung cancer for clinical trials.

Several minimally invasive techniques including transbronchial fine needle aspiration (TBNA), cervical mediastinoscopy (CM), anterior mediastinotomy, scalene node biopsy, and video-assisted thoracoscopic surgery (VATS) are available for staging of lung cancer. Among them, standard cervical mediastinoscopy (CM) is the classic staging procedure, and it is still the most widely used procedure. It is well tolerated, and can be performed in an outpatient setting with minimal morbidity. This is an important advantage of CM because it does not delay the beginning of systemic therapy once the pathologic diagnosis is established. The efficacy of CM in staging the mediastinum in lung cancer is well established, with a procedural sensitivity of well over 90% and specificity of 100%.[2] It is also a safe procedure. In experienced hands, the morbidity and mortality rates are as low as 0.6% and 0.05%, respectively.[3,4] Although cervical mediastinoscopy is the procedure of choice for invasive staging of lung cancer, it has some limitations. (Table 1) The left upper lobe mass provides a unique challenge for CM staging because the lymphatic drainage includes both the aorto-pulmonary (AP) window and the paratracheal lymph nodes (LN). Standard CM is unable to reach AP window. This problem is usually solved by either extended mediastinoscopy,[5] or mediastinoscopy combined with left mediastinotomy.[6] Such procedures, however, are cumbersome, and may lead to morbidity including wound infection, laceration of the innominate artery, and cerebrovascular accident.[7] CM also has the limitation of inability to evaluate the pleural space or evaluate chest wall invasion. With the development of video-assisted thoracoscopic surgery, this technique has been used for staging of lung cancer, and it provides an exciting alternative staging procedure to compensate for the limitations of CM.

TABLE 1 Comparison of VATS and CM in staging of lung cancer.

	Advantages	Limitations
VATS	• Access to lymph nodes at special locations including AP window (levels 5, 6), posterior subcarina (level 7), and inferior mediastinum (levels 8, 9) • Evaluation of the primary tumor (T stage) to determine resectability and appropriate operation approach; Diagnosis of unknown primary lesion or intrapulmonary metastases • Differetiation diagnosis of pleural effusion found by imaging examinatons; Diagnosis of pleural studding, or "radiographic silent" small malignant pleural effusion; Detection of occult pleural dissemination by VATS-PLC (pleural lavage cytology)	• Need general anesthesia with single-lung ventilation and one-night hospital stay • Unable to access the contralateral mediastinal lymph nodes • Generally need a chest tube
CM	• No need of single-lung ventilation • Can be done in out-clinic setting • Diagnosis of bilateral mediastinal lymph nodes	• Difficult or unable to access AP window (LN5, 6), and inferior mediastinum (LN8, 9) • Difficult or unable to evaluate the local regional invasion of the primary tumor • Unable to detect pleural dissemination

VATS has the advantages of the ability to view and explore the entire hemithorax (hilum, mediastinum, visceral pleura, and chest wall), using limited incisions with low morbidity.[8] The sensitivity and accuracy of the procedure is very high (up to 100%), and is equivalent to open thoracotomy for the purposes of staging of lung cancer.[9,10]

VATS is especially useful in evaluation of left anterior mediastinal lymph nodes of the subaortic nodes (level 5) and para-aortic nodes (level 6). Potential advantages are better visibility (especially of the left phrenic nerve), less wound infection, and a better cosmetic result. It can also provides useful information in a subset of right lower lobe tumors who will develop selective lymph node enlargement in the inferior pulmonary ligament (Level 9). These lymph nodes are not accessible by cervical mediastinoscopy, and can only be sampled by thoracoscopy.

Differential diagnosis of pleural effusion is very difficult in some patients. VATS is the procedure of choice for these patients. It can collect samples of both pleural effusion and suspicious pieces of pleura for cytology and pathology. The efficacy of VATS in diagnosing pleural effusions is well established, and it is especially useful for recurrent undiagnosed pleural effusions.[11,12,13] VATS can also identify malignant pleural effusions too small to be seen on CT. With the aid of pleural lavage cytology (PLC), it can detect occult pleural dissemination before an attempt at resection.[14] This has particular significance because positive PLC is found to indicate subclinical T4 disease, and is associated with poor survival.[15] The detection of such occult pleural dissemination provides a chance for systemic treatment instead of surgery for this subgroup of patients.

So far, most research in preoperative clinical staging has been directed toward determining the status of mediastinal nodes (or the N descriptor), whether diagnosed by mediastinoscopy, CT, or PET scanning. There has been little evaluation of the relative accuracy of staging of the T descriptor. On the contrary, VATS can not only determine the N stage, but also can evaluate the local-regional invasion of the primary tumor (T stage), and subsequently determine the resectability.[16] The routine use of VATS in lung cancer can identify unresectability in 7% of patients (range from 3.3% to 11.9%), and prevent unnecessary exploration thoracotomy or unrewarding resection in this subgroup of patients.[17,18,19]

Complications of VATS vary according to the type and extent of procedure performed and include pneumothorax, air embolism, bleeding, lung injury, and implantation of tumor cells.[20] The overall complications rate is 14%, and the rate of complications leading to emergency thoracotomy is around 1% to

3%. The mortality rate is 0% to 4.5% depending on the patient's medical condition and the specific procedure done.[10]

Surgical techniques

We have described the techniques of thoracoscopic staging in our previous publications.[17,21,22,23] In general, VATS staging is performed under gerneral anesthesia, using a double-lumen endotracheal tube. The patient is placed in the lateral decubitus position and is prepared as for standard thoracotomy. Placing the patient in Trendelenburg position also improves exposure. A 10 mm trocar cannula is inserted through the sixth intersoctal space in the posterior axillary line. An operating thoracoscope is used to rule out malignant pleural effusion or pleural implants first. The use of CO_2 inflation may facilitate decompression of the lung and improve visibility. This can be done safely with low flows and low pressures.[24] Having explored the hemithorax, two additional incisions are then made, one in the third intercostals space in the midclavicular line and the other in the seventh intercostals space in the anterior axillary line in the line of a future thoracotomy. The three ports are thus placed in a "baseball diamond" configuration. Such triangular orientation of ports can greatly facilitate the sampling of mediastinal lymph nodes (Figure 1, 2). A further systematic exploration of the chest should be performed to search for metastatic nodules on the parietal pleura, pericardium, or diaphragm. The lung should be examined for synchronous lesions and also for iatrogenic injury from the trocar insertion. Efforts should be made to differentiate benign adesion from local regional invasion to chest wall and mediastinal structures, and subsequently to determine resectability. Presence of effusion should be noted and fluid sent for cytologic analysis. Pleural lavage cytology can also be performed for detection of occult pleural dissemination at this point. Lymph nodes are then biopsied. At the end of the procedure, a single 28F chest tube is placed through the

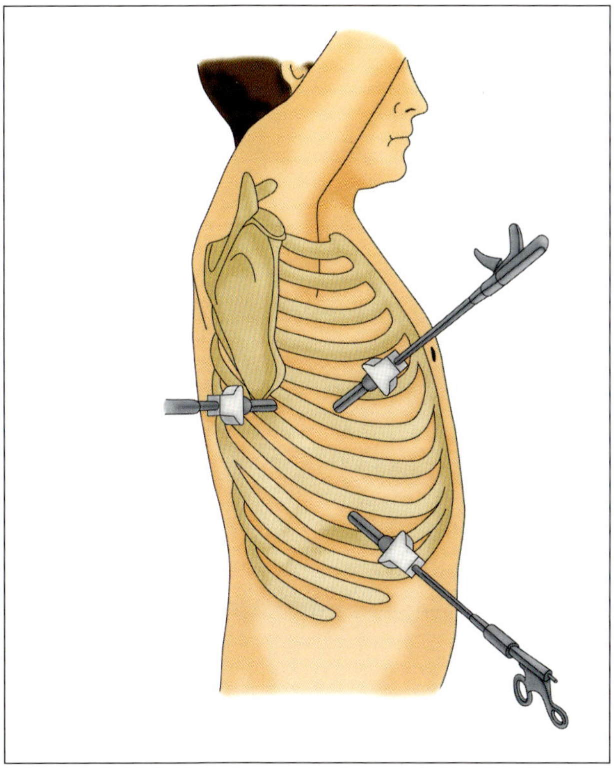

FIGURE 1. Port sites for right thoracoscopic staging for lung cancer.

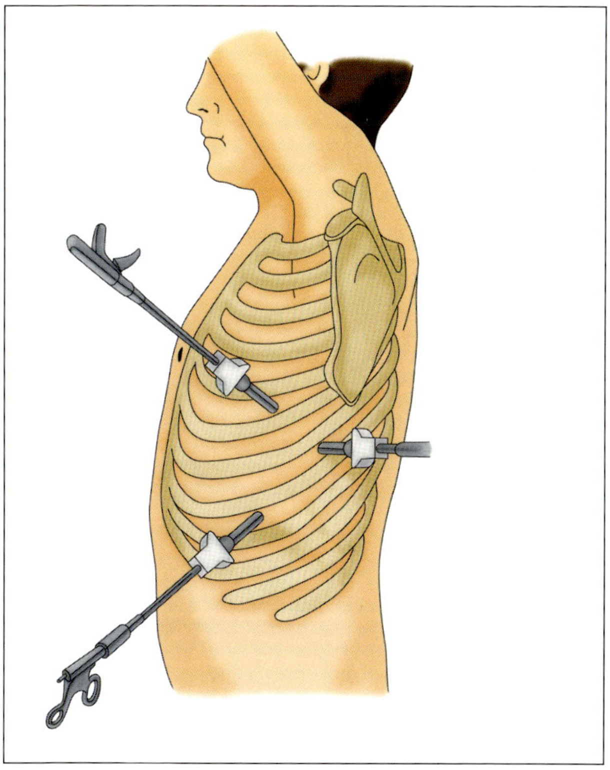

FIGURE 2. Port sites for left thoracoscopic staging for lung cancer.

most inferior trocar site for drainage. The thoracoscope confirms that the chest tube is placed posteriorly for optimal drainage and that incisions are hemostatic. Two-lung ventilation should then be resumed and the ipsilateral lung inspected for full re-expansion.

Right-sided lymph node dissection

Lymph node dissection on the right requires adequate exposure of the right paratracheal area, which requires mobilization of the azygos vein. This provides access to the level 2 and level 4 nodes superior to the azygos vein and also to level 10 nodes that are inferior to the azygos vein. Additionally, the subcarinal (level 7), paraesophageal (level 8), and inferior pulmonary ligament (level 9) nodes should be sampled for complete staging. An inverted pyramid arrangement of 3 ports provides the access to all of these nodes after initial exploration shows no metastases. For dissection of the subazygos region the right lung is collapsed and the apex of the superior segment of the lower lobe or posterior segment of the upper lobe is grapsed with a Duval-type lung retractor. The retractor is pulled anteriorly to expose the azygos region. It is best to insert the retractor through the lowest port. A grasper is used to lift up the mediastinal pleura over the azygos vein. The mediastinal pleura is dissected by using of a cautery scissors, and the azygos arch is skeletonized. It can then be divided with an endoscopic vascular stapler if additional exposure is necessary. The mediastinal pleura is again incised inferior to the arch down to the level of the inferior pulmonary ligament, exposing the carinal bifucation and subcarinal lymph nodes in this region. When taking biopsy of the subcarinal lymph nodes (level 7), it is often necessary to clip or ligate small bronchial artery branches. The mediastinal fat under the azygos arch and all of the lymph nodes in this region are then sharply dissected and the nodes removed with clips to ensure hemostasis.

Left-sided lymph node dissection

The left chest is explored and the phrenic and vagus nerves are followed from the apex inferiorly to the point where they cross the pulmonary artery and form the triangle. Enlarged lymph nodes are easily identified in the AP window. The remainder of the hemithorax is examined for any evidence of gross metastatic disease and the extent of direct spread of the pulmonary tumor is evaluated. A Babcock/Allis-type grasper is used to elevate the mediastinal pleura overlying the lymph nodes and an electrocautery probe is used to incise the pleura. The lymph nodes are bluntly dissected from the surrounding connective tissue and the vascular pedicle is ligated with an endoscopic clip applier. The clip applier can be used as a dissecting instrument as well. The nodes are removed and the area irrigated with saline solution. Dissection of the inferior pulmonary ligament is undertaken next. The basal segments of the lower lobe are grasped with an atraumatic endoscopic lung grasper (Duval-type retractor), and are retracted apically and toward the chest wall. The inferior pulmonary ligament is sharply incised with scissors, and the cautery attachement is used to ensure hemostasis. The lymph nodes are biopsied after the dissection.

Summary

CM remains the most sensitive and most specific way of pathologic staging of the mediastinum. VATS has the advantage that it can provide both N stage and T stage information. It is especially usefully in staging of tumor located in left upper lobe, and in evaluation of resectability before operation. Currently, the main indications of VATS in staging of lung cancer include: 1. Diagnosis of mediastinal lymph node metastases in special areas including the AP window, posterior-subcarina, and inferior mediastinum, or in patiens who are not able to undergo mediastinoscopy (status post tracheostomy, status post mediastinoscopy, severe cervical kyphosis, etc.); 2. Diagnosis of unknown pulmonary lesions, or evaluation of the tumor invasion to the chest wall, the main mediastinal structures, and pleural space dissemination (combined with VATS-PLC); 3. Routine use in all patients before resection to determine the resectability and appropriate surgical approach. Nevertheless, VATS and CM can be used as complementary procedures to provide tissue biopsies for diagnosis and staging information. The appropriate application of these techniques can improve diagnostic accuracy while limiting surgical morbidity. Whether using one technique alone or using them in combination should be determined based on the individual's clinical characteristics, imaging examinations, and the treatment protocol requirements.

References

1. Krasna MJ, Reed CE, Nugent WC, et al. Lung cancer staging and treatment in multidisciplinary trials: Cancer and Leukemia Group B cooperative group approach. Ann Thorac Surg 1999; 68:201-7
2. Park BJ, Louie O, Altorki N. Staging and the surgical management of lung cancer. Radiol Clin North Am 2000;38:545-61
3. Hammoud ZT, Anderson RC, Meyers BF, et al: The current role of mediastinoscopy in the evaluation of thoracic disease. J Thorac Cardiovasc Surg 1999;118:894-899
4. Goldstraw P. Mediastinal exploration by mediastinoscopy and mediastinotomy Br J Dis Chest. 1988;82:111-20.
5. Ginsberg RJ, Rice TW, Goldberg M, et al. Extended cervical mediastinoscopy: a single staging procedure for bronchial carcinoma of the left upper lobe. J Thorac Cardiovasc Surg 1987;94:673-678
6. Jiao X, Magistrelli P, Goldstraw P. The value of cervical mediastinoscopy combined with anterior mediastinotomy in the preoperative evaluation of bronchogenic carcinoma of the left upper lobe. Eur J Cardiothorac Surg. 1997;11:450-4.
7. Urschel JD, Vretenar DF, Dickout WJ, Nakai SS. Cerebrovascular accident complicating extended cervical mediastinoscopy. Ann Thorac Surg. 1994;57:740-1
8. Rendina EA, Venura F, DeGiaconio T, et al: Comparative merits of thoracoscopy, mediastinoscopy, and mediastinotomy for mediastinal biopsy. Ann Thorac Surg. 1994;57:992-5
9. Champion JK, McKernan JB. Comparison of minimally invasive thoracoscopy versus open thoracotomy for staging lung cancer. Int Surg 1996;81:235-6
10. Bogot NR, Shaham D. Semi-invasive and invasive procedures for the diagnosis and staging of lung cancer II. Bronchoscopic and surgical procedures. Radiol clin North Am 2000;38:535-44
11. Boutin C, Rey F, Gouvernet J, et al. Thoracoscopy in pleural malignant mesothelioma: A prospective study of 188 consecutive patients. Part 2: Prognosis and staging. Cancer 1993; 72: 394-404
12. Menzies R, Charbonneau M: Thoracoscopy for the diagnosis of pleural disease. Ann Intern Med 1991;114:271-6
13. Sharma S, D'Cruz A: Thoracoscopy in the diagnosis of pleural effusion of ambiguous etiology. J Surg Oncol 1991;48:133-5
14. Roberts JR, Blum MG, Arildsen R, Drinkwater DC, Christian KR, Powers TA, Merrill WH. Prospective comparison of radiologic, thoracoscopic, and pathologic staging in patients with early non-small cell lung cancer. Ann Thorac Surg. 1999; 68: 1154-8
15. Jiao X, Krasna MJ. Clinical significance of micrometastasis in lung and esophageal cancer: A new paradigm in thoracic surgery. Ann Thorac Surg. 2001, in press
16. De Giacomo T, Rendina EA, Venuta F, Della Rocca G, Ricci C. Thoracoscopic staging of IIIb non-small cell lung cancer before neoadjuvant therapy. Ann Thorac Surg 1997;64:1409-11
17. Sonett JR, Krasna MJ. Thoracoscopic staging for intrathoracic malignancy. In Yim AP, Hazelrigg SR, Izzat MB et al eds. Minimal access cardiothoracic surgery. W.B. Saunders Company 2000
18. Roviaro GC, Varoli F, Rebuffat C, et al. Videothoracoscopic operative staging for lung cancer. Int Surg 1996;81:252-254
19. Roberts JR, Matthew GB, Arildsen R, et al. Prospective comparison of radiologic, thoracoscopic, and pathologic staigng in patients with early non-small cell lung cancer. Ann Thorac Surg 1999;68:1154-8
20. Nakamoto K, Maeda M, Okamoto T, et al. Preoperative diagnosis with video-assisted thoracoscopy with miniaturized endoscopes in general thoracic surgery. Chest. 1998;114:1749-1755
21. Krasna MJ. Introduction to thoracoscopic surgery: Indications, basic techniques and instrumentation. In Cuschieri A, MacFadyen BV eds: Seminars in Laparoscopic Surgery. Philadelphia, WB Saunders. 1996;3:201-210
22. Krasna MJ, McLaughlin JS: Efficacy and safety of thoracoscopy for diagnosis and treatment of intrathoracic disease: The University of Maryland experience. Sur Laparosc Endosc. 1994;4:182-188
23. Krasna MJ, Mack MJ. Lymph node dissection and staging. In Krasna MJ, Mack MJ eds: Atlas of Thoracoscopic Surgery. Quality Medical Publishing, Inc., St. Louis, Missouri, 1994
24. Wolfer RD, Krasna MJ, Hasnain JU, et al. Hemodynamic effects of carbon dioxide insufflation during thoracoscopy. Ann Thorac Surg 1994;58:404-408

CHAPTER

Video-assisted thoracic surgery in the management of pulmonary metastases

17

X. Jiao, M.J. Krasna

The lung is the second most frequent site of metastases after the liver. Almost 30% of patients who have curative resection of a malignancy will develop pulmonary metastases.[1] Despite advances in systemic therapies for lung metastases, these modalities have yet to provide consistent long-term survival rates in patients with documented lung metastases. Surgical resection has come to be accepted as standard treatment for patients with isolated pulmonary metastases. Although no prospective studies have ever been performed to clearly assess the benefit of pulmonary metastasectomy, there is an abundance of retrospective data that indicates long term survival benefits of complete pulmonary metastasectomy over historical controls without resection. The general criteria in selecting patients for pulmonary metastasectomy is well established. Standard criteria for therapeutic metastasectomy include local control of the primary tumor or ability to completely resect the primary with synchronous presentations; radiological findings consistent with metastatic disease; absence of extrathoracic metastases; ability to perform a complete resection of the metastases; no significant comorbidity that would preclude surgery; no alternative therapy that is superior to surgery.[2] Using these criteria with the open pulmonary resection technique, either unilateral or bilateral, long-term survival rates of 30% to 58% can be achieved for patients with soft tissue and osteogenic sarcomas respectively,[3,4] with a 0.8% overall mortality, and only 0.5% mortality in the subset of solitary lesions less than 2 cm diameter treated by sublobar resection.[5] Many factors may affect the survival after metastasectomy. These include tumor doubling time, the histology of the primary tumor, number of lung metastatic lesions (solitary versus multiple), disease-free interval, nodal status, and complete resectability. Among them, the most important prognostic indicator, as well as the most constant single variable reflecting prolonged post-thoracotomy survival, is complete resectability of pulmonary metastases.

Surgical approaches and resection techniques for pulmonary metastases include median sternotomy, trans-sternal bilateral (clamshell) thoracotomies, posterolateral thoracotomy, and more recently, video-assisted thoracic surgery (VATS). The choice of approach depends on the individual patient, tumor histology, number of lesions, location of nodules, and laterality of the disease. Each approach is associated with various advantages and disadvantages (Table 1). If all metastases are resected, however, patient survival is not influenced by the choice of incisions.[6]

Although open surgery has been the standard approach to pulmonary metastasectomy, with the advances of video equipment and endoscopic instruments, VATS has realized an expanded role in the diagnosis and management of solitary pulmonary metastasis in recent years. The first case of

TABLE 1 Advantages and limitations of different surgical approaches for pulmonary metastasectomy.

Approaches	Advantages	Limitations
Median Sternotomy	• Bilateral thoracic explorations with one incision • Less pain	• Difficult in exposure and resection of posterior lesions, medial lesions, and especially lesions in left lower lobe • Contraindicated to patients with radiation therapy, diabetes, obesity, chronic obstructive pulmonary disease, previous median sternotomy, etc.
Posterolateral Thoracotomy	• Standard approach to the hemithorax • Excellent exposure	• Unable to explore the contralateral lung • Increased postoperative pain
Extended thoracotomy (Clamshell or hemi-clamshell)	• Bilateral exploration • Excellent exposure of lower lobe as well as mediastinum	• Sacrifice of the internal mammary artery • Increased pain and discomfort
Video-Assisted Thoracic Surgery (VATS)	• Excellent visualization of pleural surfaces • Minimal morbidity and discomfort • Short hospital stay • Excellent cosmetic results	• Difficult or unable to bimanually palpate lung parenchyma • Increased risk of incomplete resection • Need special endoscopic instruments • Difficulty in resection of deep lesions or big lesions (>3 cm)

a thoracoscopic pulmonary metastasectomy was reported by Dowling and associates in 1992,[7] followed by their first large series using VATS to perform metastasectomy in 1993.[8] Since then, studies on the role of VATS in diagnosis and treatment of pulmonary metastases have been performed world widely with cautious enthusiasm.

The role of VATS in diagnosis of pulmonary metastases

At the time of presentation, an isolated pulmonary nodule does not necessarily represent the systemic or untreatable spread of a primary neoplasm. It must first be diagnosed as a metastasis, a primary neoplasm, or other primary pathology. Although current imaging techniques can provide initial diagnostic information, their accuracy is questionable. The most commonly used imaging technique, computed tomography (CT), rarely detects lung lesions greater than 3 mm in diameter and occasionally misses larger lesions, whereas central lesions may be obscured by the pulmonary vasculature. Spiral CT overcomes several disadvantages of conventional CT, because continuous transport of the patient through the scanner allows rapid acquisition of CT data. Within the scanned volume, spiral CT provides complete contiguity of slices, improving diagnostic accuracy and reducing the need for repeat scans. Spiral CT as an imaging modality for pulmonary metastasectomy appears to yield more detail than standard CT. It can significantly detect more lesions than conventional CT, and is regarded as the technique of choice for assessing pulmonary metastases.[9,10] High-resolution positron emission tomography (PET) is a technique that can usually distinguish benign from malignant processes.[11,12] The current applications of PET in oncology include characterizing tumor lesions, differentiating recurrent disease form treatment effects, tumor staging, evaluating the extent of disease, and monitoring therapy.[13] When assessing the resectability of pulmonary metastases, PET may prove particularly useful in excluding other sites of metastatic disease. Another significant benefit of FDG-PET in evaluating chest masses is its high negative predictive value.[14]

Despite the development of imaging techniques,

tissue diagnosis remains the final and important diagnostic method, as the presence of metastatic disease will provide information about the adequacy of previous or ongoing treatment and often dictate further therapy. VATS provides an ideal minimally invasive approach for this purpose. The role of VATS in "diagnostic" resections has been well accepted. It has been proved to be safe and efficacious for the evaluation of primary indeterminate nodules, as well as for evaluation of pulmonary nodules in patients with a previous malignant condition. VATS for excisional biopsy has a sensitivity and specificity approaching 100%.[15,16,17,18] Currently, VATS biopsy may be indicated for diagnostic intention when conventional methods (percutaneous or transbronchial needle biopsy) are unsuccessful or if the lesion is a small discrete lesion in the peripheral lung parenchyma. Also, under appropriate circumstances, it may be therapeutic and diagnostic in that the nodules can be completely excised.[19]

The role of VATS in the treatment of pulmonary metastases

In the 1990s, advances in endoscopic surgical instrumentation and refinements in VATS provided surgeons the ability to perform VATS parenchyma-sparing wedge resections for peripheral lung lesions. Since most metastatic disease to the lung is found peripherally in the outer third,[20] these lesions are often amenable to VATS wedge resection. The clinical criteria for VATS metastasectomy are similar to that for open approach. In addition, the lesion must be in the peripheral one third of the lung parenchyma and be no larger than 3 cm in diameter for VATS resection. Ideally, there should only be 1 or 2 metastatic lesions to be resected, although resection of higher numbers of lesions have been achieved. Multiple lesions generally need thoracotomy to assure complete resection of all tumors. An additional application of VATS in pulmonary metastasectomy is that it can be used to assisted median sternotomy. In this setting, VATS offers increased exposure by visualizing the retrocardiac left lower lobe.[21]

The advantage of thoracoscopic removal of solitary metastases is the limited surgical trauma, which results in an improved postoperative recovery, shorter hospital stay, and decreased long-term morbidity. These effects, however, should be counterbalanced by the risk of incomplete resection of metastatic disease that is assured by thoracotomy and direct palpation.[22,23,24] McCormack and associates demonstrated that without manual palpation, the probability of missing occult metastases during VATS procedures is very high.[25] Nevertheless, this study is questioned given the technique of conventional CT scanning they used. It makes sense that, with the development of newer imaging techniques including spiral CT and positron emission tomography (PET), more small nodules that are usually occult with conventional chest x-ray examination or CT scan will be found and located before resection. This will greatly facilitate VATS resection and decrease the risk of missing nodules.

Surgical techniques

The surgical techniques are similar to the standard VATS procedure. Resection types include stapled wedge resection, laser eradication, or occasionally major lobectomy. Generally, a 1-cm gross margin is required during resection to assure complete resection and minimize excision of normal lung tissue. Due to the close gross surgical margins obtained with wedge excision, the staple line should be confirmed to be free of disease by pathology. Handling of the lesion itself should be kept to a minimum, and the stapling device must be carefully applied to avoid crushing or dividing the lesion. Trocars should be routinely used, and a retrieval device such as a sterile glove or a commercially produced retrieval bag should be implemented to reduce to possibility of "seeding" the intercostals access site, although it's a rare complication.[26,27,28] Conversion to thoracotomy is indicated when lesions identified preoperatively are not found or when technical problems encountered may compromise surgical margins when resecting lung metastases for potential cure.

Since it is difficult to do a complete instrument palpation of the pulmonary parenchyma with the VATS approach, several techniques to locate small or deeply seated lesions before or during the operation have been developed to overcome this limitation. Preoperative CT-guided needle localization and methylene blue injection or the introduction of a hooked-wire can be performed under the radiological vision before surgery.[29,30,31,32] Marking the lesions under the CT-scan with water-soluble barium sulfate or 99m Tc-labeled human serum albumn microspheres were also found to be helpful.[33,34] Intraoperative ultrasound is another safe and effective method in detection of invisible or nonpalpable pulmonary nodules at the time of thoracoscopy.[35,36] All these methods may help surgeons perform minimally invasive lung resections with clear surgical margins. More recently, Mineo TC and associates developed a unique transxiphoid approach that allows bilateral manual palpation of the lung at VATS metastasectomy.[37] They found that this approach can facilitates bilateral VATS metastasectomy, and can find occult metastases. With this method, they found that even with helical computed tomography, occult metastases may still be identified in about one-third of the patients by bilateral palpation.[38] However, the real prognostic value of the resection of these occult additional lesions is as yet undefined.

Results of VATS pulmonary metastasectomy

An early report by Yim and associates demonstrated a high rate of early recurrence following VATS pulmonary metastasectomy. The result led them to conclude that VATS should not be used for therapeutic metastasectomy.[39] However, their conclusion was limited by the small size of the group (7 patients), the short term of follow-up, and unfavorable VATS candidates (multiple lesions or bilateral lesions). The histologic type may also have contributed to the high recurrence rate since patients with metastatic osteogenic sarcomas have a high risk of recurrence even after open pulmonary metastasectomy.[40]

With careful patient selection for VATS pulmonary metastasectomy, based on high-resolution spiral CT scanning, survival comparable to that of open procedures has been reported with shorter hospital stay and less postoperative pain. In an international multi center study, Lin et al reported that with the VATS technique, resection of peripheral pulmonary metastases for diagnostic (78 patients) and potentially curative (99 patients) intentions appeared comparable to historical results by "open" thoracotomy.[18] In this study, the vast majority of recurrent disease (69%) occurred distant from the site of the first lung metastases, while 26% of recurrences developed within the ipsilateral hemithorax but away from the site of the original metastasis; only 5% had local recurrence that would be attributed to technical failure to clear the tumor sufficiently by VATS. This may suggest that the biology of the tumor, rather than the surgical technique, may predispose the patient to a more disseminated course. The concern about the inability to bimanually palpate the lung to search for lesions "missed" by CT seems unsubstantiated by this pattern of recurrent disease.

The risk of missing lesions in VATS resection seems to be lower in patients with solitary lesion on preoperative CT scan. Mutsaerts and associate compared thoracoscopic pulmonary metastasectomy with confirmatory thoracotomy. They found that with a VATS resection, a complete resection rate of 92% was achieved in patients with one lesion, while it dropped to 20% in patients with more than one lesion by preoperative CT scan. They concluded that VATS is a viable treatment option for patients who present with a solitary pulmonary metastasis with a diameter of 3 cm or less.[41] Other studies on colorectal pulmonary metastases also support this conclusion. Giacomo et al reported a 5-year survival 49.5% in patients with solitary lung metastases from colorectal cancer with thoracoscopic resection, which is similar to the data in the literature. The incidence of local recurrence after thoracoscopic metastasectomy (21.7%) is similar or even lower than observed after the open approach.[42] Watanabe et al also found that thoracoscopic resection of one or two colorectal cancer lung metastases resulted in a survival rate similar to standard thoracotomy.[43] Landreneau et al recently reported a series of 80 patients with colorectal pulmonary metastases who underwent VATS resection. The majority of patients (60) had solitary lesions and 20 patients had multiple lesions (2-7). Thin cut computed tomography (CT) was used to identify lesions. The 5-year survival was 30.8%. The mean survival of patients with one lesion was longer than that of patients with multiple lesions (34.8 vs. 26.5 months), although the difference was not significant (P = 0.37). Sixty-nine percent of patients developed a recurrence: 8% local, 24% regional, and 38% distant.[44] Their results suggest that with careful patients selection with high resolution CT scan, therapeutic pulmonary metastasectomy may result in a survival that is comparable to open resection.

Generally, the morbidity of VATS pulmonary metastasectomy is very low, although complications may include atelectasis, pneumonia, air leak lasting more than 1 week, and failure to resect all metastases, leaving positive margins or pleural seeding or port seeding with extraction of the metastasis.[6] No mortality associated with the VATS technique in pulmonary metastasectomy has been reported, but conversion to open thoracotomy may occasionally be needed when lesions identified preoperatively are not found or when technical problems encountered may compromise surgical margins when resecting lung metastases for potential cure.

General considerations and future study

The role of VATS in the diagnosis of pulmonary metastases is well established, while its role in the treatment of pulmonary metastases remains less defined. Studies on VATS resection of colorectal pulmonary metastases demonstrated that VATS is an effective and less invasive approach. A survival comparable to that of open procedure can be expected, especially in patients with solitary nodule or no more than 2 lesions. However, its application to patients with other primary malignancies remains unclear, and its application in patients with multiple or bilateral lesions has been a controversial issue.

An argument against VATS pulmonary mastastectomy is that it's difficult or impossible to palpate pulmonary parenchyma with VATS procedure, and consequently may increase the risk of incomplete resection because additional lesions which are "radiographic silent" can often be found by intraoperative palpation of the lung with open thoracotomy. Nevertheless, there is no evidence that resection of pulmonary metastases at the time that they become radiographically apparent is any less efficacious than open procedures that remove all nodules, benign and malignant, before their radiological identification.[45,46]

Although routine mediastinal lymph node dissection accompanying pulmonary metastasectomy is not an accepted standard curative concept in patients with pulmonary metastases, some recent studies support radical lymphatic dissection since lymph node metastasis was found to be associated with high risk of local recurrence and poor survival.[47,48,49] These results remind us of another argument against the resection of pulmonary metastases by video-assisted techniques since it is difficult to do radical lymphatic dissection with VATS. Another concern is the increasing risk of circulating tumor cell dissemination during VATS resection. Yamashita and associates demonstrated that VATS might increase the circulating tumor cells in lung cancer resection.[50] This may be partly due to the more frequent and stronger retraction and manipulation of the pulmonary lobes containing the tumor on all sides by forceps to attain better fields of vision during video-assisted lobectomy. Whether it is true in pulmonary metastases resection is unknown, although theoretically, the likelihood is low because usually a simple stapled wedge resection is done without too much manipulation of the lung and the lesion. Finally, one should be very cautious about the real benefit to be expected from VATS metastasectomy. Kirby et al compared VATS lobectomy and muscle-sparing thoracotomy in lung cancer patients in a randomized trial, and found no differences between the groups regarding operating time, intraoperative blood loss, duration of chest tube drainage, or length of hospital stay, although more postoperative complications occurred in the thoracotomy group.[51]

In summary, the role of VATS in diagnosis of pulmonary metastases is well established, while its role in treatment of pulmonary metastases is still controversial, especially in patients with in patients with multiple or bilateral lesions. Only a prospective randomized trial may determine the efficiency and eligibility of VATS in the management of pulmonary metastases. Unfortunately, a recent prospective randomized trial to compare open resection (thoracotomy or median sternotomy) to minimally invasive (video-assisted) resection was ceased prematurely due to poor accrual.[52] Nevertheless, with the development of imaging and lesion location techniques, as well as the new surgical techniques and endoscopic instruments, VATS may find its role in therapeutic resection for lung metastasis.

References

1. Roberts DG, Lepore V, Cardllo G, etal. Long-term follow-up of operative treatment for pulmonary metastases. Eur J Cardiothorac Surg 1989;3:292-6
2. Rusch VW. Pulmonary metastasectomy: current indications. Chest 1995;107:322s-31s
3. Putnam JB, Roth JA. Surgical treatment for pulmonary metastases from sarcoma. Hematol Oncol Clin North Am 1995;9:869-887
4. Pastorino U, Gasparini M, Tavecchio L, Azzarelli A, Mapelli S, Zucchi V, et al. The contribution of salvage surgery to the management of childhood osteosarcoma. J Clin Oncol 1991;9:1357-1362
5. Pastorino U. Commentary. Eur J Cardio-thorac Surg 1999;16:s15-s16
6. Zwischenberger JB, Alpard SK. Resection for pulmonary metastases. In Yim AP, Hazelrigg SR, Izzat MB et al ed. Minimal access cardiothoracic surgery. W.B. Saunders Company 2000
7. Dowling RD, Wachs ME, Ferson PF, et al. Thoracoscopic Nd:YAG laser resection of a pulmonary metastasis. Cancer 1992;70:1873-75
8. Dowling RD, Keenan RJ, Ferson PF, et al. Video assisted thoracoscopic surgery of pulmonary metastases. Ann Thorac Surg 1993;56:772-75
9. Kauczor HU, Hnasen M, Schweden F, et al. Computerized tomography in diagnosis of lung metastases: Improvement with the spiral technique. Radiology 1994;34:569-575
10. Collie DA, Wright AR, Williams JR, et al. Comparison of spiral-acquisition computed tomography and conventional computed tomograhpy in the assessment of pulmonary metastatic disease. Br J Radiol 1994;67:436-444
11. Kubota K, Matsuzawa T, Fujiwara T, et al. Differential diagnosis of lung tumor with positron emission tomography: A prospective study. J Nucl Med 1990;31:1927-1932
12. Strauss LG, Conti PS. The applications of PET in clinical oncology. J Nucl Med 1991;32:623-648
13. Hoh CK, Schiepers C, Seltzer MA, et al. PET in oncology: Will it replace the other modalities? Semin Nucl Med 1997;27:94-106
14. Hubner KF, Buonocore E, Singh SK, et al. Characterizatrion of chest masses by FDG positron emission tomography. Clin Nuci Med 1995;20:293-298
15. DeCamp MM Jr, Jaklitsch MT, Mentzer SJ, et al. The safety and versatility of video-thoracoscopy: A prospective analysis of 895 consecutive cases. J Am Coll Surg 1995;181:165-167
16. Mack MJ, Hazelrigg SR, Landreneau RJ, et al. Thoracoscopy for the diagnosis of the indeterminate solitary pulmonary nodule. Ann Thorac Surg 1993;56:830-832
17. Mitruka S, Landreneau RJ, Mack MJ, et al. Diagnosing the indeterminate pulmonary nodule: Percutaneous biopsy versus thoracoscopy. Surgery 1995;118:676-684
18. Lin JC, Wiechmann RJ, Szwerc MF, Hazelrigg ST, et al. Diagnostic and therapeutic video-assisted thoracic surgery resection of pulmonary metastases. Surgery 1999;126:636-42
19. Greelish JP, Friedberg JS. Secondary pulmonary malignancy. Surg Clin N Am 2000;80:633-657
20. Crow J, Slavin G, Kreel L. Pulmonary metastasis: A pathologic and radiologic study. Cancer 1981;47:2595-2601
21. Hazelrigg SR, Naunheim K, Auer JE, et al. Combined median sternotomy and video-assisted thoracoscopic resection of pulmonary metastases. Chest 1993;104:956-958
22. Hazelrigg SR, Nunchuck SK, Landreneau RJ, et al. Cost analysis for thoracoscopy: thoracoscopic wedge resection. Ann Thorac Surg 1993;56:633-5
23. Landreneau RJ, Wiechmann RJ, Hazerigg SR, et al. Effect of minimally invasive thoracic surgical approaches on acute and chronic postoperative pain. Chest Surg Clin N Am. 1998;8:891-906
24. Forster R, Heinecke A, Leschber G, et al. Thoracoscopy versus thoracotomy. The dilemma of the comparison and its meaning for quality assurance in thoracic surgery. Zentralbl Chir. 1999;124:120-7
25. McCormack P, Bains MS, Begg CB, et al. Role of video-assisted thoracic surgery in the treatment of pulmonary metastases: Results of a prospective trial. Ann Thorac Suge 1996;62:213-217
26. Downey RJ, McCormack P, LoCicero J. Dissemination of malignant tumors after video-assisted thoracic surgery. J Thorac Cardiovasc Surg 1996;111:954-60
27. Mutsaerts EL, Zoetmulder FA, Rutgers EJ. Port site metastasis as a complication of thoracoscopic metastasectomy. Eur J Surg Oncol 2001;27:327-8
28. Parekh K, Rusch V, Bains M, et al. VATS port site recurrence: a technique dependent problem. Ann Surg Oncol 2001;8:175-8
29. Landreneau RJ, Mack MJ, Hazelrigg SR, et al. Video assisted thoracic surgery: basic technical concepts and intercostals approach strategies. Ann Thorac Surg 1992;54:800-7
30. Mack MJ, Shennib H, Landreneau RJ, Hazelrigg SR. Techniques for localization of pulmonaryu nodules for thoracoscopic resection. J Thorac Cardiovasc Surg 1993;106:550-3
31. Templeton P, Krasna MJ. Needle/wire lung nodule localization for thoracoscopic resection. Chest 1993;104:953-954
32. Shah RM, Spim PW, Salazar AM, et al. Localization of peripheral pulmonary nodules for thoracoscopic excision: Value of CT-guided wire placement. AJR Am J Roentgenol. 1993; 161: 279-283

33. Moon SW, Wang YP, Jo KH, et al. Fluoroscopy-aided thoracoscopic resection of pulmonary nodule localized with contrast media. Ann Thorac Surg 1999;68:1815-20
34. Chella A, Lucchi M, Ambrogi MC, et al. A pilot study of the role of TC-99 radionuclide in localization of pulmonary nodular lesions forthoracoscopic resection. Eur J Cardiothorac Surg. 2000;18:17-21
35. Santambrogio R; Montorsi M; Bianchi P; Mantovani A; Ghelma F; Mezzetti M. Intraoperative ultrasound during thoracoscopic procedures for solitary pulmonary nodules. Ann Thorac Surg 1999; 68: 218-22
36. Hida Y, Kato H, Nishibe T, et al. Value of intraoperative intrathoracic ultrasonography during video-assisted thoracoscopy pulmonary resection. Surg Laparosc Endosc 1996; 6: 472-475
37. Mineo TC, Pompeo E, Ambrogi V, Pistolese C. Video-assisted approach for transxiphoid bilateral lung metastasectomy. Ann Thorac Surg 1999;67:1808-10
38. Ambrogi V, Paci M, Pompeo E, Mineo TC. Transxiphoid video-assisted pulmonary metastasectomy: relevance of helical computed tomograhpy occult lesions. Ann Thorac Surg 2000;70:1847-52
39. Yim AP, Lin J, Chan AT, et al. Video-assisted thoracoscopic wedge resections of pulmonary metastatic osteosarcoma: Should it be performed? Aust N Z J Surg 1995;65:737-739
40. Roth J, Putnam J, Wesley M, et al. Differing determinants of prognosis following resection of pulmonary metastases from osteogenic and soft-tissue sarcoma patients. Cancer 1985; 55: 1361-66
41. Mutsaerts EL, Zoetmulder FA, Meijer S, et al. Outcome of thoracoscopic pulmonary metastasectomy evaluated by confirmatory thoracotomy. Ann Thorac Surg 2001;72:230-3
42. De Giacomo T, Rendina EA, Venuta F, et al. Thoracoscopic resection of solitary lung metstases from colorectal cancer is a viable therapeutic option. Chest 1999;115:1441-3
43. Watanabe M, Deguchi H, Sato M, et al. Midterm results of thoracoscopic surgery for pulmonary metastases especially from colorectal cancers. J Laparoendosc Adv Surg Tech A. 1998;8:195-200
44. Landreneau RJ, De Giacomo T, Mack MJ, et al. Therapeutic video-assisted thoracoscopic surgical resection of colorectal pulmonary metastases. Eur J Cardiothorac Surg. 2000; 18: 671-6
45. Roth JA, Pass HI, Wesley MN, et al. Comparison of median sternotomy and thoracotomy for resection of pulmonary metastases in patients with adult soft-tissue sarcomas. Ann Thorac Sug 1986;42:134-8
46. Sonett JR. VATS and thoracic oncology:Anathema or opportunity. Ann Thorac Surg 1999;68:795-6
47. Kamiyoshihara M, Hirai T, Kawashima O, et al. The surgical treatment of metastatic tumors in the lung: is lobectomy with mediastinal lymph node dissection suitable treatment? Oncol Rep 1998;5:453-7
48. Loehe F, Kobinger S, Hatz RA, et al. Value of systematic mediastinao lymph node dissection during pulmonary metastasectomy. Ann Thorac Surg 2001; 72: 225-9
49. Ercan S, Nichols FC, Trastek VF, Allen MS, Deschamps C, et al. Prognosis of mediastinal lymph node metastasis found during pulmonary metastasectomy for extrapulmonary carcinoma. STS proceedings, San Antonin, Nov. 4-6, 2001
50. Yamashita J, Kurusu Y, Fujino N, et al. Detection of circulating tumor cells in patients with non-small cell lung cancer undergoing lobectomy by video-assisted thoracic surgery: a potential hazard for intraoperative hematogenous tumor cell dissemination. J Thorac Cardiovasc Surg. 2000;119:899-905
51. Kirby TJ, Mack MJ, Landreneau RJ, Rice TW. Lobectomy-video-assisted thoracic surgery versus muscle-sparing thoracotomy. A randomized Trial. J Thorac Cardiovasc Surg 1995; 109:997-1001
52. Sonett JR. Pulmonary metastases: biologic and historical justification for VATS. Eur J Cardio-thorac Surg 1999; 16: S13-S16

CHAPTER

Role of laparoscopy in hematologic malignancies

18

R. Matthew Walsh

Abstract

Surgery continues to play an important role in the diagnosis and treatment of hematologic malignancies. Laparoscopic techniques expand our capabilities in the diagnosis and therapy for Hodgkin's disease, non-Hodgkin's lymphom and leukemias. Laparoscopic strategies include retroperitoneal lymph node biopsy, staging of Hodgkin's disease, and splenectomy for splenomegaly. Therapy typically involves splenectomy for primary splenic lymphoma, symptomatic splenomegaly, and cytopenias. Over a six year period, 177 laparosocpic splenectomies have been performed, 60 (34%) for hematologic malignancies. The principle indication was definitive diagnosis of splenomegaly in 32 patients (53%), and lymphoma was subsequently found in 17 (53%). Cytopenias were common in patients operated for hematologic malignancies, prseent in 38 patients (63%). In summary, laparoscopic approaches to patients with hematologic malignancies, especially laparoscopic splenectomy are safe and effective.

Introduction

Hematologic malignancies encompass a wide spectrum of lymphoproliferative disorders. Advances in molecular cytogenics have improved our ability to characterize, treat and predict patient outcome.[1-4] The advent and proliferation of novel chemotherapeutic treatments based on recent molecular discoveries has not diminished the role of surgeons in the management of these diseases. Surgery has retained its traditional, valuable role in diagnosis and treatment of selected patients with hematologic malignancies. Surgery is typically required in the diagnosis of these malignancies to obtain an adequate tissue sample requisite for subtype determination. The attainment of an adequate tissue sample is essential, and usually mundane when it involves excision of a peripheral node. A far greater quandry may exist when the dominant disease resides in the retroperitoneum or spleen. Less well appreciated is the therapeutic role of surgery, principally splenectomy. Splenectomy can positively effect the treatment of associated cytopenias and low grade lymphocytic diseases which predominate in the spleen.[5-7]

Laparoscopy represents a powerful surgical tool in the management of patient with predominantly abdominal hematologic malignancy. The surgical contributions in diagnosis and treatment have been expanded by the application of laparoscopic techniques.[8,9] Laparoscopy facilitates a minimally invasive portal to the retroperitoneum for diagnostic lymph node biopsies. Laparoscopic splenectomy also offers both diagnostic and therapeutic potential even in the setting of massive splenomegaly.[10] This review will focus on the role of laparoscopic techniques in the specific management of Hodgkin's disease, non-Hodgkin's lymphoma, and chronic B-cell leukemias. The potential and nuanced role of laparoscopic splenectomy in hematologic malignancies will be highlighted.

An extensive experience has been gained at the Cleveland Clinic with laparoscopic splenectomy over the last six years, beginning in August, 1995. A total of 177 laparoscopic splenectomies have been performed during that time period. The indications for splenectomy included idiopathic immune thrombocytopenia (ITP) in 68 patients (38%), hematologic malignancies in 60 patients (34%), and other splenic processes in 49 patients (28%). Removal of the spleen for hematologic malignancy is primarily indicated for diagnosis in patients with splenomegaly, or therapy for cytopenias. Cytopenia may be present in patients with known splenomegaly or associated with leukemias. Of the 60 patients operated for hematologic malignancy, a diagnosis for splenomegaly was the principle indication in 32 patients (53%), lymphoma was known preoperatively in 12 (20%), chronic B-cell lymphocytic leukemia in 12 (20%) and hairy cell leukemia in 4 (7%). Associated cytopenias were present in 38 patients (63%). The principle indication for splenectomy was considered diagnostic in 32 patients (53%) and therapeutic in 28 patients (47%). A subsequent diagnosis of lymphoma was determined in 17 patients (53%) operated for a definitive diagnosis of splenomegaly. The subsequent discussion will be disease specific, and a summary of the operative approach to laparoscopic splenectomy will be detailed.

Laparoscopic Staging of Hodgkin's Disease

Thomas Hodgkin first described the clinical and postmortem features of the disease that would bear his name in 18321,[11] and the approach to treatment of patients with Hodgkin's disease has changed markedly, and continues to evolve. Initially, all treatments were considered palliative, including the first treatments with radiation therapy. The encouraging preliminary results of radiation therapy led to progressively higher and, ultimately, curative doses of radiation.[12] The addition of chemotherapeutic agents in combined treatment modalities has resulted in curative therapy for the majority of patients with an initial treatment regimen.[13] The achievements made in treatment have not been devoid of significant late sequelae, which include cardiac failure, infectious diseases and most importantly, second malignancy. The current emphasis in treating Hodgkin's is to maintain a long disease free interval while reducing adverse long-term effects.[14] A more tailored approach to treatment with less aggressive chemotherapy and/or radiation therapy is being considered for early-stage Hodgkin's disease in patients with favorable prognostic indicators.

Critical in treatment decisions is an accurate staging of the disease. The Ann Arbor System has served clinicians well for over 25 years, and Cotswold's modifications also have proven useful in incorporating the bulk of disease.[15,16] The stage of disease has had a strong prognostic value and two prognostic groups can be identified: those with favorable Ann Arbor Stage I, II, and IIIA, and those with unfavorable Stages IIIB and IV.[13] Additional independent prognostic factors include age, gender, presence of systemic symptoms ("B" symptoms: fever >38°, drenching night sweats and weight loss > 10% in 6 months), erythrocyte sedimentation rate (ESR), and blood lymphocyte count.

Favorable groups include female patients under 40 years of age with "B: symptoms, an ESR <30, and lymphocyte count >1,000.[12] The prognostic value of histologic subtype is of little current value although lymphocyte-predominant, nodular patients have a greater risk of disease recurrence.

Fundamental in an effective strategy towards a tailored, less aggressive treatment protocol is an accurate determination of disease stage. Non-invasive procedures predominate in the work-up, but are variably applied. Investigational studies include computer tomography (CT) of chest/abdomen, magnetic resonance imaging (MRI) of spleen/bone marrow, gallium scanning, technetium bone scanning, immunoscintigraphy, and positron emission tomography (PET) with ftuorodeoxy-glucose (FDG).[17,18] Lymphangiography is rarely valuable in the evaluation of patients with Hodgkin's.[19] The goal of the staging studies is to determine the presence of infradiaphragmatic disease. Staging laparotomy remains the most precise means of determining the presence and extent of abdominal involvement in patients with clinical Stage I-II supradiaphragmatic

Hodgkin's disease.[14] Of all patients with clinical Stage I-II disease, 20% to 35% will have occult splenic or upper abdominal nodal involvement not detected by non-invasive studies.[20,21] Combining prognostic variables can be useful in predicting patients with the lowest risk for occult abdominal involvement, this is commonly done in Europe to determine treatment groups.[12] Patients should be considered for staging laparotomy and splenectomy only if the outcome of the procedure influences treatment. This approach continues in the United States based on the philosophy that extensive staging reduces both the initial treatment needed in some patients and the subsequent treatment- related short- and long-term complications. Laparoscopic staging with splenectomy can further substantiate this philosophy by reducing surgical morbidity through utilization of minimally invasive techniques while assuring comparable pathologic staging. The operative staging for Hodgkin's disease should include complete splenectomy, wedge biopsy of the liver, and three core needle liver biopsies. In addition, lymph node biopsies should be obtained and individually labeled from the left and right para-aortic and iliac nodes, celiac, porta hepatis, and mesenteric regions with all operative sites marked by metallic clips.[22] Staging laparotomy or laparoscopy is not justified unless care is taken to ensure that patients are staged completely. The most significant finding gained from abdominal staging is the presence of absence of splenic involvement. Further, in patients with clinical Stage I and II are found to have positive nodes at operation, the nodes are typically located at the para-aortic region, and only 4% will have occult disease in the porta hepatis. The complications of staging laparotomy are not innocuous and may be an important factor in considering its role in the evaluation of patients. Overwhelming post-splenectomy infection and postoperative small bowel obstruction have each been reported in up to 10% of patients.[23] Hopefully, staging laparoscopy can positively impact on the rate of some postoperative complications.

Non-Hodgkin's Lymphoma

In contrast to Hodgkin's disease, non-Hodgkin's lymphoma (NHL) does not spread in a predictable fashion. Patients with non-Hodgkin's lymphoma may present without peripheral lymphadenopathy yet prominent retroperitoneal lymphadenopathy and/or hypersplenism that may require laparoscopy for diagnosis. Isolated and suspicious retroperitoneal lymphadenopathy is readily amenable to laparoscopic biopsy and an expeditious evaluation and prompt treatment should be facilitated with the advantages of minimal surgical trauma. The approach to patients with hypersplenism may be more problematic.

The spleen is involved in 30% to 40% of patients with NHL, usually as a consequence of advanced disease.[24] Manifested by splenomegaly, this may be a consequence of lymphomatous infiltration and/or increased sequestration of cellular blood components. Treatment is directed at the local symptoms attributable to splenomegaly or the hematologic consequences of sequestration. Splenomegaly may cause abdominal or pleuritic pain, and early satiety. Hematologic manifestations include thrombocytopenia, neutropenia, and anemia that are difficult to treat medically and may prevent the administration of adequate chemotherapy.[25] Splenectomy can reliably alleviate local symptoms of splenomegaly and reverse cytopenias, which may predict improved survival.[24-26] These benefits can be achieved with an acceptable morbidity of <30%, and mortality <5%, even with advanced disease.[24,25,27] Infections are the most commonly reported complications of splenectomy and include overwhelming sepsis, wound infection, and subphrenic abscess. The use of preoperative pneumoccal vaccines and prophylactic antibiotics, meticulous surgical technique and avoidance of intra-abdommal drains can decrease infectious complications.[28]

Primary splenic lymphoma refers to lymphoma confined to the spleen, with or without hilar adenopathy. When strictly defined, this is an uncommon manifestation of NHL, representing 1% of all patients with malignant lymphoma.[27] The presentation of primary splenic lymphoma commonly includes left upper quadrant abdominal pain, weight loss, fatigue, anorexia, fever, and night sweats. Although splenomegaly is discernible on physical exam, asymptomatic splenomegaly is not typical of the disease. Non-invasive radiological investigations with liver-spleen and gallium scanning and ultrasound are useful in documenting splenomegaly, but they are not accurate in diagnosing lymphomatous splenic involvement.[29] Lymphatous nodules of 5 to 9 mm can be adequately visualized with high-resolution CT scans. The differential diagnosis of large solitary or multiple splenic masses with low attenuation foci includes abscesses, hematomas, cysts, Hodgkin's disease, angiosarcoma, and metastatic carcinoma. The mean weight of spleens primarily involved with lymphoma is over 1 kg,[27] which does not necessarily preclude consideration of laparoscopic splenectomy. The mean morcellated splenic weight in the 60 patients operated for hematologic malignancy was 734 gms, and the largest spleen 3.3 kg. The mean operative time was 168 minutes with a mean blood loss of 260 cc. A pre-operative measurement of cranial-caudal splenic size may be useful in predicting the feasibility of laparoscopic splenectomy. A CT-measured length under 20 cm is considered amenable to standard laparoscopic removal. Additional important parameters include a palpable margin that does not cross the midline or extend further than the iliac crest. Splenectomy is indicated for suspected isolated splenic lymphoma to alleviate symptoms, confirm the diagnosis and treat the disease. Splenectomy alone for primary splenic lymphoma is associated with improved survival as compared to patients with diffuse NHL and splenomegaly.[27,30]

Leukemias

Splenectomy is occasionally indicated for patients with chronic B-cell lymphocytic leukemia (CLL) and hairy cell leukemia.[31-33] The indications for splenectomy are rarely diagnostic, and typically for treatment of cytopenias, or pain from splenomegaly. The cytopenias associated with these leukemias are variable and include autoimmune hemolytic anemia in hairy cell leukemia.[34] Improvement in critical cytopenias may be required prior to treatment with chemotherapeutic agents or to reduce transfusion requirements. Laparoscopic splenectomy for leukemia was performed in 16 (27%) of the 60 patients operated for hematologic malignancy.

Operative Technique

The challenging operative component of laparoscopic staging procedures involves the splenectomy, especially in primary splenic lymphoma when splenomegaly is present. Therefore, when splenectomy is planned as part of the procedure, it should be performed first: this is an important consideration in our operative planning since it affects how patients are positioned. We advise the lateral approach to laparoscopic splenectomy, which is similar to the positioning for laparoscopic adrenalectomy. The advantages to the lateral approach include fewer port sites, easier manipulation of the spleen to reduce capsular injury, improved access to all peritoneal attachments, and superior exposure to the hilum.[35,36] All patients receive peri-operative antibiotics, typically a first generation cephalosporin. Patient positioning is performed following endotracheal intubation and securing of the endotracheal tube, placement of an orogastric tube and urinary catheter. It is important to note that appropriate cushioning includes rolls placed at the level of the umbilicus, beneath the right axilla, and between the legs. Both arms are extended and supported. The operative table is broken to expand the distance between the iliac crest and costal margin. Positioning of personnel and equipment is equally important. The table is also placed in reverse-Trendelenburg position which allows blood and irrigation fluid to flow into the pelvis, out of the operative field. The lateral approach is well suited for an operation performed by the surgeon and one assistant, both facing the patient's abdomen. Surgeon and assistant direct their attention at one monitor positioned over the patients left shoulder for in-line operating.

Typically, three 10 mm port sites are required for laparoscopic splenectomy. Port sites are tentatively marked so that after insufflation the optimal positions of the trocars will be 4 cm below the inferior tip of the spleen but within reach of the diaphragm. The approximate position of the most lateral port site is at the level of the eleventh rib, the medial site is in close proximity to the midline, and the middle port is halfway between. The middle trocar is placed first, with an open technique and the other two are placed under direct visualization. A 10 mm, 30° or 45° laparoscope is a requirement.

Dissection is begun by mobilizing the splenic

flexure of the colon inferiorly only as necessary. Proceeding caudal to cranial, the peritoneal attachments are sharply divided close to the spleen. The dissection then proceeds lateral to medial with minimal retraction required by a blunt laparoscopic grasper due to the assistance of gravity. The pancreas and splenic vessels in the hilum are rapidly visualized. Mobilization of the inferior pole, including the branch from the epiploic vessels, can be divided between clips or harmonic scalpel. The operation proceeds best when the laparoscope is exchanged between the medial and lateral trocars, and the surgeon operates with both hands. Care should be taken when mobilizing the superior pole to identify the greater curvative of the stomach and short gastric vessels. The final division of the hilum is usually done with a vascular gastrointestinal anastomosis (GIA) stapler.[37] Several firings of the stapler are usually required, and may be utilized to divide the short gastric vessels. If preferable, a right-angled clamp may be used to individually dissect the hilar and short gastric vessels,. Which can then be clipped and divided. Next, the spleen is placed into an impermeable retrieval bag of appropriate size. This bag should be strong yet flexible so that it is easy to manipulate but not rupture during extraction. Placing a large spleen in the bag - often the most difficult aspect of the procedure - is facilitated by placing the end of the bag at the diaphragm, opening the bag widely toward the lateral trocar, holding the posterior lip of the bag with the left hand while gasping the splenic hilum with the right hand and sliding ("surfing") it into the bag. The bag is delivered through the middle port and excised in chunks with a ringed forceps.

Hand-assisted laparoscopic splenectomy is infrequently required, even in patients with splenomegaly. This adaptation was required in eight patients (13%) with hematologic malignancy, all in patients with cranio-caudal length greater than 20 cm. Although uncommon, this technical modification is important to utilize to decrease the chance of conversion, reduce overall operative time, facilitate retraction and placement in the specimen retrieval bag. Essentially, the medial port is substituted with the left hand through an appropriately sized midline incision. A commercially available kit is required and is easy to use.[38] The important point is to use this technique early in the course of the operation when its use is predictable.[39]

Following completion of the splenectomy, the patient can be placed more supine if staging is being performed for Hodgkin's disease. The remainder of the staging can be performed with a small midline incision[40] or laparoscopically. Continued laparoscopic staging may require additional trocar(s) and placement of the monitors at the feet with visualization from the medial, subxiphoid port. Core liver biopsies can be performed percutaneously under laparoscopic guidance. The vascular GIA stapler or harmonic scalpel also be used to obtain a wedge biopsy of the liver.[41] The additional lymph node biopsies of the para-aortic, para-iliac and portal lymph nodes can be accessed after division of the peritoneum using two-handed technique similar to open surgery.[42] All biopsy sites should be individually marked with clips and specimens sent to pathology on saline for processing. The abdomen is generously irrigated and all surgical sites are checked for hemostasis. A drain is placed in the splenic bed only if there is serious concern that a pancreatic injury may have occurred.

The orogastric tube and, typically, the urinary catheter are removed in the operating room unless the patient is older or infirm. A liquid diet is started the evening after surgery and a regular tray is given on the following morning. Patients are encouraged to ambulate beginning on the day of surgery. Serum amylase and hemoglobin levels are checked the first postoperative day. Discharge occurs on the first, or more typically, second postoperative day.

The potential complications of laparoscopic splenectomy do not differ from those of the traditional operation; they include bleeding, pancreatic and gastric injury, intra-abdominal abscess, and post-splenectomy sepsis. In our experience, minor complications occurred in four patients (7%) with hematologic malignancies, compared to complications in seven patients (10%) operated for ITP. Greater than 80% of cases should be completed laparoscopically, with bleeding being the most common reason for conversion to open splenectomy.[43,44] The results of laparoscopic splenectomy compare favorably with open operation in terms of incidence of wound infection, length of stay, return of bowel function, and postoperative pain.[45-48] It is anticipated that the risk of adhesive small bowel obstruction also will be improved with all laparoscopic procedures. The feasibility and improved outcome of laparoscopic splenectomy and retroperitoneal lymph node biopsies will expand its utilization for a variety of hematologic malignancies.

References

1. Muller-Hermelink HK, Zettl A, Pfeifer W, Ott G: Pathology of lymphoma Progression. Histopathology 38(4):285-3306, 2001.
2. De Wolf-Peeters C: Marginal zone lymphomas, MALT and splenic types. Advances in Clinical Pathology: the Official Journal of Adriatic Society of Pathology. 4(4): 190-2, 2000.
3. Caligaris-Cappio F: How immunology is reshaping clinical disciplines: the Example of haematology. Lancet 358(9275):49-55, 2001.
4. Stetler-Stevenson M, Braylan RC: Flow cytometric analysis of lymphomas and lymphoproliferative disorders. Seminars in Hematology 38(2):111-23, 2001.
5. Coon WW: Surgical aspects of splenic disease and lymphoma. Current Problems In Surgery 35(7):543-646, 1998.
6. Williams SF, Golomb HM. Perspective on staging approaches in the malignant Lymphomas. Surgery, Gyneclogy & Obstetrics 163(2): 193-201, 1986.
7. Morel P, Dupriez B, Goselin B, Fenaux P, Estienne MH, Facon T, Jouet JP, Bauters F: Role of early splenectomy in malignant lymphomas with prominent splenic involvement (primary lymphomas of the spleen). Cancer 71(1):207-15, 1993.
8. Cuschieri A: Role of video-laparoscopy in the staging of intra-abdominal Lymphomas and gastrointestinal cancer. Seminars in Surgical Oncology 20(2): 167-72, 2001.
9. Pratt BL, Greene FL: Role of laparoscopy in the staging of malignant disease. Surgical Clinics of North America 80(4): 1111-26, 2000.
10. Hemford BT, Park A, Walsh RM, Kercher KW, Matthews BD, Frenette G, Sing RF: Laparoscopic splenectomy in patients with normal-sized spleens versus splenomegaly: does size matter? American Surgeon 67(9):854-7; discussion 857-8, 2001.
11. Hodgkin T: On some morbid appearances of the absorbent glands and spleen. Medico-Chir Trans 1832:17-68-114.
12. Tubiana M: Hodgkin's disease: historical perspective and clinical presentation. In Baillieres' clinical haematology." Philadelphia: Balliere Tindall (9):503-530, 1996.
13. Rosenberg SA: The manangement of Hodgkin's disease: Half a century of change. The Kaplan Memorial Lecture. Ann Oncol 1996:7:555-560.
14. Mauch PM: Management of early stage Hodgkin's disease: The role of radiation Therapy and/or chemotherapy. In "Baillieres' clinical haematology.: Philadelphia: Balliere Tindall; 1996,(9):531-541.
15. Lister TA, Crowther D, Sutcliffe SB, et al: Report of a committee convened to Discuss the evaluation and staging of patients with Hodgkin's disease. Cotswolds meeting [published erratum in J Clin Oncol 1990;8:1602]. J Clin Oncol 1989;7:1630-1636.
16. Specht L, Lauritzen AF, Nordentoft AM, et al: Tumor cell concentration and Tumor burden in relation to histopathologic subtype and other prognostic factors in early stage Hodgkin's disease. The Danish National Hodgkin Study Group. Cancer 1990;65:2594-2601.
17. Bangerter M, Griesshammer M, Binder T, et al: New diagnostic imaging Procedures in Hodgkin's disease. Annals of oncology. 7 Suppl 4:55-9, 1996.
18. Carde P: Diagnostic procedures. In "Baillieres'clinical haematology." Philadelphia: Balliere Tindall; 1996 (9):479-501.
19. Libson E, Polliack A, Bloom RA: Value of lymphangiography in the staging Of Hodgkin lymphoma. Radiology 1994;193-757-759.
20. Leibenhaut M, Hoppe RT, Efron B, et al: Prognostic indicators of laparotomy Findings in clinical stage I-II supradiaphragmatic Hodgkin's disease. J Clin Oncol 1989;7:81-91.
21. Mauch P, Larson D, Osteen R, et al: Prognostic facotrs for positive surgical Staging in patients with Hodgkin's disease. J Clin Oncol 1990;8.257-265.
22. De Vita VT Jr, Jaffe ES, Hellman S: Diagnosis and staging of lymphomas. In De Vita VT Jr, Hellman S, Rosenberg SA (eds): "Cancer: principles and practice of oncology." 2nded. Philadelphia: Lippmcott; 1985. P. 1648-1653.
23. Jockovich M, Mendenhall NP, Sombeck MD, et al: Long-term complications of Laparotomy in Hodgkin's disease [Review]. Ann Surg 1994;219:615-624.
24. Lehne G, Hannisdal E, Langholm R, Nome O: A 10-year experience with splenectomy in patients with malignant non-Hodgkin's lymphoma at the Norwegian Radium Hospital. Cancer 1994;74:933-939.
25. Delpero JR, Houvenaeghel G, Gastaut JA, et al: Splenectomy for hypersplenism In chronic lymphocytic leukaemia and malignant non-Hodgkin's lymphoma [published erratum in Br J Surg 1990;77-957. Br J Surg 1990;77-443-449.
26. Morel P, Dupriez B, Gosselin B, et al: Role of early splenectomy in malignant Lymphomas with prominent splenic involvement (primary lymphomas of the Spleen). A study of 59 cases. Cancer 1993;71:207-215.
27. Brox A, Bishinsky JI, Berry G: Primary non-Hodgkin's lymphoma of the spleen. Am J Hematol 1991;38-95-100.
28. Brodsky J, Abcar A, Styler M: Splenectomy for non-Hodgkin's lymphoma. Am J Clin Oncol 1996;19-558-561.
29. Piekarski T, Federle MP, Moss AA, London SS: Computed tomography of the spleen. Radiology 1980;135:683-689.
30. Kehoe J, Straus DJ; Primary lymphoma of the spleen. Clinical features and Outcome after splenectomy. Cancer 1988; 62: 1433-1438.

31. Cheson BD: Chronic lymphocytic leukemia and hairy-cell leukemia. Current Opinion in Oncology 3(1):54-62, 1991.
32. Montserrat E: Chronic lymphoproliferative disorders. Current Opinion in Oncology 9(1):34-41, 1997.
33. Molica S, De Rossi G, Luciani M, Levato D: Prognostic features and Therapeutical approaches in B-cell chronic lymphocytic leukemia: an update. Haematologica 80(2):176-93, 1995.
34. Binet JL: Treatment of chronic lymphocytic leukaemia. French Co-operative Group on CLL. Baillieres Clinical haematology 6(4).867-78, 1993.
35. Park A, Gagner M, Pomp A: The lateral approach to laparoscopic splenectomy. Am J Surg 1997,173:126-130.
36. Trias M, Targarona EM, Balague C: Laparoscopic splenectomy: An evolving Technique. A comparison between anterior and lateral approaches. Surg Endosc 1996;10:389-392.
37. Miles WF, Greig JD, Wilson RG, Nixon SJ: Technique of laparoscopic Splenectomhy with a powered vascular linear stapler. Br J Surg 1996;83:1212-1214.
38. Litwin DE, Darzi A, Jakimowicz J, Kelly JJ, Arvidsson D, Hansen P, Gallery MP, Denis R, Fowler DL, Medich DS, O'Reilly MJU, Atlas H, Himpens JM, Swanstrom LL, Arous EJ, Pattyne P, Yood SM, Ricciardi R, Sandor A, Meyers WC: Hand-assisted laparoscopic surgery (HALS) with the Hand-Port system: Initial experience with 68 patients. Annals of Surgery 231(5):715-23, 2000.
39. Heniford BT, Matthews BD, Answini GA, Walsh RM: Laparoscopic splenectomy for malignant diseases. Seminars in Laparoscopic Surgery 7(2):93-100, 2000.
40. Lefor AT, Flowers JL, Heyman MR: Laparoscopic staging of Hodgkin's disease. Surg Oncol 1993;2:217-220.
41. Lefor AT, Flowers JL: Laparoscopic wedge biopsy of the liver. J Am Coll Surg 1993;178-307-308.
42. Rhodes M, Rudd M, O'Rourke N, et al: Laparoscopic splenectomy and lymph node biopsy for hematologic disorders. Ann Surg 1995;222:43-46.
43. Emmermann A, Zornig C, Peiper M, et al: Laparoscopic splenectomy. Technique and results in a series of 27 cases. Surg Endosc 1995;9:924-927.
44. Friedman RL, Hiatt JR, Korman JL, et al: Laparoscopic or open splenectomy for Hematologic disease: which approach is superior? J Am Coll Surg 1997;185:49-54.
45. Gigot JF, Legrand M, Cadiere GB, et al: Is laparoscopic splenectomy a justified approach in henmatologic disorders? Preliminary results of a prospective multicenter study. Belgian Group for Endoscopic Surgery. Int Surg 1995;80:299-303.
46. Delaitre B, Pitre J. Laparoscopic splenectomy versus open splenectomy. A Comparative study. Hepatogastroenterology 1997;44:45-49.
47. Glasgow RE, Yee LF, Mulvihill SJ: Laparoscopic splenectomy. The emerging Standard. Surg Endosc 1997;11:108-112.
48. Walsh RM, Heniford BT, Brody F, Ponsky J: The ascendance of laparoscopic Splenectomy. American Surgeon 67(1):48-53, 2001.

CHAPTER

Endoscopic surgery to the axilla: a substitute for "open" surgery?

19

E. Leandros, N. Alexakis

Axillary treatment remains an integral part of the management of primary invasive breast cancer even though there are controversies.

Long-term follow-up studies of axillary node-negative breast cancer patients revealed that 30% died of metastatic disease. Regional lymph node metastases are not considered a prerequisite for distant metastases. The effect of axillary management on survival, local control, and staging is still the objective of numerous studies.

Surgical treatment to the axilla generally involves an axillary lymph node dissection (ALND), undertaken with mastectomy or breast-sparing surgery.

With the rapid evolution in the field, MIS procedures on the axilla are becoming important.

Axillary Lymph Node Dissection (ALND)

ALND is the extirpation of lymph nodes in the axilla. To standardize the extent of axillary dissection, the axillary space is arbitrarily divided into three levels. Level 1 nodes are those in the external mammary, scapular, axillary vein and central axillary groups, which lie lateral to the lateral border of the pectoralis, minor muscle. Level 2 nodes are those in the central axillary group, which lie under the pectoralis minor muscle. The level 3 nodes are those subclavicular nodes that lie medial to the minor muscle. The costoclavicular ligament, at which point the axillary vein passes into the thorax and becomes the subclavian vein, defines the apex of the axilla. Lymph nodes in the space between the pectoralis major muscle and minor muscles are known as the interpectoral group (Rotter nodes).

The lymphatic drainage of the breast is rich. Three principal pathways are identified The major site of drainage is to central axillary nodes. The internal mammary and interpectoral nodes, although primary routes of lymph flow, are rarely the sides of nodal metastases from breast cancer in the absence of simultaneous axillary disease Secondarily the lymphatic spread of breast cancer is into the high axillary nodes in the subclavicular chain and henceforth into the supraclavicular fossa. A keen knowledge of the nerve structures in the axilla is required to avoid their sacrifice. Coursing close to the chest wall on the medial aspect of the axilla is the long thoracic nerve (Bell), which innervates the serratus anterior muscle. This muscle is important to the fixation of the scapula to the chest wall during adduction of the shoulder and extension of the arm, and its denervation results in the winged scapula formation. The second major nerve encountered during axillary dissection is the thoracodorsal nerve to the latissimus dorci muscle at the lateral border of the axilla. This nerve arises from the posterior cord of the brachial plexus and enters the axillary space under the axillary vein, close to the entrance of the long thoracic nerve, and then crosses the axilla to the medial surface of the latissimus dorci muscle. It is usually preserved during axillary dissection unless its sacrifice is required for complete removal of tumor-containing nodes. The lateral pectoral n. travels around the lateral margin of the pectoralis minor m. and is in a vulnerable position during the division of the clavipectoral fascia and exposure of the axillary space. It supplies the pectoralis major m. Loss of innervation results in a flaccid and atrophic muscle. If possible, this branch can be saved. Finally there are the large sensory intercostal brachial or brachial cutaneous nerves that supply sensation to the undersurface of the upper arm and skin of the chest wall along the posterior margin of the axilla. Cutting these nerves causes cutaneous anesthesia to these areas and sometimes chronic pain syndromes. Many advocate preservation of the most superior brachial cutaneous n. which crosses the central axilla.

Complete ANLD is dissection of nodes from level 1 to 3. Partial ALND is dissection of nodes from levels 1 and 2. Axillary sampling is removal of level 1 nodes. In most cases, metastases to the axillary lymph nodes occur sequentially: level 1 nodes are involved first, followed by involvement of level 2 and level 3 nodes. Skip metastases occur occasionally. Most authorities recommend a level 1 and 2 dissection, which correctly stages 96% of patients with primary breast cancer and has acceptable morbidity. Removal of level 3 nodes provides little additional information and has high morbidity.

Sentinel Lymph Node Biopsy (SLNB)

It is a diagnostic test that determines the status of regional lymph nodes. It is studied with the ultimate goal to avoid the morbidity of ALND. The sentinel node is the lymph node first receiving lymphatic fluid from the tumor containing area. The surgeon injects bleu dye or radioactive colloidal particles intradermally, peritumorally The sentinel node is visualized by lymphoscintigraphy and its general location marked on the skin. During surgery it is identified visually/with a gamma probe, and removed The bleu dye method is simple, cost effective but requires extensive dissection of the axilla and the detection rate of the sentinel node appears to be slightly lower. The radioactive colloidal particles method is more costly and requires more experience. However the predictive value for both methods seems identical. In a review of 12 published series on with a total of 1945 patients the sentinel node was found in up to 98% of patients [range 68.7%-98.2%], and accurately predicted the state of the axilla in 95% of patients, with a false-negative finding of up to 6.7% (range 0%-25%, sensitivity 75%-100%).

The disadvantages of SLNB include the presence of multicentric carcinoma, vascular/lymphatic invasion; invasion of the sentinel node by tumor cells and therefore appears the question of oncologic security. Other risks are the inability to detect the sentinel node and the possibility of false negative results.

Endoscopic approach

There is a trend towards minimally invasive techniques with the use of endoscopic technology.

Today, only about 30% to 40% of all invasive breast cancers are node-positive. Thus in most cases, the potential morbidity of ALND could be avoided if the status of the axillary nodes were ascertained with a less invasive procedure

Technique

Preoperative evaluation. Patients with palpable lymph nodes or a primary tumor in the direct vicinity of the axilla or a large [>3 cm] tumor, are **excluded.** Most use liposuction first and then axilloscopy but others not (because it may destroy the integrity of lymph nodes, which could lead to the spread of tumor cells).

Patient and operative team positioning. Patients are placed in the supine position with the ipsilateral arm abducted at 90 degrees. The lumpectomy is performed after 20min of the injection of dye/radiolebeled colloids but others perform the axillary dissection first.

Port placement (Figure 1). 1 cm skin incision at the superior aspect of the axilla. The clavicopectoral fascia is incised. A balloon distention device is in-

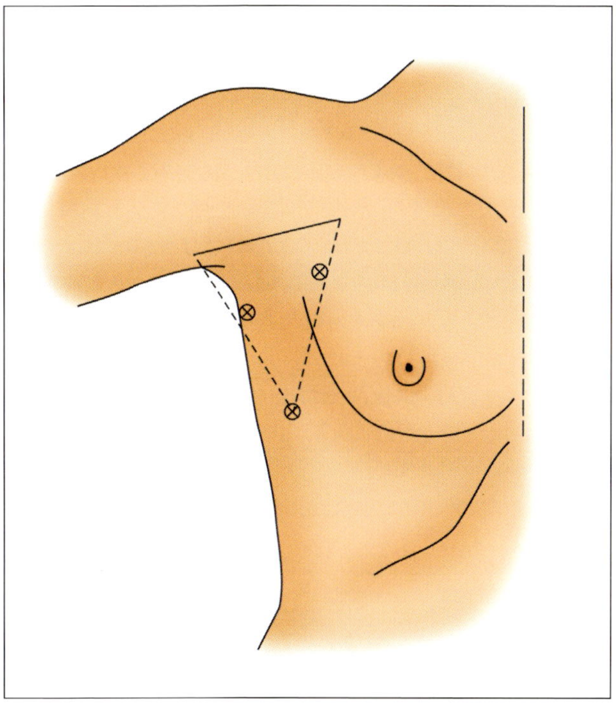

FIGURE 1.

serted and distended. The main effect is a lateral and upward displacement of the axillary contents (fat and lymph nodes) whereas the long thoracic n. is driven from the thoracic wall in a posteromedial direction. The intercostobrachial n. is similarly separated from the lymph node and fat bulk. The balloon is removed and the 10mm trocar is placed at the lowest caudal point at the anterior axillary line. Others use lipoapiration of the axillary fat. CO_2 insufflation is initiated [with <1lt/min flow] up to a pressure of 7-9 mmHg. (although that the CO_2 may cause extensive subcutaneous emphysema and the concern that gas inssufflation may increase the risk of tumor implantation). A 30 degrees laparoscope is introduced. Dissection is carried out bluntly with the 10 mm optic. Two additional trocars are placed in the anterior (5mm) and posterior (5 mm) axillary line (lateral to the latisimmus dorci and the pectoralis major). The sentinel node is identified using a combination of forceps and monopolar scissors or the harmonic scalpel, removed and send for histologic examination.

If the surgeon decides to continue, the dissection is carried with a combination of atraumatic forceps, bipolar forceps, scissors and suction. The lymphatic and fat tissue is mobilized en-block up to the second level with identification of the long thoracic nerve., the axillary vein, the thoracodorsal vessels and nerve. The lymphatic-fat tissue is then removed through the 10mm trocar. The use of an endobag is feasible but technically difficult. The site is irrigated with saline. Most surgeons insert a closed drain.

Results

Clinical examination of the axilla is inaccurate. Approximately 30% of patients with palpable axillary nodes prove to be node-negative following ALND and about 30% of clinically node-negative patients have nodal involvement. Axillary lymph node status is the single most important prognostic factor in patients with primary breast cancer. Node positive patients have a worse prognosis than node-negative patients. Lymph node status does not predict response to therapy. Adjuvant systemic therapy reduces the annual odds of relapse and death by approximately 30% and 25% respectively, for node negative and node positive patients. The prognostic information derived from nodal status may help a patient decide an appropriate treatment. But with the new approach to administer adjuvant systemic therapy to all patients with the addition of tamoxifen for those with estrogen receptor -positive tumors may reduce the importance of axillary staging.

The prognostic significance of nodal status is poorly understood. Nodal status perhaps serves as a marker of both tumor chronology and phenotype. About 35%-40% of patients with clinically detected invasive breast cancer prove to be node-positive following ALND. The NSABP-04 and Kings/Cambridge trials indicate that if the axilla is not treated with either ALND or radiotherapy, 15%-20% of patients will experience a relapse in the axilla within 5 years, but only l%-2% of patients develop axillary recurrence after treatment of the axilla. Several retrospective studies emphasize the importance of axillary treatment on local control. The risk of axillary relapse correlates with the size of the primary tumor. The extent of ALND influences the risk of axillary relapse.

Local recurrence often causes morbidity: pain

and lymphedema develops if the nerves and the vessels are invaded.

Axillary recurrences are a marker of tumor biology, indicating an increased risk for distant metastases and death.

The effect of axillary treatment on breast cancer mortality remains controversial. The results of the NSABP-04 and Kings/Cambridge trials suggest that the delayed treatment of the axilla does not adversely affect breast cancer mortality, and thus that axillary treatment has no effect on breast cancer mortality.

It seems unlikely that the extent of the ALND has any effect on overall survival, other than stage a patient for adjuvant therapy.

Substantial morbidity still follows this procedure [ALND]: wound complications, lymphedema, arm pain, decreased shoulder mobility, in up to 5-20% of patients.

Wound infection rates of up to 19% have been reported, although this is considered a clean operation, with no clear reasons for that.

Paresthesia is reported at up 70% of patients and this is attributed to the sacrifice of the intercostobrachial n.

Pain has been reported to up 33% of patients and this is independent from the sacrifice of the intercostobrachial n.

Weakness is reported to up 25%.

Arm lymphedema is a common and troublesome complication. It can occur any time following ALND, with an incidence of 2-27% The arm is edematous, often painful with limited movement. There is no specific therapy for this condition.

The incidence of significant morbidity (i.e. potential arm edema) with the endoscopic technique of the axillary dissection is probably similar to the open technique. Thus the use of endoscopic approach with minimal tissue manipulation and disturbance will be much better.

The technique of axillary dissection with a laparoscope was first described by Brunt and al. in 1996 (fifth world congress -SAGES Philadelphia 1996) They use pediatric instruments in cadavers through several ports, while a lifting device maintained a patent axillary space.

In 1997 and 1998 three reports were published, who evaluated the technical feasibility and safety of endoscopic -ALND in human cadavers (Toronto, St. Louis, Israel). All used a balloon dissector for expansion of the subcutaneous axillary. All agreed that endoscopic ALND is feasible with available technology, was easy to perform, offered easy access to the axilla and clear visualization of the axillary vein, long thoracic n., thoracodorsal n., and intercostobrachial n.

The first published reports of the above method with various modifications, in live patients appeared in 1998.

The results from up today published papers are as follows:

Operative time: double with the laparoscopic approach (61 - 110 min [mean] in various reports, range 30-150 min)

Perioperative complications: Seromas from 3-25%. The seroma rate for open surgery is 2.3-59%.

Sensibility disorders after open surgery occur in 20-60%. Thus the intercostobrachial nerve must be preserved to prevent paresthesia and sensibility loss at dermatome C5.

This nerve is better seen with the endoscope and can be preserved.

Hematoma occurs after open surgery in 0.8-4% and wound complications (hematoma, wound dehiscence) in 0.4-8%. With the endoscopic technique 5%. Rarely an abscess. (Two abscesses were described in 7 series of 269 pts [0,7%] who had undergone endoscopic dissection).

Mobility of the arm after axillary surgery is important. After conventional surgery 4- 17% of patients have impaired shoulder joint mobility and 30% shoulder stiffness at 3 mo and 4% at 12 months. With the endoscopic approach 21% immediately post-op have reduced shoulder mobility but none at 4.6 months or in another report 8% had restricted joint mobility at 6 mo but none at 18 mo. Thus the endoscopic approach may allow earlier and better arm mobility.

Lymphedema: effectiveness unknown with the endoscopy Up to 20% with the open surgery.

No. of dissected nodes: from 13 to 17[median] (Range 1-28). Equals those with the open technique.

Duration of drainage: [mean] 4-6 days

Esthetic results: better

Node histology: Same pathologic information

Node alteration: A cellular crush is more frequently seen with the endoscopic approach. Savat and al. reported a 13.4% incidence of morphologic lymph nodes defects after liposuction as compared with a 6.6% rate with open surgery. Therefore the switch to blunt dissection over liposuction.

Trocar site metastases: The fear of some surgeons of tumor spillage is argued by others that trocar site metastases is an indication of aggressive tumor biology and is not related to mechanical spread.

Recurrence: In the small number of cases of local recurrence, extensive axillary involvement has been observed.

Conclusions

The above findings and results suggest that endoscopic axillary surgery is safe for tumor control and adequate staging and may be used not only for the resection of the sentinel node but also to complete ALND.

References

1. Iglehart JD. The Breast. In Sabiston, Textbook of surgery, W B Saunders 1997. pp555-593
2. Orr RK. The impact of prophylactic axillary node dissection on breast cancer survival. Ann Surg Oncol 1999; 6:109-16
3. Dent: axillary lymphadenectomy for breast cancer. Arch Surg 131:1125-1127, 1996
4. CRC Working Party (Kings/Cambridge) trial for early breast cancer: a detailed update at the tenth year. Lancet 2:55-60, 1980
5. Fisher, Redmont, Fisher: Ten year results of a randomized trial comparing radical mastectomy and total mastectomy with or without radiation. N Engl J Med 312: 674-681,1985
6. Gelber, Goldhirsch, Coates: Adjuvant therapy for breast cancer: Understanding the overview. J Clin Oncol 11:580-585, 1993
7. Goldhirsch, Click, Gelber,: Meeting highlights: International consensus panel on the treatment of primary breast cancer. J Natl Cancer Inst 90: 1601-1608, 1998
8. Henderson, Patek: The relationship between prognostic and predictive factors in the management of breast cancer. Breast Cancer Res Treat 52:261-288,1998
9. Jatoi, Hilsenbeck, Clark,: The significance of axillary lymph node metastasis in primary breast cancer. J Clin Oncol 17:2334-2340, 1999
10. Koscielny, Le,Tubiana: The natural history of breast cancer. The relationship between involvement of axillary nodes and the initiation of distant metastases. Br J Cancer 59:775-782, 1989
11. Morrow:Axillary dissection: When and how radical? Semin Surg Oncol 12:321-327, 1996
12. Rotstein, Ferguson, Cummmings: Determinants of clean surgical wound infections for breast procedures at an oncology center. Infect Control Hosp Epidemiol 13:207-214, 1992
13. Sacks, Baum: Primary management of carcinoma of the breast. Lancet 342: 1402-1408, 1993
14. Veronesi, Rilke, Luini,: Distribution of axillary node metastases by level of invasion. Cancer 59: 682-687, 1987
15. Salvat, Knopf, Ayoubi, Slamani, Vincent-Genod, Guilbert, Walker:Endoscopic exploration and lymph node sampling of the axilla. Eur J Obstet Gynecol Reprod Biol 1996 Dec 27; 70(2): 165-73
16. Avrahami, Nudelman, Watenberg, Lando, Hiss, lelchuk. Minimally invasive surgery for axillary dissection. Cadaveric feasibility study. Surg Endosc 1998 May ; 12(5):466-8
17. Brunt, Jones, Wu, Brunt, Radford. Endoscopic axillary lymph node dissection: an experimental study in human cadavers. J Am Coll Surg 187 (2) 158-163, 1998
18. Wilmot, Watemberg, Landau, Litwin: Of balloon axilloscopy and avoidance of iatrogenic injury to the long thoracic nerve. Arch Surg 1997;132:1121-1124
19. Harder, Zuber, Kocher, Torhorst: Endoscopic surgery to the axilla. Recent Results Cancer Res 1998; 152:180-89
20. Tsangaris, Trad, Brody, Jacobs, Tsagaris, Sackier: Endoscopic axillary exploration and sentinel lymphadenectomy. Surg Endosc 13,43 (1999)
21. Kamprath, Bechler, Kuhne, Knause, Schneider:Endoscopic axillary lymphadenectomy without prior liposuction. Surg Endosc 13, 1226 (1999)
22. Reynaud, Abbey-Toby, Albuisson, Wattiez, Suzanne, Dechelotte: Histologic comparison between endoscopic axillary lymphadenectomy after liposuction and classical surgical technique. Ann Pathol 1999 Sept;19(4):289-93
23. Kuhn, Santjohanser, Koretz, Bohm, Kreienberg: Endoscopic axillary lymph node excision.Zentralbl Gynakol 1999; 121(2): 82-7
24. Epstein: Routine or delayed axillary dissection for primary breast cancer? Eur J Cancer 31A: 1570-1573, 1995
25. Suzzane F, Emering C, Wattiez A, Bournazaux JA, Bruhat MA, Jacquetin B. Axillary lymphadenectomy by liposuction and endoscopic picking: apropos of 72 cases. Chirurgie (1997) 122:138-142

26. Kuhn T, Santjohanser C, Koretz K, Bohm W, Kreienberg R. Axilloscopy and endoscopic sentinel node detection in breast cancer patients. Surg Endosc (2000) 14:573-577

27. Kuhn T, Santjohanser C, Grab D, Klauss W, Koretz K, Kreienberg R. Endoscopic axillary surgery in breast cancer. Br J Surg 2001,88:698-703.

CHAPTER

Robotic technology in laparoscopic surgery 20

M.K. Smith, J. Marescaux

At the end of the last century the introduction of laparoscopic surgery into routine use revolutionized the practice of surgery. The next revolution for the new millennium may prove to be the introduction of robotics into the field of surgery. Laparoscopic surgery is a modality that for the first time allowed the surgeon to operate on organs without being in direct contact with the organ itself using information about anatomical structures viewed on a monitor and not directly visualized by the surgeon. In this way, laparoscopy served to distance the surgeon from the direct performance of the surgery. The benefits given by performing the procedure laparoscopically came at the expense of the loss of tactile sense and precision of the surgeon. The development of robotics occurred in part as an attempt to improve these inadequacies of laparoscopy. The computer was introduced as an interface between the movements of the surgeon and the effect of the instruments. This resulted in the digitization of the surgical gest by the computer. Once digitized, this information could be altered by the computer in various ways in an effort to aid the surgeon. A secondary benefit of the digitization was the ability to transfer this information over distances and thus making telesurgery possible. Taken together, these new technologies, such as robotics and telemedicine, have the potential to improve many aspects in the surgical domain including surgical technique, training, education as well as the realization of telesurgery. These advancements have occurred largely through the integration of computer capabilities with the surgical act enabling the computer to augment, enhance or change the perception and/or performance of the procedure. With the use of the computer, it is possible to incorporate other computer generated data such as that from the patient's own CT or MRI scans into its database which then can be used by the surgeon either preoperatively or intraoperatively to plan and perform surgical interventions. Thus computer-assisted surgery (CAS) has become a new entity which may progress beyond the limitations of human capabilites and has allowed surgery to enter into the realm of augmented reality.

The development of the field of robotics has focused on a robot's ability to aid a human to perform a certain task. In the area of surgery, a field that benefits from the increased precision and reproducibility gained by the use of robotics, the development of computer-assisted surgery has moved from theory into clinical trials. As early as 1968, a "robotic" retractor was described and by the end of the century surgical robotic devices are actively being used in clinical trials in many areas of surgery and subspecialty surgery.[1-7]

The advantages of computer-assisted surgery, including the use of robots in surgery, are the increase in 3 dimensional accuracy, the reproducibility of repeated procedures, the increased precision of movements, and the ability to perform surgery over a distance. The robotics engineering enhances the ability of the surgeon to perform technically precise suturing techniques through a combination of reduction of physiologic tremor, enhanced visualization, and augmentation or reduction (scaling) of the surgeon's instrument manipulation. The surgeon is therefore assisted by the computer interface to perform intricate intracorporeal suturing using computer-driven laparoscopic instruments which when used in the conventional laparoscopic surgery are generally seen as too cumbersome to perform such precise work. Thus, robotic surgery has now allowed the field of minimally invasive surgery to progress into the field of microsurgical techniques. Computer assisted surgery has already been used to perform such microsurgeries as tubal reanastomosis in gynecologic surgery[1,2] or coronary artery bypass grafting.[3-6]

Robotics can be used in many different aspects of surgical procedures either to assist in guiding the surgeon or to be more actively involved in the procedure itself. Consistent with the former aspect is the use of the robot for retraction or camera-holding only. These robotic systems, such as Aesop TM (Computer Motion, Galeta, CA), a pre-programmed voice-controlled camera holder with both active and passive movement capabilities, are used to reduce fatigue of the surgical assistant and to provide memory capacity to stored camera positioning. It also makes "solo surgery" possible by allowing the operating surgeon to control the movement of the camera by voice, obviating the need for a second assistant. In trials, the robotic camera holders appear to be superior and cost-effective compared with their human counterparts[8] and robotic retractors possibly cause less pressure and thus less trauma to organs. The control of such robotic camera holders remotely by an operator kilometers away has also been reported.[9,10]

Most of the surgical robots in use today use computer-assisted "passive" manipulation where the robot is under the direct control of an operating surgeon. All of such robotic systems currently work on a "master-slave" principle,which involves the use of a "master" computer console operated by the surgeon that integrates computer input, manipulation of the master instruments that control the endoscopic instruments, and the "slave" instruments that are attached to and manipulated by the robotic control arms. This principle is the basis for the robotic systems currently in use including ZEUS TM (Computer Motion), Da VinciTM (Intuitive Surgical, Inc, Mountain View, CA). The computer controller translates the manipulations of the surgical instruments into electronic signals, ie digitization, which then relays the information to the actual instruments, which are driven by a motor drive and are placed intracorporally. This ability to digitize the manipulation of surgical instruments is the basis for dexterity enhancement as well as the possibility of performing remote surgery since the signals once digitized can be transmitted over greater distances.

Other aspects of robotic surgery include robot guided by digital imaging, used mainly in the fields of neurosurgery and orthopaedic surgery, where imaging is combined with robotic use to spatially orient the robot in the surgical field. This is used in the RoboDocTM (Integrated Surgical Systems, Sacramento, CA) that shapes the proximal femur for hip replacement;[11] and in neurosurgery for biopsy and surgery with stereotaxis.[12] Prostatic biopsy by robots using images from transrectal ultrasound is also described.[13] In eye surgery, retinal surgery and vessel injection are performed using image-robot interfaces.[14]

As mentioned above, there are several available surgical robotic systems. Our institute has been actively involved in the initial trials using ZEUS Robotic Surgical SystemTM for gastrointestinal interventions. Zeus consists of three major components: the surgeon-computer interface consisting of a video monitor and two surgical instrument manipulators, a computer controller, and two robotic arms that control the instruments. In addition, "Aesop" is used simultaneously for camera manipulation, which allows the operating surgeon to control all aspects of the surgery from the computer console, positioned a distance from the patient (Figures 1, 2).

The advantages of any surgical robotic system must include the practicality of its use, including the time involved to set-up the robot, the ease of its use and the need for technical support. The ZEUS system is installed on the operating table sidearms after positioning of the patient. During 25 performed procedures at our institution, the median time for assembly and takedown of ZEUS by op-

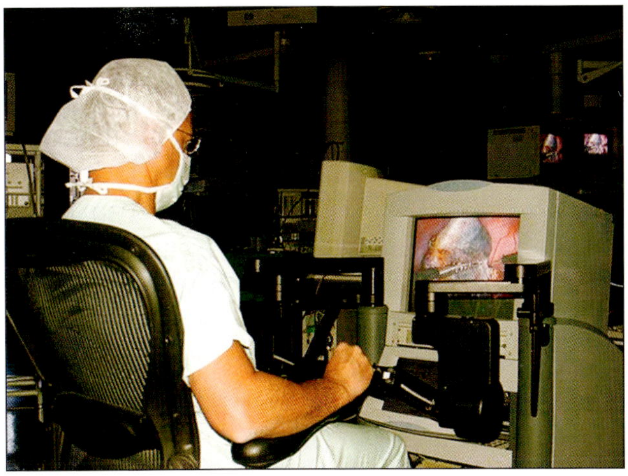

FIGURE 1. Surgeon at the computer-interface of ZEUS.

erating room staff was 18 minutes.[15] Other systems, such as the DaVinci, are free – standing units that can be quite large in size and remain independent from the operating table itself. The need for an engineer in the operating theatre has been seen as a drawback and added cost to the interventions. Although the master-slave systems of ZEUS and DaVinci have negated this need to an extent, the early procedures done with the robotics have had an engineer present during the surgery. However, as experience with the robots increase this need has decreased.

Due to the robot's increased precision, many of the initial clinical trials of robotic surgery have been performed in surgical subspecialty procedures requiring a high degree of precision to perform microanastomoses. In the field of urology, pyeloplasties in experimental animals have been performed using ZEUS, with good results.[16] In gynecologic infertility surgery, successful human[1,2] tubal anastomosis have been performed. In one study of reanastomosis in 19 Fallopian tubes using ZEUS, 17 were patent and pregnancy occurred in 5 patients so far.

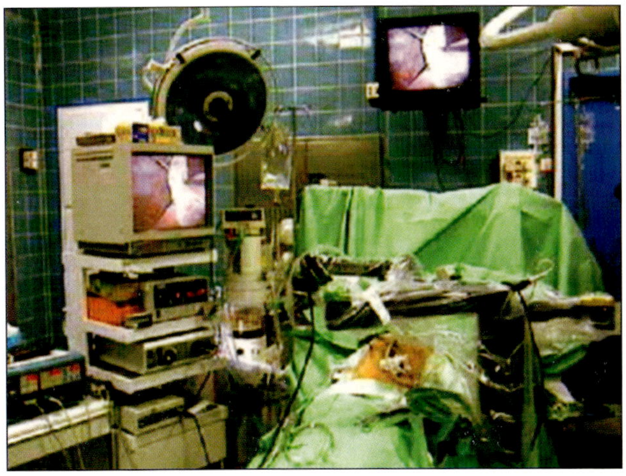

FIGURE 2. OR set-up with robotic arms in place.

Most of the human studies of robotic surgery to date have involved cardiac surgery.[3-6] The first robotically assisted beating heart coronary artery bypass graft was performed using ZEUS. Robotic dissection of only the internal thoracic artery, or a coronary bypass graft to the LAD has been described for ZEUS[3,5] and DaVinci.[4] In a prospective trial using ZEUS to perform left internal thoracic artery-left descending artery bypass grafting, Damiano et al have successfully performed in 8 patients with 100% patency rate at 6 weeks after surgery.[3]

Fewer studies have been done in general surgery with the use of robotics. The first robotic cholecystectomy was reported in 1998.[17] As mentioned above, in our own clinical series of the first 25 cholecystectomies performed with ZEUS, we have demonstrated operative times (median time for dissection of 25 minutes) similar to those of conventional laparoscopic surgery. Operating room staff was easily trained to install and disassemble the robot. There were no complications due to the use of the robot.[15] Other procedures such as Nissen fundoplication and hernia repair have also been reported.[18]

Future areas of research for advances in robotic technology are the development of tactile feedback systems to restore the tactile sense that is lost in laparoscopic surgery. Two aspects of tactile sensation include 1) the sense of how firmly the tissue is held (force feedback) and 2) the sense of change of elasticity and firmness of the tissue (for example, in the presence of a tumor). At our own institute, we have used a computer based force feedback system during simulated surgical procedures for training purposes.[19] This computerized system may in the future be integrated into the robotic computer program itself. Other modalities to provide such information are currently under investigation including integrating forceps with microsensors or the use of vibration to enhance tactile sensibility.[20]

The development of the intraoperative use of the robot is only one field of robotic surgery which is making its impact on the practice of surgery. Another area is in the development of teleeducation, telementoring as well as telesurgery, or the performance of surgery where the surgeon is physically separated from the patient, is made possible by the computer interface's digitization of the surgeon's movements. It has many practical applications for the education of surgery, for example to obtain expert advice from a consulting surgeon in another part of the world during the actual procedure or to provide telementoring where an more experienced surgeon can mentor a novice throughout a procedure. In a recent study,[21] surgical trainees already trained in the basics of laparoscopic cholecystectomy,were mentored by a supervising surgeon in an adjacent room who was watching the surgery performed live in the operating room. In 31 of 33 cases the procedure was completed by the trainee with only mentoring by the supervising surgeon. In another study, five laparoscopic inguinal hernia repairs were performed aboard a naval vessel at sea by a surgeon being mentored by a more experienced laparoscopic surgeon thousands of miles distant from the operation.[22] In these and other recent studies, the utility of training less experienced surgeons by those more experienced by transmission of live video images from the operation proved effective. In the case of the naval ship, the expertise available via telementoring for consultations and intraoperative advise may greatly reduce the costs and risks incurred by transporting crewman to land facilities for lack of expertise on the ship itself. The further development of such technology will allow in the near future, transmission of the signals across greater distances such that a surgeon, with the aid of the robot, will be able to perform the surgery on a patient who is in another hospital on another continent.

While CAS has led to advances in microsurgery, ergonomics, solo-surgery and telesurgery, the real potential of CAS rests in the computer's ability to integrate information from preoperative imaging studies and planned virtual reality dissection planes during real-time surgery. At the present time, the surgeon controls the telemanipulated procedure with information projected onto the imaging screen in similar fashion to that of the conventional laparoscopic technique. However, in the future, this video image may be augmented by projection of anatomical information obtained from computer generated 3 –dimensional pre- or intraoperative imaging studies that in the case of the liver for example, define vascular and biliary branches as well as exact location of the pathology. In our institute, we have created an automated 3D imaging of anatomical and pathological hepatic structures from a patient's own spiral CT scan to aid in preoperative planning for hepatic resection.[19] (Figure 3) This system is also able to delineate portal vein anatomy and automatically give segmental anatomy based on Couinand principles for each patient's unique anatomy. By taking the digital information generated by the CT images and processing it, a 3 – dimensional representation of the patient's liver is automatically created. Once reconstructed, the view of the liver can be manipulated on the computer screen by the surgeon to be oriented in many different directions and directly compared to the original CT scan images. This offers a more complete anatomical view of the liver and of the pathology. It is also possible to use this information to plan virtual reality liver dissections before the actual surgical procedure to determine the most advantageous dissection planes

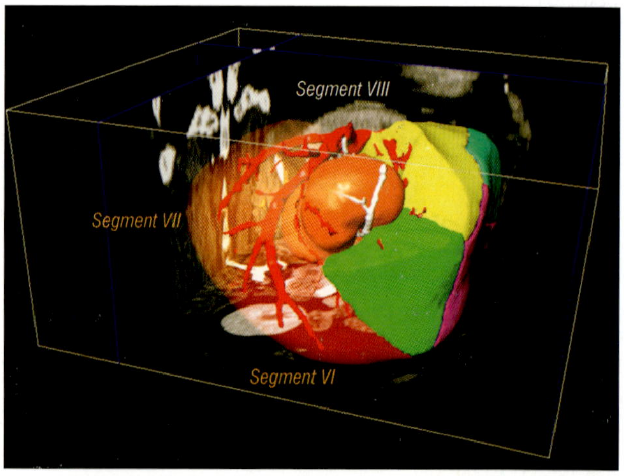

FIGURE 3. 3-D reconstruction of the liver anatomy.

and to anticipate possible difficulties such as aberrant anatomy. This technology will be of even more benefit if information from the surgical procedure itself is able to interact with the anatomical information given by the preoperative imaging. This link is provided by the use of CAS. In the future, integration of 3D imaging and virtual reality gives the possibility to directly incorporate this information into a computer system which can project radiographic studies onto organs while they are being operated on to accurately delineate pathology intraoperatively and guide robotic interventions. (Figure 4) Thus this technology allows the surgeon to transform the surgical procedure into an augmented-reality one. In addition, it will be possible to integrate the surgeon's preoperative simulated procedure into the robotics' computer system for guidance during surgery. Although preliminary in nature, the technology already exists to perform such data integration. It presents an advantage to both patient and surgeon to intraoperatively clearly define pathology, margins of resection as well as vasculature of the organ by projection of the preoperative images, identifying structures that would not otherwise be seen, for example, a liver tumor deep in the parenchyma.

In conclusion, the instruments used in modern day surgery will no longer just consist of those present in the operating room itself but will include many outside resources aimed at assisiting the surgeon preoperatively to plan the most advantageous procedure possible. To accomplish this, technologic advances will be employed at every aspect of the surgical procedure from 3-D preoperative imaging to the intraoperative use of robotics for technically demanding procedures and the ability to incorporate the patient's own imaging studies into the computer to augment the image of the procedure. This new technology will have a growing influence on surgical decision-making and patient management in the immediate future. As new advancements are made in the area of virtual reality and robotics, its utility in the operating room will need to be defined by surgeons according to its ability to improve patient care and maximize the benefits rendered to the patient. While the ultimate role of robotics in the operating room has yet to be defined, it is certain that the advancement of the technology will continue into the new millennium, creating newer, less invasive techniques with the potential to greatly benefit the management of our patients.

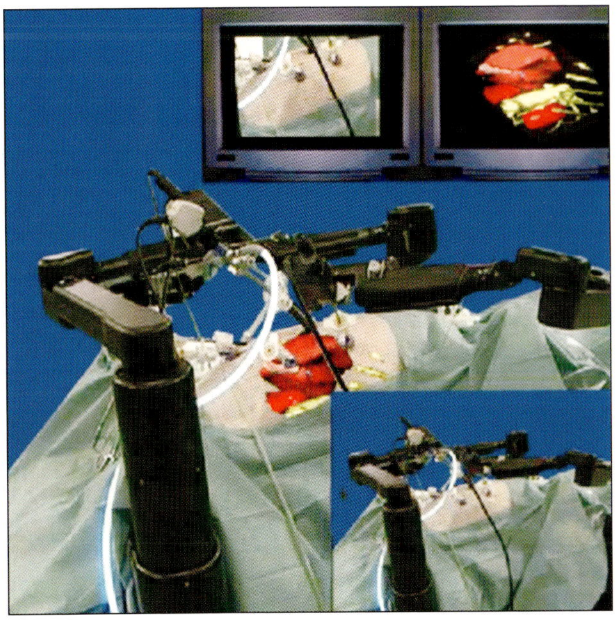

FIGURE 4. Augmented reality surgery.

References

1. Falcone T, Goldberg J, Garcia-Ruiz A, Margossian H, Stevens L. Full robotic assistance for laparoscopic tubal anastomosis: a case report. J Laparoendosc Adv Surg Tech A 1999 Feb; 9(1):107-13
2. Falcone T, Goldberg JM, Margossian H, Stevens L. Robotic-assisted laparoscopic microsurgical tubal anastomosis: a human pilot study. Fertil Steril 2000 May 1;73(5):1040-1042
3. Damiano RJ Jr, Ehrman WJ, Ducko CT, Tabaie HA, Stephenson ER Jr, Kingsley CP, Chambers CE. Initial United States clinical trial of robotically assisted endoscopic coronary artery bypass grafting. J Thorac Cardiovasc Surg 2000 Jan; 119(1):77-82
4. Falk V, Diegeler A, Walther T, Banusch J, Brucerius J, Raumans J, Autschbach R, Mohr FW. Total endoscopic computer enhanced coronary artery bypass grafting. Eur J Cardiothorac Surg 2000 Jan;17(1):38-45
5. Reichenspurner H, Damiano RJ, Mack M, Boehm DH, Gulbins H, Detter C, Meiser B, Ellgass R, Reichart B. Use of the voice-controlled and computer-assisted surgical system ZEUS for endoscopic coronary artery bypass graft. J Thorac Cardiovasc Surg 1999 Jul;118(1):11-6

6. Stephenson ER Jr, Sankholkar S, Ducko CT, Damiano RJ Jr. Robotically assisted microsurgery for endoscopic coronary artery bypass grafting. Ann Thorac Surg 1998 Sep; 66(3): 1064-7
7. Glauser D, Fankhauser H, Epitaux M, Hefti JL, Jaccottet A. Neurosurgical robot Minerva: first results and current developments. J Image Guid Surg 1995;1(5):266-72
8. Kavoussi LR, Moore RG, Adams JB, Partin AW. Comparison of robotic versus human laparoscopic camera control. J Urol 1995 Dec;154(6):2134-6 Published erratum appears in J Urol 1997 Oct;158(4):153
9. Satava RM, Simon IB. Teleoperation, telerobotics, and telepresence in surgery. Endosc Surg Allied Technol 1993 Jun; 1(3):151-3
10. Kavoussi LR, Moore RG, Partin AW, Bender JS, Zenilman ME, Satava RM. Telerobotic assisted laparoscopic surgery: initial laboratory and clinical experience. Urology 1994 Jul; 44(1): 15-9
11. Paul HA, Bargar WL, Mittlestadt B, Musits B, Taylor RH, Kazanzides P, Zuhars J, Williamson B, Hanson W. Development of a surgical robot for cementless total hip arthroplasty. Clin Orthop 1992 Dec;(285):57-66
12. Benabid AL, Hoffmann D, Le Bas JF, Lavallee S.[Value of image guided neurosurgery in neuro-oncology]. [Article in French] Bull Cancer (Paris) 1995 Dec;82 Suppl 5:573s-580s
13. A. Tests on reliability of a prostate biopsy telerobotic system. Stud Health Technol Inform 1999;62:302-7
14. Yu DY, Cringle SJ, Constable IJ. Robotic ocular ultramicrosurgery. Aust N Z J Ophthalmol 1998 May;26 Suppl 1:S6-8
15. Marescaux J, Smith M, Forbes L, Jamali F, Malassagne B, Leroy J. Robotic Laparoscopic Cholecystectomy: Initial Clinical Experience with 25 Patients. Annals of Surgery (in press).
16. Sung GT, Gill IS, Hsu TH. Robotic-assisted laparoscopic pyeloplasty: a pilot study. Urology 1999 Jun;53(6):1099-103
17. Himpens J, Leman G, Cadiθre. Telesurgical laparoscopic cholecystectomy. Surg Endosc1998;12:1091.
18. Cadiθre GB, Himpens J, Germay O, Lupinc N, Degueldre M, Vandromme J, IzizaBruyns. Chirurgie laparoscopique par robot: faisabilitι. A propos de 78 cas.Le Journal de Coelio-Chirurgie 2000(33):42-48.
19. Marescaux J, Clement JM, Tassetti, C Koehl,S Cotin, Y Russier, D Mutter, H Delingette, N Ayache.Virtual reality applied to hepatic surgery simulation: the next revolution.Ann Surg 1998; 228: 627-34.
20. Buess, GF, M Schurr, S Fischer. Robotics and allied technologies in endoscopic surgery. Arch Surg 2000 Feb;(135): 229-235.
21. Byrne, JP, Mughal MM. Telementoring in laparoscopic cholecystectomy: a useful adjunct in training and assessment of higher surgical trainees. BR J Surg 2000 Mar; 87(3): 362-73.
22. Cubano, M, BK Poulouse, MA Talamini, R Stewart, LE Antosek, R Lentz, R Nibe, MF Kutka, M Mendoza- Sagaon; Long distance telementoring: A novel tool for laparoscopy aboard the USS Abraham Lincoln. Surg Endosc 1999(13): 673- 78.

INDEX

A

B

C

D

E

F

G

H

I

J

K

L

M

N

O

P

Q

R

S

T

U

V

W

X

Y

Z